Care-giving in dementia

Publicity about neuroscientific research into the dementias spreads quickly compared to the advances made in the field of care-giving. *Care-Giving in Dementia* has been written to counterbalance that trend, and to promote care-giving in dementia as a specialization in its own right. Contributors from England, Europe, America and Australia, representing all the major health care professions, have joined together to provide a rich source of information on the most up-to-date developments in care-giving in dementia for those working in the field.

Presented here are four sections dealing with models and theories for research and practice; interpersonal interventions in care facilities; interventions in the community; and interventions in the family. The final chapter recommends that all health care professionals working with persons with dementia should receive a joint 'core' training programme to which professional-specific training could be added. Common themes running through the chapters are that care must be stage-specific; that professionals must work with the abilities that are spared; that lifespan information is needed to plan optimal individualized care; that the results of using interpersonal approaches on a sustained basis can be a useful source of information for continuous assessment; and that optimal care of the person with dementia requires care for their family.

Care-Giving in Dementia emphasizes that, in the absence of cures or treatments for dementia, happiness and stimulation of the individual's capacity for it are more acceptable goals for care-giving than improved cognition.

Gemma Jones is a research psychologist in the Departments of Psychology and Old Age Psychiatry at the Institute of Psychiatry, London; **Bère Miesen** is a clinical psychogerontologist at the Psychogeriatric Center 'Marienhaven', Warmond, the Netherlands.

Care-giving in dementia

Research and applications

Edited by

Gemma M.M. Jones

and

Bère M.L. Miesen

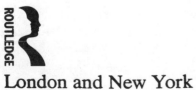

London and New York

First published in 1992
by Routledge
11 New Fetter Lane, London EC4P 4EE

Simultaneously published in the USA and Canada
by Routledge
29 West 35th Street, New York, NY 10001

First published in paperback in 1993

Typeset in Times Roman by Leaper & Gard Ltd, Bristol
Printed and bound in Great Britain by
Mackays of Chatham PLC, Chatham, Kent

A Tavistock/Routledge publication

British Library Cataloguing in Publication Data
Care-giving in dementia : research and applications.
  1. Humans. Dementia. Care
  I. Jones, Gemma M.M. *1957–*   II. Miesen, Bère M.L. *1946–*
362.2

Library of Congress Cataloging-in-Publication Data
Care-giving in dementia : research and applications / [editors] Gemma
  M.M. Jones and Bère M.L. Miesen.
  p.   cm.
Includes bibliographical references and index.
  1. Senile dementia.   2. Psychotherapy in old age.   3. Senile
dementia–Patients–Care.   4. Community mental health services.
  I. Jones, Gemma M.M., 1957–   .   II. Miesen, Bère M.L., 1946–
[DNLM: 1. Community Mental Health Services–in old age.
2. Dementia, Senile.   3. Dementia, Senile–rehabilitation.
4. Family.   5. Models, Theoretical.   6. Psychotherapy–in old age.
WT 150 C271]
RC524.C37   1991
618.97′6898306–dc20
DNLM/DLC
for Library of Congress   91-459
                                                                                CIP

ISBN 0-415-04265-8
     0-415-10168-9 (pbk)

This book is dedicated to four pioneers who have promoted new concepts for the well-being of elderly persons upon which providing care for persons with dementia is based. These four pioneers are:

Sr.St. Michael Guinan, who has challenged society to consider the quality of life in the third age, and to provide the financial, social and spiritual support for those whose third age is a dark one;

Irene Burnside, who has made gerontological nursing a new specialty in its own right, within which care-giving for dementia will be a new sub-specialty;

Joep Munnichs, who has persistently and stubbornly promoted the relevance of life-span psychology for understanding old age;

John Bowlby, who unknowingly provided the concept of attachment history which turned out to be a fundamental key to be able to relate to the inner world of the demented elderly.

Contents

Figures and tables

Figures

Tables

Contributors

Marja A. Abbenhuis studied psychology at the University of Nijmegen in the Netherlands. She works at the Geriatric Hospital in Weert and conducts neuropsychological research primarily with Alzheimer's disease patients at the University of Limburg.

Dr Thomas Arendt is a psychiatrist and neuropathologist who works in the Department of Neurochemistry at the Paul Flechsig Institute for Brain Research, Karl Marx University, Leipzig, Germany. His work has primarily involved the description and quantification of lesions associated with normal aging and dementias. During his sabbatical at the Institute of Psychiatry in London, he worked on developing animal models of Alzheimer's disease and cholinergic neural implants.

Ruth Bright is a music graduate who has worked as a music therapist for over 30 years. Because of her special interest in the health of the elderly and problems associated with old age, particularly Alzheimer's disease, she went on to develop a method of conducting music therapy specifically for persons with dementia. She has published widely on music therapy and lectures throughout the world.

Dr Alistair Burns graduated from Glasgow University in Medicine. He held posts in general medicine and psychiatry at the Maudsley Hospital in London, before becoming Senior Registrar and Honourary Lecturer in old age psychiatry in the section of Old Age Psychiatry, Institute of Psychiatry, London. His interests are in the biological research in old age psychiatry, especially dementia of the Alzheimer type.

Cathy Conroy graduated with an SS in occupational therapy in 1961, in Michigan, USA and has had an interest in working with the elderly ever since. She moved to the UK later that year and started working at Moorgreen Hospital in 1976. She commenced M Phil studies at the University of Southampton in 1985. She has published several articles on reality orientation and is currently focusing on research pertaining to interventions for dementia which can be used by occupational therapists.

Pam Dawson RN, MSN is a Clinical Nurse Specialist in the Department of Extended Care, Sunnybrook Medical Centre and a Clinical Associate, Faculty of Nursing, University of Toronto, Canada. Her clinical and research interests are in the areas of care for the cognitively impaired and their families. Her publications have appeared in *The Canadian Nurse, Geriatric Nursing* and *The Gerontologist* among other journals.

Dr Han Diesfeldt is a psychologist, Director of Research and Head of the Department of Psychogeriatrics of the Stichting Verpleeghuizen Nederland, in Laren. His clinical work is in the assessment and treatment of psycho-geriatric patients. In 1985 he was awarded the Professor Schreuder Prize (a biennial prize for outstanding research in gerontology). He has published widely about the language and memory impairments in dementia, and he is editor of the Dutch *Journal of Gerontology and Geriatrics* (*Tijdschrift voor Gerontologie en Geriatrie*).

Mia Duijnstee has been working in health care for the past 20 years, first as a nurse, and then as a psychologist. She is currently the Coordinator of the Care for the Elderly section of the Netherlands Institute on Care and Welfare. She has published extensively, both theoretical and clinical articles on her experience with patients and their family members. Her special concerns have been the living and working climate in nursing homes and home care services for the demented elderly. She is completing her doctorate on the burden of family members of elderly people with dementia.

Naomi Feil ACSW received her Master's degree in 1956 from Columbia University, New York School of Social Work. She began validation therapy in 1963 and has continued to develop and research its application ever since. In addition, she has been writing, lecturing, scripting-writing, producing films and giving workshops internationally, to promote her approach to care for the disoriented elderly. She is also an actress and uses her acting skills in her films and teaching.

Dr Chris J. Gilleard studied psychology at Sheffield University and took his MSc in Clinical Psychology at the University of Leeds. He has worked with the elderly since then in York, Edinburgh, Ankara (Turkey) and now works as a clinical psychologist at Springfield Hospital in London, UK. Together with Anne Pattie he developed the Clifton assessment procedures for the elderly. In addition to research on day care, he has researched psychotropic drug use in institutions for the elderly. His current research interests include aspects of care and services for the elderly mentally impaired, the cognitive pathology of dementia, and the development of assessment instruments for use with the elderly and neuropsychiatrically impaired patients. He is the author/co-author of several books, chapters and articles about the impaired elderly.

Dr Barbara K. Haight is an Associate Professor of Nursing at the College of Nursing, Medical University of South Carolina. She received her Doctorate of Public Health from the University of South Carolina. She is also the Programme Director for the gerontologic nursing speciality area in the graduate programme. Her primary research interest is in life review and she has written and presented internationally on the subject. She is the Vice Chairperson for the Council of Gerontological Nursing in the American Nurses Association and is active consulting for local nursing homes and the South Carolina Commission on Aging.

Dr Carol P. Hausman has a private practice in clinical psychology and gerontology in Washington, D.C. She is a clinical instructor in psychiatry at the Georgetown University Medical School and a faculty member in the Graduate Department of Psychology at the American University. She is a graduate of Wellesley College, and received her Masters degree from George Washington University and her PhD from the University of Maryland.

Donna Head is a clinical psychologist at St George's Hospital in London. Her research work on reminiscing was completed during her training in work with the elderly while training in clinical psychology at the Institute of Psychiatry.

Dr Pearl D.J. Hettiaratchy FRCPsych is a consultant psychiatrist in psychogeriatrics at St Paul's Hospital in Winchester, UK. She has been working in geriatric psychiatry since 1975 and has special interests in services for the ethnic elderly, support groups for families of persons with dementia and multidisciplinary training for professionals working with dementia.

Dr Eena Job published her first novel in 1947, wrote freelance for radio primarily for the next 15 years, and then graduated in Honours Sociology from the University of Queensland in 1970. She completed her MA in 1976 and her PhD, on the study of people aged 80 and over in 1982. She had conducted a series of courses on memory for the University of Queensland Continuing Education Department and other educational bodies. *Fending Off Forgetfulness: A Practical Guide to Improving Memory* was published in 1985.

Dr Gemma M.M. Jones was born in Canada and is currently living in the UK. She is a research psychologist in the Departments of Psychology and Old Age Psychiatry at the Institute of Psychiatry, London. Her HBSc in Zoology is from the University of Western Ontario; thereafter she obtained a BSN in nursing at the University of British Columbia and her PhD in the neuropsychopharmacology of Alzheimer's disease with the University of London, UK. She has worked extensively with persons with dementia and their families. She lectures, researches, writes, makes educational video tapes and conducts workshops about her theoretical and clinical work with dementia.

Jill Manthorpe MA is a graduate of the University of York and the University of Hull. She is the author of *Elderly People: Rights and Opportunities* (1985) and *Grandparents' Rights* (1989) (with Celia Atherton) and numerous articles on retirement, services for older people and the voluntary sector. She is currently lecturing part-time at the University of Hull to students in nursing, social work and social sciences degree programmes.

Dr Bère M.L. Miesen is a clinical psychogerontologist at the Psychogeriatric Center 'Marienhaven', Warmond, the Netherlands, where he is involved in clinical work, education and research. His PhD is from the University of Nijmegen. He is the author/co-author of many books and publications pertaining to lifespan psychology, gerontology and psychogeriatrics. His first book of poems was published in 1979. He is a co-producer of several video tapes related to his work with dementia.

Sarah Portnoy is a clinical psychologist at the Institute of Psychiatry. She works with persons who have learning difficulties. Her research work on reminiscing was completed during her training in work with the elderly while training in clinical psychology at the Institute of Psychiatry.

Dr Jeroen G.W. Raaijmakers studied psychology at the University of Nijmegen, the Netherlands, and is currently the Head of the Cognitive Psychology Group at the TNO Institute for Perception, Soesterberg, the Netherlands. He has published mostly on memory retrieval, was a consulting editor for the *Journal of Experimental Psychology: Learning, Memory and Cognition*, and is currently the Managing Editor of *Acta Psychologica*.

Dr Carolyn J. Rosenthal is an Associate Professor in the Department of Behavioural Science, University of Toronto, Canada. She obtained her PhD in Sociology from McMaster University. Her research interests include intergenerational relations in families and how these change as members age, health professionals' perceptions and interactions with older patients, and familial social support to institutionalized elderly. Dr Rosenthal is the author of the book *Nurses, Patients and Families* and of numerous articles in aging and family journals. She is the former chairperson of the Canadian Association on Gerontology, Social Sciences division.

Dr Sarah J. Saunders is President of the Board of Directors, and Head of the Community Older Persons Alcohol Program (COPA), Queen Elizabeth Hospital, Toronto, Canada. She is a Physician in the Hospital Outreach Service of the Addiction Research Foundation. **Kathryn Graham BA, MA, Margaret Flower RN,** and **Marilyn White-Campbell BA** are the COPA project co-ordinators and field workers.

Dr Forrest Scogin received his BA from the University of Tennessee, USA, his MA and PhD in Clinical Psychology from Washington University in Missouri. He completed a one-year post-doctoral fellowship in psychotherapy prior to joining the Department of Psychology at the University of Alabama in 1984. His research interests are in geriatric depression, psychosocial interventions for older adults and police psychology.

Janice E. Whittick MPhil is a Chartered Clinical Psychologist, formerly at the Keil Centre in Edinburgh, Scotland. She graduated from Strathclyde University in 1980, and since then has been involved in research projects on community care of the dementing elderly and their family carers. She has combined her research interest with a clinical career since graduating from Edinburgh University in 1985.

Robert T. Woods is a Clinical Psychologist and Senior Lecturer in Clinical Psychology at the Institute of Psychiatry in London, UK. He is a member of the Maudsley Hospital Community Support Team for the Elderly. Since 1975 he has been working with elderly people, co-ordinating psychological services, teaching, conducting research and clinical assessments. He has published numerous papers on work with the elderly, family relationships, depression and cognitive assessment. He conducts workshops and lectures internationally, and is the author and co-author of several books including *Reality Orientation: Psychological Approaches to the Confused Elderly*, *Clinical Psychology with the Elderly*, and most recently; *Alzheimer's Disease: Coping with a Living Death (1989)*. He is a member of the Medical and Scientific Advisory Panel for the Alzheimer's Disease Association.

Foreword

We have received in the 20th century the gift of long life, made possible by rising standards of living and the fruits of scientific advances. More people are living longer and well, than ever before in history. This has prompted some to call for 'a fresh map of life' to guide us in exploring and exploiting this gift of a new age, which begins after the work life has ended and the children have left home (P. Laslett (1989) *A Fresh Map of Life*, London: Weidenfeld & Nicolson).

Not all who arrive at old age are able to meet its challenges with vigour and competence, or to enjoy new learning and the pursuit of leisure. Some are demented and have lost their memories for family members' identities, have lost contact with their own former identities and cannot get through a day without the help of care-givers. The present book is a new map of the other side of aging, a map for professional and family providers to follow in caring for the many people who have a dementing illness.

There have been advances in diagnosis, treatment and care of dementing illnesses. While the advances have not been as large as we would like, we have learned much about the care of the bodies, minds and the heartaches caused by dementing illness. *Care-Giving in Dementia: Research and Applications* passes on the new learning of the authors and fills the gap between research and knowledge gained by university centres and its application by institutions, staff members and family care-givers. In filling this gap, the book has necessarily been multidisciplinary and multi-professional. No single profession has all the answers to problems of taking care of dementing individuals. *Care-Giving in Dementia: Research and Applications* shares at a very practical level, what we know so we can bring light to the underside of growing old, the care and treatment of those who grow old but in their dementia leave their knowing to others. The editors and authors deserve our thanks for shining a bright light on the dark side of growing old.

James E. Birren

Chapter 1

Introduction

Gemma Jones

This is a practical book for practical people; it is aimed at health care professionals and students who spend time doing 'hands on' care with elderly persons who are mentally fragile because of having a dementing illness. It is also a covert plea that the area of care-giving in dementia be seen as a speciality area in its own right, and that the reader join in the advancement and promotion of this speciality area. All ideas for change and innovation in health care come from persons in practice, who are angry and discontent enough to sustain the motivation and energy to look for new solutions or means of improvement.

The contributors to this book come from a range of health care professions and countries and are exceptionally dedicated to their work. Hopefully this dedication will be apparent and inspire you as you read through the chapters.

This book had an interesting beginning, arising from discussions amongst a number of us who presented papers at the 13th International Congress on Gerontology, in New York, July, 1985. We were expressing concerns that there seemed to be a disproportionate amount of funding and publicity for neurobiological research into dementia compared with research about 'care-giving in dementia'. To counterbalance this tendency, we initially undertook to write a joint article about the various approaches to care-giving that we were using individually, and to have it published in a journal. The response was so overwhelming that we had to change to a book format before the original article was ever compiled. As the range of topics continued to increase, we were forced to restrain our content to the following categories: models and theories, interventions for persons with dementia in care facilities, interventions for persons with dementia in the community, interventions for family and, educational approaches to multi-disciplinary care. (Behaviour modification is not included as an intervention in this book because of the consensus of opinion that persons with attentional, short- and long-term memory deficits are not helped by traditional reward and punishment regimens. Remotivation therapy is not included in this book because we could not find anyone who was still using it, or had experience in using it, to contribute a chapter.)

Just as the fields of psychology and nursing are now becoming established as evolving 'sciences' in their own right, so too is *care-giving in dementia*. A brief history of the advances in care-giving might be helpful if you are not used to thinking in terms of this evolution.

Prior to the turn of this century mentally frail and disabled young and old were relegated to workhouses and asylums. (Dementia was not a separately diagnosable condition and persons with aberrant behaviours were thought of as being merely 'crazy' or 'possessed'.) Care in such places was barely custodial. The first study on the results of sensory deprivation in the disoriented elderly was only done in the 1940s. With the advent of space travel there was a spate of research on sensory deprivation. In a nutshell, this research showed that even healthy young adults develop visual and auditory hallucinations within a few hours in conditions of darkness and silence, and even more surprisingly, in the presence of diffuse noise and diffuse light. The comparison of these conditions of sensory deprivation to those existing in many care facilities is a natural one to make.

By the 1950s the first studies of actual stimulation programmes with persons diagnosed as having 'chronic brain syndrome' (what we call dementia today), showed that groups which received intensive personalized attention from staff, in addition to receiving occupational and recreational therapy, improved, whereas control groups who did not receive additional attention, generally deteriorated. At about the same time Folsom developed reality orientation therapy (ROT). ROT assumes that persons with dementia can still learn and participate in present reality, as opposed to 'living in the past', if family and care-givers repeatedly give them the cues about the environment that they can no longer remember themselves. In ROT, the date, time, season and current events are discussed daily with the dementia sufferer in the hope that this will provide them with the frame-work to remain present in reality. ROT is used both in the context of providing such information consistently, 24 hours a day, and in group settings.

The limitations of ROT have only recently been critically evaluated. Some people have nothing but physical and psychological pain left in their present reality and they do not want to remain in it, they feel happier reliving pleasant, safe moments in the past. Second, as brain damage in dementia increases, it becomes increasingly difficult, if not impossible, to remain orientated and learn factual kinds of information (see Chapter 5). ROT is now recognized as being helpful in working with persons in the early stage of dementia, but not thereafter. This is because ROT was based on early psychological models of memory, which maintained that if an item of information was repeated often enough, it would move from short-term into long-term memory. (Research has now shown that this 'two-stage model of memory' is not correct and that there are many types of memory. These may be differentially affected and spared in various types of dementia. Moreover, only recently have the contributions of visual and attentional deficits to memory failure begun to be examined.) ROT was a laudable beginning to providing personal interventions for persons with dementia, but it was not an end point. Other approaches such as sensory stimulation, resocialization, remotivation and behaviour modification were developed in the 1960s and 1970s. In this book, the even newer methods of reminiscing, life review, music therapy, memory retraining and validation therapy are described. These are not end points in the evolution of care-giving in dementia either; simply developmental milestones. So you see, we have come a long way in developing care strategies and approaches, and there is a long way to go if we seriously want to incorporate new multi-disciplinary research into practice.

With the enormous advances in information about the neurobiology and neuropsychology of dementia comes a new understanding about the different types and subtypes of dementia; how perception, attention and memory are affected; and what abilities are spared. This new information undoubtedly has implications for care-giving but it is not commonly disseminated by academics to professionals who do the daily, practical work.

The problems involved in translating research into practice are well known to all of us. In the field of care-giving for dementia they are more challenging than usual because of the multidiscipinary nature of the research. Collaborative, multidisciplinary research and care-giving has only become a realistic goal with recent advances in diagnostics. Chapter 1 emphasizes how difficult it has been to diagnose and understand dementia processes.

This book does not pretend to fill in the entire gap between research and practice, but it does attempt to demonstrate that many persons are tackling the gap. Hopefully, it will encourage other health care professionals and students who have new ideas and observations from their own practice to contribute to the field of care-giving by openly talking and writing about them. Moreover, this book demonstrates that there are many similarities between the approaches used by persons in different countries and professions. Slow though it may seem, our knowledge in care-giving is evolving, and in a common direction.

The overall key observation we had in editing this book is that many researchers and clinicians around the world have independently come to identify similar types of approaches and techniques for working with the dementing elderly. It is especially encouraging that the care-giving strategies described in this book assume that the behaviours exhibited in dementia still express meaning, symbolically if not explicitly.

The threads that run through these chapters are that: care must be stage-specific; that we must work with the abilities that are 'spared' of disease; that lifespan information is needed for individualized care; and, that the results of interpersonal approaches can be a useful source of information for continuous assessment. In the absence of cures or treatments, the 'happiness' and 'optimal stimulation' of the person, rather than miraculous hopes for restoration of lost functions, are acceptable goals for care-giving interventions at this point in time. (Bère Miesen discusses these and other themes and threads common to the chapters in this book in more detail in Chapter 25.)

While the causes of dementia, its diagnosis, progression, cure and treatment, continue to puzzle and elude us, we must respond to the demographic predictions for an expanded elderly population and plan to meet the needs of those persons who will become demented before effective treatments or cures are available. Given the shortage of trained staff in geriatric settings already, it is difficult to imagine how these enormous future needs will be met.

It is our hope that *care-giving in dementia* will become a more attractive field to work in if: it is seen as a speciality in its own right; the myth is dispelled that all that is required to work with the elderly 'comes naturally', without specific training; care-giving in dementia is not seen as pointless and hopeless; and professionals realize that there are a variety of inter-personal approaches and techniques that can be used effectively to the satisfaction of both the elderly person affected and the care-giver. The feeling of 'second-class status' often associated with the care of the elderly should diminish as professional care-givers become involved in the con-tinued evolution of their speciality.

Part I

Models and theories

Chapter 2

Clinicopathologic correlations and the brain–behaviour relationship in Alzheimer's disease

Thomas Arendt and Gemma Jones

SUMMARY

This chapter starts with a general description of dementia, its epidemiology, and distinguishes it from the physiological process of aging. Current definitions of dementia and clinicopathologic correlations in dementia are considered before the historical aspects of the use of the term 'Alzheimer's disease' are discussed. The basic pathology of Alzheimer's disease is described and then the major brain areas are discussed in terms of a neuropsychological view of cognitive and behavioural functioning. The concluding section appeals for professional care-givers to work with those functions that are spared, for as long as they are spared, i.e. to provide stage-specific care, and to make the environments for care-giving as rich and stimulating as possible.

INTRODUCTION

The chapter was intended to be a simple, clear guide to the neuropathology of dementia, describing how it relates to behaviour, with the ultimate aim that perhaps this information will be of use to persons involved in developing new methods of care-giving for dementia. This is a difficult task because oversimplification is potentially as harmful as writing with so much technical detail that the chapter cannot be understood. The dementing illnesses are extremely complex. They show patterns of great variability and are not easily diagnosed, or distinguishable from one another.

This chapter tries to synthesize the current knowledge as systematically as possible, with particular attention to the historical events relating to the discovery of the dementing illnesses. It is very important to understand this history, because the term Alzheimer's disease has referred to different aspects of the disease at different times. It started out referring persons who had the early onset form of the illness, and it now encompasses both early- and late-onset forms. The literature of the past 30 years cannot be properly understood unless one is familiar with this history.

Dementing disorders are the most common disorders of later life associated with increasing medical, social and economic problems. There are several reasons for the increasing incidence of dementia, which today has reached epidemic proportions, as well as for increased professional and public awareness of it.

Major demographic changes have occurred in the industrial countries throughout the world during the last one hundred years. Whereas at the beginning of this century only about 25 per cent of the population lived beyond 65 years, in our days more than 70 per cent do so (Siegel, 1980). According to the World Health Organization (WHO) this increase in average life expectancy will continue, resulting in a doubling of the number of people aged more than 60 years, within the next 20 years. Whereas this aging phenomenon is already well under way in the more developed parts of the world, it has been predicted that the less developed countries will have reached a situation comparable to that of Europe in 1950 by the year 2025 which means the epidemic of dementia will reach developing countries about half a century later (Table 2.1).

Aging in and of itself is a physiological process, without pathological features. However, aging can influence the onset and course of disorders. Among these, are namely disorders of the cardiovascular system, cancer and disorders affecting the central nervous system, leading to an impairment of intellectual abilities. The most important disorders of the central nervous system in later life are stroke, Parkinson's disease and senile dementia (WHO, 1986). During the last decades there has been a decrease in mortality from the most frequent life-limiting disorders, namely disorders of the cardiovascular system. Some success has been achieved in symptomatological treatment of Parkinsonian patients (Marsden and Parkes, 1977). For senile dementia, the factors which cause the disease and the mechanisms by which it develops, and, therefore, an approach for its prevention and treatment, still remains obscure.

Table 2.1 Expected increase in percentage of elderly people

	Percentage aged 60 years and over		
	1950	*1980*	*2025*
World	8.5	8.5	13.7
Europe	12.8	17.0	24.6
Northern America	12.0	14.7	22.0
East Asia	7.5	8.7	19.4
Latin America	5.5	6.3	10.8
Africa	5.5	5.0	6.8

Source: World Health Organization, 1982.

EPIDEMIOLOGY OF DEMENTIA

Epidemiological surveys carried out in Northern and Western European countries, in the United States, as well as in the Soviet Union, China, Japan, Australia and New Zealand, report an average frequency of about 1.5 to 14.0 per cent of the general population for people who suffer from a severe dementia and 4 to 53 per cent for those who have a less severe form of dementia (Akesson, 1969; Cooper and Sosna, 1983; Kay *et al.*, 1964; Pasamanick *et al.*, 1957). These surveys did not reveal major geographic or ethnic differences in patterns of dementia. The incidence of dementia shows a clear-cut age dependency (Table 2.2). Whereas the prevalence of severe cases of dementia in the age group between 30 and 60 amounts to only about 0.1 per cent (Kokman, 1984) it is increased in the seventh decade to 2 to 3 per cent, and reaches an average of 17 to 50 per cent in the ninth decade (Sulkava *et al.*, 1985).

DEFINING DEMENTIA

Dementia is not a disorder in its own right, it is rather a syndrome or a grouping of symptoms which can be manifested in a variable combination.

Since we are dealing with a very complex deterioration of elaborate functions of the nervous system, many different attempts have been made to give a definition of the disturbances collectively referred to as dementia. Following a suggestion of the WHO we can define dementia in the following way:

> Dementia is the global impairment of higher cortical functions, including memory, the capacity to solve the problems of day-to-day living, the performance of learned perceptuo-motor skills, the correct use of social skills and control of emotional reactions, in the absence of gross 'clouding of consciousness'. The condition is often irreversible and progressive.

(WHO, 1986)

Table 2.2 Prevalence of dementia by age and sex (percentage)

Age	Males	Females	Overall
65–69	3.9	0.5	2.1
70–74	4.1	2.7	3.3
75–79	8.0	7.9	8.0
80+	13.2	20.9	17.7

Source: Kay and Bergmann, 1980:43.

The absence of 'clouding of consciousness' is important to note since this refers to the awareness of a person to what is happening to him.

Dementia usually starts with relatively slight impairments but can progress to a point where all skills of communication and self-care are lost. This process might be regarded as a quantitative and qualitative continuum with stages labelled as mild, moderate or severe, depending on the degree of dementia. As happens with other kinds of disorders, the progression of dementia can be dependent on internal as well as external factors. Several rating scales have been developed for assessing the severity of dementia. With the help of such scales, for example, the clinical dementia rating scale (Hughes *et al.*, 1982), it is possible to place the patient in one of five stages along a continuum from healthy to severely demented. Within each stage of severity, the typical features of dementia are described in terms of memory, orientation, judgement, problem-solving, participation in community affairs, life at home, hobbies and personal care (Table 2.3).

CLINICOPATHOLOGIC CORRELATIONS IN DEMENTIA

A variety of disorders can each produce the syndrome of dementia. Alzheimer's disease is by far the most common form of dementia in later life and accounts for 40 to 55 per cent of all cases. Table 2.4 shows a list of dementing disorders grouped according to what we know today about the cause of the disease (aetiological classification). Such classification is of particular heuristic value for the investigation of the mechanisms under-lying the pathological process and for the development of approaches for prevention and treatment. There is no cure for the two most frequent forms of dementia: Alzheimer's disease (AD) and multi-infarct dementia. Some of the more rare forms of dementia, however, which together amount to about 20 per cent of all cases, are reversible.

An aetiological diagnosis of dementia, however, cannot be derived from the clinical appearance of the disorder alone; further investigations such as neurological investigation, testing blood samples and CT scan need to be carried out. For practical reasons it might, therefore, be helpful to classify dementing disorders according to the prominent pattern of mental dysfunc-tion. One possibility is to discriminate according to the behavioural pattern, as reflected by classification of 'cortical' or 'subcortical' dementia (Albert *et al.*, 1974; Cummings, 1986) (Tables 2.5 and 2.6). Although somewhat simplistic, these characteristic patterns of behaviour can be matched to some extent to patterns of pathological changes in the brain, as the terms cortical and subcortical already imply. As the cerebral cortex is the centre for various complex mental processes such as initiating voluntary actions, language, speech and perceiving the world, damage to the cortex can produce problems with language, perceptual skills, performance of actions on command and recognition of familiar objects (Cummings, 1986). On the other hand, damage to the striatum and thalamus, subcortical brain structures, involved mainly in the pathology of disorders characterized by a 'subcortical pattern' of mental impairment, can result in a general slowing down of intellectual activity, some form of memory deficit, alterations of personality, and impaired ability to manipulate acquired knowledge (Albert *et al.*, 1974).

Conceptually, cortical and subcortical abilities can be categorized as instrumental functions and fundamental functions, respectively (Table 2.7) (Albert, 1978; Cummings, 1986). Instrumental functions include language, praxis, perceptual recognition, memory and calculation. Abnormalities of instrumental functions produce aphasia, apraxia, agnosia, amnesia and acalculia deficits associated with the 'cortical dementias'. Instrumental abilities are the most highly evolved of human activities and depend on phylogenetically recent and ontogenetically late developing structures (Yakovlev, 1948). Fundamental functions, on the other hand, include arousal, activation, attention, sequencing, motivation and mood. These functions are much less discreetly organized and involve subcortical nuclei (basal ganglia and thalamus) that are interconnected with the cerebral cortex. The major projections are reciprocal connections with the frontal lobe and afferent connections from the limbic system. Fundamental functions are crucial for survival and emerge early during phylogenetic and ontogenetic development. Dysfunctions of these abilities produce the cardinal features of subcortical dementia including slowing down of information processing, dilapidation of memory and cognition, and disturbances of mood and motivation (Cummings, 1986).

HISTORICAL ASPECTS OF CLINICOPATHOLOGIC CORRELATIONS IN ALZHEIMER'S DISEASE

Alzheimer's disease is named after the German physician Alois Alzheimer who in 1904 discovered 'senile plaques' in the cerebral cortex of the brain of a patient over 65 years, who had suffered from dementia (Alzheimer, 1904). Similar changes had already been described 6 years earlier following observations of the brains of two patients over 65 years (Redlich, 1898) as well as in brains of epileptics (Blocq and Marinesco, 1892). In 1906 Alzheimer described the occurrence of senile plaques and neurofibrillary tangles in the brain of a patient of 51 years who had been demented for four and a half years (Alzheimer, 1907). Shortly after this, clinicopathological studies were published describing memory functions as the initial symptoms as well as the progressive course of this disorder. These appeared to occur in people before they had reached the conventional point of old age and were, therefore, called 'presenile dementia' (Perusini, 1909). At this time presenile dementia was believed to be a special entity, different from senile dementia. However, despite the age of onset there was never

Table 2.3 Clinical dementia rating (CDR)

	Healthy CDR 0	Questionable dementia CDR 0.5	Mild dementia CDR 1	Moderate dementia CDR 2	Severe dementia CDR 3
Memory	no memory loss or slight inconsistant forgetfulness	mild consistent forgetfulness, partial recollection of events 'benign' forgetfulness	moderate memory loss, more marked for recent events interference with everyday activities	severe memory loss, only highly learned material retained, new material rapidly lost	severe memory loss, only fragments remain
Orientation	fully oriented		some difficulty with time relationships oriented for place and person at examination but may have geographic disorientation	usually disoriented in time, often to place	oriented to person only
Judgement and problem-solving	solves everyday problems well, judgement good in relation to past performance	only doubtful impairment in solving problems, similarities, differences	moderate difficulty in handling complex problems, social judgement usually maintained	severe impairment in handling problems, similarities, differences, social judgement usually impaired	unable to make judgement or solve problems

Community affairs	independent function at usual level in job, shopping, business and financial affairs, volunteer and social groups	doubtful or mild impairment, if any in these activities	unable to function independently at these activities though may still be engaged in some; may still appear normal to casual inspection		no pretence of independent function outside home
Home and hobbies	life at home, hobbies and intellectual interests well maintained	life at home, hobbies and intellectual interests well maintained or only slightly impaired	mild but definite impairment of function at home, more difficult chores abandoned, more complicated hobbies and interests abandoned	only simple chores preserved, very restricted interests, poorly sustained	no significant function in home outside of his own room
Personal care	fully capable of self-care		needs occasional prompting	requires assistance in dressing, hygiene, keeping of personal effects	requires much help with personal care, often incontinent

Source: Hughes *et al.*, 1982.

Table 2.4 Classification of dementing disorders according to the causes of the disease ('aetiological classification')

Aetiology	Illness	Treatment
Unknown	Alzheimer's disease	—
Multiple infarcts	Multi-infarct dementia	—
Genetic disorder	Down's syndrome	—
	Parkinson's disease	(antiParkinsonian drugs do not help the dementia)
	Huntington's disease	—
	Wilson's disease	penicillamine
Physical damage	normal pressure hydrocephalus	operation
	boxing dementia	—
	brain tumour	operation
Toxic damage	postalcoholic amnesia/ dementia	stop drinking
Infections	Creutzfeldt–Jakob disease	—
	AIDS	—
Endocrine disorder	hypothyroidism	thyroxine
	parathyroid disorder	pharmacological or surgical treatment
Nutritional deficiencies	vitamin deficiencies	vitamins

clear-cut evidence that this type of presenile dementia could be differentiated in any way from 'senile dementia'. Thus, the distinction between presenile and senile forms of Alzheimer's disease, as we call it today, was always more a question of terminology rather than nosology. Since then, many physicians, being aware of the similarities between these two forms of dementia regarded them as two distinct types of manifestation of one disorder. This viewpoint was supported later by the demonstration of many similarities in morphological and biochemical changes in the brain (Albert, 1964).

Due to the methods which were available for the investigation of the brain in the early years of this century, the biological approach to psychiatric illness was mainly a structural one. In 1912, when Wilson described a disorder which was later named after him, he pointed out that this disorder could also be associated with dementia although the neuropsychological changes were different than those of Alzheimer's disease.

Table 2.5 Contrasting features of cortical and subcortical dementia

Aspect	Cortical dementia	Subcortical dementia
Neuropsychological features		
Severity	more severe deficits earlier in the disease course	mild to moderate throughout the course
Speed of cognition	normal	slowed
Memory short term	encoding deficit, aided little by clues	recall partially facilitated clues and recognition tasks
Remote recall	normal in early stages temporal gradient	no temporal gradient
Language	anomia, comprehension deficit, paraphasia	normal or mild anomia
Visuospatial skill	impaired, poor model copying	impaired, poor manipulation of egocentric space (map reading, judgement of horizontal and vertical)
Cognition	impaired early, late untestable	poor abstraction and categorization
Neuropsychiatric features		
Personality	indifference, occasional disinhibition	apathy, irritability
Depression	uncommon	common
Mania	absent	infrequent
Psychosis	common, simple delusions	common in some disorders may have complex delusion
Motor system		
Speech	no dysarthria	dysarthria
Posture	normal (flexed late)	flexed or extended
Gait	normal (until late)	hypo- or hyperkinetic
Speed	normal (until late)	slow
Adventitious movements	none or myoclonus	tremor, chorea, dystonia
Tone	normal early, rigid in later stages	abnormal (hypotonic in choreic disorders, hypertonia in Parkinsonian conditions)

Source: Cummings, 1986.

Table 2.6 Classification of dementing disorders according to the preferential pattern of neuropsychiatric impairment ('clinicopathological classification')

Cortical pattern	Subcortical pattern
Alzheimer's disease	Wilson's disease
Pick's disease	Parkinson's disease
Creutzfeldt–Jakob disease	Huntington's disease
Dementia associated with large vessel stroke	Progressive supranuclear palsy

Table 2.7 Characteristics of instrumental and fundamental functions

Aspect	Instrumental functions	Fundamental functions
Neuropsychological activities	language, memory, perceptual recognition, praxis, calculation	timing, arousal, attention, motor programming, motivation, mood
Neuropsychological deficits	aphasia, amnesia, agnosia, apraxia, acalculia	slowing, forgetfulness, dilapidation of cognition, depression, apathy
Associated type of dementia	cortical	subcortical
Principal grey matter structures	neopallidal association, cortex and hippocampus	basal ganglia, thalamus, brainstem
White matter connections	discrete well myelinated intra- and interhemispheric tracts	more diffuse, shorter, less-well-myelinated projections
Organizational composition	parallel connection of functional units, lateral dominance well developed	serial connection of structures with overlapping functions, poorly lateralized
Phylogeny	recent evolutionary acquisition, most well developed in humans	more primitive
Ontogeny	incompletely developed at birth, myelination and dendritic growth continue through childhood	functional at birth or soon after

Source: Cummings, 1986.

Whereas Alzheimer's disease is mainly characterized by a 'cortical pattern' of psychopathology which involves qualities like perception and language, Wilson's disease is mainly characterized by deficiencies in motivation, emotion, arousal and attention summarized as 'subcortical pattern'. This distinction between 'cortical' and 'subcortical' refers to the brain areas known at this time to be involved in the pathology of these disorders and reflects early attempts to establish clinicopathological relationships. This structural approach to psychiatry was enhanced by the investigation of cerebral damage to soldiers during the First World War. It added knowledge to the understanding of the relationship of certain brain areas to psychological functions. At this time, however, the psychoanalytical approach started its triumphant advance around the world and the biological approach was only 'rediscovered' 40 years later, when modern neuropharmacology was developed. Influenced by the increasing knowledge about the mechanisms that neurons use to exchange signals by means of chemical compounds termed neurotransmitters, the biological understanding of the brain at this time was mainly influenced by a chemical approach rather than a structural one such as in the beginning of the century. As a consequence of this, many neurochemical aspects of neuropsychiatric disorders were discovered. The most important one being probably the description of dopaminergic dysfunction in Parkinson's disease subsequently leading to the possibility of symptomatic treatment (Ehringer and Hornykiewicz, 1960). Today we observe the beginning of a synthesis of the structural and chemical approaches to the understanding of the brain. Much has been added to this eclectic understanding of brain function from the investigation of Alzheimer's disease.

In terms of a structural equivalent of a neuropsychiatric deficiency Alzheimer's disease can best be described by means of a 'cortical pattern of dementia', although usually it is accompanied by features of the 'subcortical pattern', too. This already shows the limitation of a pure structural approach and leads to the biochemical aspects of the disorder which have been best described in terms of the dysfunction of the cholinergic neurotransmitter system.

THE BRAIN–BEHAVIOUR RELATIONSHIP IN ALZHEIMER'S DISEASE

The diagnosis of Alzheimer's disease is mainly one of systematic exclusion of other possible causes of dementia. This careful exclusion is particularly important for identifying those forms of dementia which are treatable and, therefore, at least partially reversible. With certainty the diagnosis of Alzheimer's disease can only be established after post-mortem examination, which confirms the clinical diagnosis in about 85 to 90 per cent of all cases (Mölsä et al., 1984).

The appearance of senile plaques and neurofibrillary tangles in the cerebral cortex and hippocampus is typical for Alzheimer's disease, and on the basis of their number the post-mortem diagnosis is made. The number of both these changes correlates with the severity of dementia (Blessed *et al.*, 1968; Wilcock and Esiri, 1982); they are, however, not absolutely specific for Alzheimer's disease and can be observed in other dementing disorders such as in elderly patients with Down's syndrome (Schwartz, 1967) and in boxing dementia (Corsellis *et al.*, 1973) and to a lesser extent even in normal elderly without mental impairment (Tomlinson *et al.*, 1968). Senile plaques consist of a conglomerate of processes of neurons which have been damaged, intermingled with glial cells and a protein which is called amyloid (Wesniewski *et al.*, 1981).

Neurofibrillary tangles are localized in the cell bodies of neurons. They consist of twisted filaments which may derive from the neurofilaments of normal neurons which are believed to play a role in the transport of chemical compounds along neuronal processes called axons. The formation of neurofibrillary tangles, therefore, likely interferes with the transport function in a neuron (Gajdusek, 1985). The amyloid protein probably takes part in the formation of tangles, too.

This amyloid protein which does not occur naturally in the body is derived from a larger protein which is normally distributed throughout the brain and other organs (Kang *et al.*, 1987). The amyloid itself, is probably the result of the impaired metabolism of this larger precursor protein. The gene which codes for this amyloid-precursor protein is found on chromsome 21 (Goldgabe *et al.*, 1987). As Down's patients have three copies of this chromosome, an overexpression of this gene might be a plausible cause for the deposition of amyloid observed in elderly Down's syndrome patients. The gene, however, is present in normal people and whether its expression is affected in Alzheimer's disease remains unclear. It seems likely that the deposition of this protein is not restricted to the brain but also occurs in other organs (Joachim *et al.*, 1989). However, the process of amyloid deposition in the brain seems to be involved in the process of cell death.

As a neurodegenerative disorder, Alzheimer's disease is characterized by a progressive loss of neurons which is irreversible. In the final stages of this disorder almost every part of the brain is affected. Early during the course of the disease, however, neuronal death is not uniformly distributed throughout the brain and certain areas seem to be more susceptible than others. Neurons with large cell bodies and long axons seem to be particularly sensitive to cell death. Some of these neurons are localized in the cerebral cortex and hippocampus, others in subcortical brain areas.

The psychopathology of Alzheimer's disease shows considerable individual differences as does the neuropathology. These differences are most pronounced for mental abilities with lateral dominance (see Table 2.7). Brain areas which are mainly affected in Alzheimer's disease and implications for deficiencies of mental abilities deriving from this brain damage will be briefly described (Chui, 1989).

Limbic system: memory and learning

In Alzheimer's disease, limbic and paralimbic systems develop a high density of neurofibrillary tangles (Ball, 1978). The location of tangles in afferent neurons of the entorhinal cortex and efferent neurons of the subiculum are believed to functionally disconnect the hippocampus from the neocortex (Hyman et al., 1984). This has been suggested as the anatomical basis of the amnesia for recent events commonly seen in early stages of Alzheimer's disease (Fuld, 1978). Recent investigations suggest that impairment in olfactory discrimination may result from lesions in the prepyriform cortex (Reyes et al., 1987). Lesions in the limbic and paralimbic system may probably contribute to the behavioural symptoms of Alzheimer's disease (Reisberg, 1986).

Temporal–parietal–occipital association cortex: visual impairment, aphasia, apraxia, agnosia and visual disorientation

Whereas the primary motor–sensory cortex is relatively spared by degenerative changes, the multimodal association cortex is highly prone to neurofibrillary degeneration (Pearson et al., 1985) which may be linked to the visual impairment, aphasia, apraxia and visual disorientation observed in Alzheimer's disease. Dysfunctions of the posterior association areas correlate with several disturbances in higher cortical function that usually follow the development of amnesia. Visuospatial impairment occurs relatively early during the course of the disease (Rosen, 1983). Disturbances of language are regarded as typical for Alzheimer's disease (Sjögren and Sjögren, 1952) and correlate with other indicators of disease severity (Martin et al., 1987). Apraxia is reported to be present in 70 to 80 per cent of cases with Alzheimer's disease, in most cases characterized by clumsiness in object manipulation and in executing complex goal-directed activities. Agnosia and psychic blindness are observed in the advanced cases of Alzheimer's disease (Sjögren and Sjögren, 1952).

Prefrontal cortex: insight, abstraction, planning, judgement, personality change, behavioural disturbance and relative preservation of social propriety

Apathy, impaired insight, and lack of judgement are common clinical observations in Alzheimer's disease (Gustafson, 1975). Concreteness, perseveration and inefficient problem solving are frequently noted in psychometric assessment. In contrast to Pick's disease, which shows a constant involvement of prefrontal cortex, social graces and appropriateness are generally well preserved in patients with AD.

Subcortical projection: memory, learning, behaviour

Several subcortical systems, such as the cholinergic basal forebrain system (Arendt *et al.*, 1983, Whitehouse *et al.*, 1982), the serotonergic raphe nuclei (Ishii, 1966), the noradrenergic locus coeruleus (Bondareff *et al.*, 1982) and, to a lesser extent, the dopaminergic substantia nigra (Ditter and Mirra, 1987) are thought to affect memory, learning and behaviour.

The cholinergic basal forebrain system (nucleus basalis of Meynert) shows a constant and severe loss of neurons in Alzheimer's disease (Arendt *et al.*, 1983; 1985; 1988a). This brain structure is localized close to the basis of the brain and the neuronal processes of its neurons reach the cerebral cortex supplying it with a neurotransmitter called acetylcholine (Wenk *et al.*, 1980). The hypothesis that cell loss in the brain area might be related to the loss of cognitive function observed in Alzheimer's disease has gained much support from pharmacological studies interfering with the metabolism of the neurotransmitter acetylcholine or its receptor (Kopelman and Corn, 1988; Drachman and Sahakian, 1979; Warburton, 1972) and from animal experiments placing artificial damage to this structure (Arendt *et al.*, 1988b; 1989; Smith, 1988). Subsequent to cell loss in this area, less acetylcholine is supplied to the cerebral cortex apparently contributing to mental dysfunction which appears as a 'cortical pattern' of neuropsychiatric involvement. However, since the nucleus basalis of Meynert also supplies structures other than the cerebral cortex, namely subcortical areas with acetylcholine (Grove, 1988a;b), such cell loss might also result in dysfunctions being part of the 'subcortical pattern' of dementia.

As the nucleus basalis of Meynert seems to be very sensitive to a variety of insults such as viral, physical, toxic and genetic damage, cell loss in this brain area occurs in several disorders which are related to the different types of causal damage (Arendt *et al.*, 1983; 1984; 1988a;b;c; Bigl *et al.*, 1989) and which all result in dementia-type behavioural damage (see Tables 2.8 and 2.4). This directly implies that damage to the nucleus basalis

Table 2.8 Dementing disorders associated with a cell loss in the cholinergic system of the basal forebrain (basal nucleus)

Alzheimer's disease	Parkinson's disease
Down's syndrome	post-alcoholic amnesia/dementia
Boxing dementia	Pick's disease
Creutzfeldt–Jakob disease	progressive supranuclear palsy

Source: Bigl *et al.*, 1989.

of Meynert is crucial for the development of dementia. Blocking signal transduction between neurons which is normally mediated by acetylcholine, by means of applying scopolamine, results in a pattern of cognitive impairment which shows some similarities to those observed in Alzheimer's disease and post-alcoholic Korsakoff's disease (Kopelman and Corn, 1988); disorders with cognitive dysfunction which both are characterized by cell loss in the nucleus basalis of Meynert (Table 2.9).

CONCLUSIONS

Many attempts have been made to improve the cognitive abilities of patients with Alzheimer's disease by pharmacological manipulation of cholinergic function in the brain. However, they all have had disappointing results so far, as have many other strategies of prevention and treatment.

The differential impairment of specific aspects of cognitive dysfunction may allow us to establish techniques to activate those functions which are spared which include motor and skill learning as well as priming (Brown and Marsden, 1988). As mechanisms of priming, for example, are relatively spared during the course of the disease, and visuospatial skills, on the other hand, are usually impaired, it might be possible to improve the spatial orientation of patients with the help of spatial cues in the environment, such as different colours for different wards of a hospital. Other approaches are discussed in detail elsewhere in this book.

The influence of the environment and other interpersonal approaches, however, may not only help to activate mental functions which are still preserved, but might even induce neurobiological processes in the brain itself which are detectable by morphological or biochemical methods. It has been demonstrated in animals that both social isolation (Oehler et al., 1987) and environments enriched with social stimuli (Greenough and Green, 1981) can induce changes in the brain biochemistry and morphology. Pilot studies on the effect of enriched environments on the progression of the cognitive impairment in demented patients indicated that patients who received intensive care (mainly directed towards psychological integrity and autonomy) were not only significantly better in their emotional, cognitive and psychomotor function than a control group but also showed biochemically detectable changes in the cerebrospinal fluid (Annerstedt et al., 1987; Karlsson et al., 1988).

It is our hope that knowledge about the neuropathology of dementia and advances in care-giving progress together. Much remains to be known about how best to utilize the functions that are spared for as long as possible, and how best to work with the various forms of dementia.

Table 2.9 Pattern of memory impairment after pharmacological blockade by scopolamine and in neuropsychiatric disorders associated with neuronal loss in the cholinergic basal forebrain

Memory aspect	Cholinergic blockade	Post-alcoholic Korsakoff syndrome	Alzheimer's disease
Primary memory (less than 30 sec)	intact	intact	impaired — intact for simple tasks, i.e. digit span, block span, simple Brown Peterson task — impaired in more complex tasks, i.e. non-verbal Brown Peterson task
Secondary anterograde memory (more than 30 sec) Explicit component (recall and recognition)	impaired	impaired	impaired
Implicit component (procedural and skill learning, priming)	intact	intact	intact
Secondary retrograde memory (remote memory)	intact	impaired (temporal gradient)	impaired

Source: Kopelman and Corn, 1988.

REFERENCES

Akesson, H.O. (1969) 'A population study of senile and arteriosclerotic psychoses', *Human Heredity* 19: 546–66.

Albert, E. (1964) 'Senile Demenz und Alzheimersche Krankheit als Ausdruck des gleichen Krankheitsgeschehens', *Fortschrille der Neurologie Psychiatie* 32: 625–73.

Albert, M.L. (1978) 'Subcortical dementia', in R. Katzman, R.D. Terry, K.L. Bick (eds) *Alzheimer's Disease: Senile Dementia and Related Disorders*, New York: Raven Press.

——,Feldman, R.G. and Willis, A.L. (1974) 'The "subcortical dementia" of progressive supranuclear palsy'. *Journal of Neurology, Neurosurgury and Psychiatry* 37: 121–30.

Alzheimer, A. (1904) 'Histologische Studien zur Differentialdiagnose der progressiven Paralyse', *Nissls Arbeiten* 1: 18.

—— (1907), 'Über eine eigenartige Erkrankung der Hirnrinde', *Allgemeine Zeitshrift für Psychiatrie* 64: 146–8.

Annerstedt, A., Alfredson, B. and Risberg, J. (1987) 'Effects of an alternative mode of care for demented elderly', Third Congress of the International Psychogeriatric Association, Chicago.

Arendt, T., Bigl, V. and Arendt, A. (1984) 'Neurone loss in the nucleus basalis of Meynert in Creutzfeldt–Jakob Disease', *Acta Neuropathologica* 65: 85–8.

——,Bigl, V., Arendt, A. and Tennstedt, A. (1983) 'Loss of neurons in the nucleus basalis of Meynert in Alzheimer's disease, paralysis agitans and Korsakoff's disease', *Acta Neuropathologica* 61: 101–8.

——,Bigl, V., Tennstedt, A. and Arendt, A. (1985) 'Neuronal loss in different parts of the nucleus basalis is related to neuritic plaque formation in cortical target areas in Alzheimer's disease', *Neuroscience* 14: 1–14.

——,Hennig, D., Gray, J.A. and Marchbanks, R. (1988c) 'Loss of neurons in the rat basal forebrain cholinergic projection system after prolonged intake of ethanol', *Brain Research Bulletin* 21: 563–70.

——,Taubert, G., Bigl, V. and Arendt, A. (1988a) 'Amyloid deposition in the nucleus basalis of Meynert complex: a topographic marker for degenerating cell clusters in Alzheimer's disease', *Acta Neuropathology* 75: 226–32.

——,Allen, Y., Marchbanks, R.M., Schugens, M.M., Sinden, J., Lantos, P.L. and Gray, J.A. (1989) 'Cholinergic system and memory in the rat: effects of chronic ethanol, embryonic basal forebrain brain transplants, and excitotoxic lesions of cholinergic basal forebrain projection system', *Neuroscience* (in press).

——, Allen, Y., Sinden, J., Schugens, M.M., Marchbanks, R.M., Lantos, P.L. and Gray, J.A. (1988b) 'Cholinergic-rich brain transplants reverse alcohol-induced memory deficits', *Nature* 332: 448–50.

Ball, M.J. (1978) 'Topographic distribution of neurofibrillary tangles and granulovacuolar degeneration in hippocampal cortex of aging and demented patients: a quantitiative study', *Acta Neuropathologica* 2: 72–80.

Bigl, V., Arendt, T. and Biesold, D. (1989) 'The nucleus basalis of Meynert during aging and in neuropsychiatric disorders', in M. Steriade and D. Biesold (eds) *Cholinergic System of the Basal Forebrain*, Oxford: Oxford University Press.

Blessed, G., Tomlinson, B.E. and Roth, M. (1968) 'The association between quantitative measures of dementia and of senile change in the grey matter of elderly subjects', *British Journal of Psychiatry* 114: 797–811.

Blocq, P. and Marinesco, G. (1892) 'Sur les lesions et la pathogenie de l'epilepsie dite essentielle', *Seminars in Medicine* 12: 445–6.

Bondareff, W., Mountjoy, R.Q. and Roth, M. (1982) 'Loss of neurons of origins of the adrenergic projection to cerebral cortex (nucleus locus ceruleus) in senile dementia', *Neurology* 32: 164–8.

Brown, R.G. and Marsden, C.D. (1988) ' "Subcortical dementia": the neuropsychological evidence', *Neuroscience* 25: 363–87.

Chui, H.Ch. (1989) 'Dementia. A review emphasizing clinicopathologic correlation and brain–behaviour relationships', *Archives of Neurology* 46: 806–14.

Cooper, B. and Sosna, U. (1983) 'Psychische Erkrankungen in der Altenbevölkerung. Eine epidemiologische Feldstudie in Mannheim', *Nervenarzt* 54: 239–49.

Corsellis, J.A.N., Bruton, C.J. and Freeman-Browne, D. (1973) 'The aftermath of boxing', *Psychology in Medicine*, 3: 270–303.

Cummings, J.L. (1986) 'Subcortical dementia. Neuropsychology, neuropsychiatry, and pathophysiology', *British Journal of Psychiatry* 149: 682–97.

Ditter, S.M. and Mirra, S.S. (1987) 'Neuropathologic and clinical features of Parkinson's disease in Alzheimer's disease patients', *Neurology* 37: 754–60.

Drachman, D.A. and Sahakian, B.J. (1979) 'Effects of cholinergic agents on human learning and memory', in A. Barbeau, J.H. Growdon and R.J. Wurtman (eds) *Nutrition and the Brain*, vol. 5, New York: Raven Press, pp. 351–66.

Ehringer, H. and Hornykiewicz, O. (1960) 'Verteilung von Noradrenalin und Dopamin (5-hydroxytyramin) im Gehirn des Menschen und ihr Verhalten bei Erkrankungen des extrapyramidalen Systems', *Klinishe Wetenshaftshritte* 38: 1236–9.

Fuld, P.A. (1978) 'Psychological testing in the differential diagnosis of the dementias', in *Alzheimer's Disease: Senile Dementia and Related Disorders*, New York: Raven Press, pp. 185–93.

Gajdusek, D.C. (1985) 'Hypothesis: interference with axonal transport of neurofilament as a common pathogenetic mechanism in certain diseases of the central nervous system', *New England Journal of Medicine* 312: 714–19.

Goldgabe, D., Lerman, M.I., McBride, O.W., Saffiotti, U. and Gajdusek, D.C. (1987) 'Characterization and chromosomal localization of a cDNA encoding brain amyloid of Alzheimer's disease', *Science* 235: 877–80.

Greenough, W.T. and Green, E.J. (1981) 'Experience and the changing brain', in J. McGaugh and S. Kiesler (eds) *Aging, Biology and Behavior*, New York: Academic Press, pp. 159–93.

Grove, E.A. (1988a) 'Neuronal associations of the substantia innominata in the rat: afferent connections', *Journal of Comparative Neurology* 277: 315–46.

—— (1988b) 'Efferent connections of the substantia innominata in the rat', *Journal of Comparative Neurology* 277: 347–64.

Gustafson, L. (1975) 'Psychiatric symptoms in dementia with onset in the presenile period', *Acta Psychiatrica Scandinavica* (Suppl.) 257: 8–35.

Hughes, C.P., Berg, L., Danziger, W.L., Coben, L.A. and Martin, R.L. (1982) 'A new clinical scale for the staging of dementia', *British Journal of Psychiatry* 140: 566–72.

Hyman, B.T., Van Hoesen, G.W., Damasio, A.R. and Barnes, C. (1984) 'Alzheimer's disease: cell-specific pathology isolates the hippocampal formation', *Science* 225: 1168–70.

Ishii, T. (1966) 'Distribution of Alzheimer's neurofibrillary changes in the brainstem and hypothalamus of senile dementia', *Acta Neuropathologica* 6: 181–7.

Joachim, C.L., Mori, H. and Selkoe, D.J. (1989) 'Amyloid β-protein deposition in tissue other than brain in Alzheimer's disease', *Nature* 341: 226–30.

Kang, J., Lemaire, H.-G., Unterbeck, A., Salbaum, J.M., Masters, C.L., Grzeschik, K.-H., Multhaup, G., Beyreuther, K. and Müller-Hill, B. (1987) 'The precursor of Alzheimer's disease amyloid A_4 protein resembles a cell surface receptor', *Nature* 325: 733–6.

Karlsson, I., Brane, G., Melin, E., Nyth, A.-L. and Rybo, E. (1988) 'Effects of environmental stimulation on biochemical and psychological variables in dementia', *Acta Psychiatrica Scandinavica* 77: 207–13.

Kay, D.W.K. and Bergmann, K. (1980) 'Epidemiology of mental disorders amongst the aged in the community', in J.E. Birren and R.B. Sloane (eds) *Handbook of Mental Health and Aging*, Englewood Cliffs, New York: Prentice Hall, pp. 34–56.

——, Beamish, P. and Roth, M. (1964) 'Old age mental disorder in Newcastle upon Tyne. Part I: a study of prevalence', *British Journal of Psychiatry* 110: 146–58.

Kokman, E. (1984) 'Delirium and dementia', in J.A. Spitell (ed.) *Clinical Medicine*, Hagerstown, MD: Harper & Row, pp. 1–24.

Kopelman, M.D. and Corn, T.H. (1988) 'Cholinergic "Blockade" as a model for cholinergic depletion. A comparison of the memory deficits with those of Alzheimer-type dementia and the alcoholic Korsakoff-syndrome', *Brain* 111: 1079–110.

Labbe, R.A., Firl, A. Jr., Mufson, E.J. and Stein, D.G. (1983) 'Fetal rat brain transplants: reduction of cognitive deficits in rats with frontal cortex lesions', *Science* 221: 470–2.

Marsden, C.D. and Parkes, J.D. (1977) 'Success and problems of long-term levodopa therapy in Parkinson's disease', *Lancet* ii: 345–9.

Martin, E.M., Wilson, R.S., Penn, R.D., Fox, J.H., Clasen, R.A. and Savoy, S.M. (1987) 'Cortical biopsy results in Alzheimer's disease: correlation with cognitive deficits', *Neurology* 37: 1201–4.

Mölsä, P.K., Paljärvi, L., Rinne, U.K. and Säkö, E. (1984) 'Accuracy of clinical diagnosis in dementia', *Acta Neurologica Scandinavica* 69 (suppl. 98): 232–3.

Oehler, J., Jähkel, M. and Schmidt, J. (1987) 'Neural transmitter sensitivity after social isolation in rats', *Physiological Behaviour* 41: 187–91.

Pasamanick, B., Roberts, D.W., Lemkau, P.V. and Krueger, D.E. (1957) 'A survey of mental disease in an urban population. I. Prevalence by age, sex, and severity of impairment', *American Journal of Public Health* 47: 923–9.

Pearson, R.C.A., Esiri, M.M., Hiorns, R.W. *et al.* (1985) 'Anatomical correlate of the distribution of the pathologic changes in the neocortex in Alzheimer's disease', *Proceedings of the National Academy of Science USA* 82: 4531–4.

Perusini, G. (1909) 'Über klinisch und histologisch eigenartige psychische Erkrankungen des höheren Lebensalters', *Nissl-Alzheimers Arbeiten* 3: 297.

Redlich, E. (1898) 'Über miliare Sclerose der Hirnrinde bei seniler Atrophie. *Jahrb Psychiat Neurol* 17: 208–16.

Reisberg, B. (1986) 'Remediable behavioral symptomatology in Alzheimer's disease', *Hospital Community Psychiatry* 37: 1199–201.

Reyes, P.G., Golden, G.T., Fagel, P.L., Fariello, R.G., Katz, L. and Karner, E. (1987) 'The periform cortex in dementia of the Alzheimer type', *Archives of Neurology* 44: 644–5.

Rosen, W.G. (1983) 'Clinical and neuropsychological assessment of Alzheimer's disease', in R. Mayeux, W.G. Rosen (eds) *The Dementias*, New York: Raven Press, pp. 51–64.

Schwartz, P. (1967) 'Systemic amyloid degeneration in mongoloid idiocy', *Journal of Neuropathology and Experimental Neurology* 26: 149–50.

Siegel, J.S. (1980) 'Recent and prospective demographic trends for the elderly population and some implications for health care', NIH Publication, no. 80–969.

Sjögren, T. and Sjögren, H. (1952) 'AGH: Morbus Alzheimer and Morbus Pick', *Acta Psychiatrica Neurologica Scandinavica* (suppl.) 82: 1–152.

Smith, G. (1988) 'Animal models of Alzheimer's disease: experimental cholinergic denervation', *Brain Research Reviews* 13: 103–118.

Sulkava, R., Wikström, J., Aromaa, A., Raitasalo, R., Lehtinen, V., Lahtela, K. and Palo, J. (1985) 'Prevalence of severe dementia in Finland', *Neurology* 35: 1025–9.

Tomlinson, B.E., Blessed, G. and Roth, M. (1968) 'Observations on the brain of non-demented old people', *Journal of Neurological Science* 7: 331–56.

Warburton, D. (1972) 'The cholinergic control of internal inhibition', in R.A. Boakes and M.S. Halliday (eds) *Inhibition and Learning*, New York: Academic Press, pp. 431–58.

Wenk, H., Bigl, V. and Meyer, U. (1980) 'Cholinergic projections from magnocellular nuclei of the basal forebrain to cortical areas in rats', *Brain Research Reviews* 2: 295–316.

Whitehouse, P.J., Price, D.L., Struble, R.G., Clark, A.W., Coyle, J.T. and DeLong, M.R. (1982) 'Alzheimer's disease and senile dementia: loss of neurons in the basal forebrain', *Science* 215: 1237–9.

Wilcock, G.K. and Esiri, M.M. (1982) 'Plaques, tangles and dementia', *Journal of Neurological Science* 56: 343–56.

Wisniewski, H.M., Sinatra, R.S., Iqbal, K. and Grundke-Iqbal, I. (1981) 'Neurofibrillary and synaptic pathology in the aged brain', in J.E. Johnson, Jr (ed) *Aging and Cell Structure*, vol. 1, New York: Plenum Press, pp. 105–42.

World Health Organization (1982) 'Special issue on public health implications of aging', *World Health Statistics Quarterly* 35: (3/4).

—— (1986) 'Dementia in later life: research and action. Report of a WHO scientific group on senile dementia', *WHO Technical Report Series 730*, Geneva: World Health Organization.

Yakovlev, P.I. (1948) 'Motility, behaviour, and the brain', *Journal of Nervous and Mental Diseases* 107: 313–25.

Chapter 3

Learning and memory in demented patients

Jeroen Raaijmakers and Marja Abbenhuis

INTRODUCTION

Due to the increase in the standards of living and the successes of medicine in the second half of this century, the life expectancy in the western world has risen substantially. Today, the over-65 population is the fastest growing segment of the population in the United States and other western nations. It is expected that the proportion of people over age 65 will almost double by the middle of the next century (Heckler, 1985). These demographic circumstances will have a number of important consequences, not the least of which is the increase in the number of patients suffering from senile dementia.

Partly because of this, there has been a tremendous increase in the research into the phenomena that accompany aging in general and senile dementia or Alzheimer's disease (DAT, dementia of the Alzheimer type) in particular. An estimated 5 per cent of the population of 65 and over is severely demented. Another 10 per cent may be mildly to moderately impaired. Although these numbers may sound alarming, they also imply that 85 per cent of the aged population does not suffer from this type of mental impairment.

Alzheimer's disease is a diffuse global deterioration of the brain which manifests itself by a loss of cognitive functions. Although the course of the disease is very idiosyncratic and may involve various intellectual and personality disturbances, problems in learning and memory are among the first symptoms. In this chapter we will discuss a number of topics that relate to the assessment of memory impairments seen in normal aging, senile dementia and other diseases that are accompanied by memory deficits.

The distinction between 'learning' and 'memory' is a subtle one. Generally speaking, learning refers to a 'systematic change in behavior or behavioral disposition that occurs as a consequence of experience in some specified situation' (Estes, 1975:9). 'Memory' is a more abstract term referring to some change in knowledge state as a result of experience that is, however, not tied to a specific type of behaviour. Thus, I can speak about a person learning to ride a bicycle but it does not make sense to say that that person remembers bicycle riding (at least this would mean something quite different). What I could say is that I remember a particular bicycle ride. Thus, 'learning' refers to a change in performance whereas 'memory' refers to a change in knowledge. In this chapter, the emphasis will be on 'memory' because memory processes (such as the storage and retrieval of information) are at the heart of the problems in learning that are observed in these patients.

Proper assessment of the memory functioning is an important aspect of the diagnostic process. Before one starts to subject people to extensive batteries of memory tests, it is vital to consider what the intended purpose is (Miller, 1984). There are a number of possibilities. A core problem is that of differential diagnosis: how to distinguish memory deficits of normal aged people – often called 'benign senescent forgetfulness' – from those of demented patients or from patients suffering from other diseases such as the amnesic syndrome or depression. For instance, the clinical picture of dementia and depression can be very similar, yet distinguishing between the two has important implications for treatment and prognosis.

A second consideration concerns the measurement of changes in performance. The validation of the diagnosis of dementia can only be verified by post-mortem examination of the brain. However, one of the core characteristics of DAT is its progressive nature. If the overall mental condition clearly deteriorates within a certain period of time, this may give some justification for the diagnosis of dementia. Moreover, careful evaluation of the course of DAT can be very important for the development of proper strategies of treatment. This brings to the fore the need for adequate tests of ongoing change.

And finally, proper assessment can have major implications in relating specific deficits of individual patients to specific modes of intervention. Although an effective treatment for DAT is not available as yet, one could strive towards strategies of management that fit the individual needs of the patient in the best possible way. Moreover, if detailed insight can be obtained into the specific impairments of the patient, consultation with the partner or family members may relieve part of the anxiety in coping with the disease. For example, if a patient forgets where he or she has put certain things, being unable to find them may result in suspicious and aggressive behaviour. A partner who does not know that this kind of behaviour has its origins in the memory deficits caused by the disease, might feel personally accused. In such cases, good advice might be of major importance in coping with the consequences of DAT.

THE PROBLEM OF DIFFERENTIAL DIAGNOSIS

One of the most difficult problems in differential diagnosis is to distinguish depression, often called pseudodementia, from DAT. Especially in the early stages of DAT, when typical symptoms are not yet as prominent as in later stages, the patient may still be aware of his or her impairments and depressive symptoms may result from this. Also, cognitive impairments may be present in a depressive illness (Huppert and Tym, 1986; Tariot and Weingartner, 1986). In the early stages of DAT, learning and memory impairments can superficially resemble those occurring in depression.

Moreover, depressive symptoms can often be observed in normal elderly people, and it can be very difficult to discern them from the apathy, loss of initiative and general decline in performance that is characteristic of the early stages of DAT (Huppert and Tym, 1986).

Another source of confusion might be the memory deficits observed in amnesia. Although several parallels can be observed between amnesia and dementia, the main characteristic of amnesia is that memory problems are the most prominent impairment while other areas of cognitive functioning remain relatively preserved, and, in general, performance on memory tests does not deteriorate over time. However, impairments of DAT patients stretch to other domains of cognitive functioning and an examination of their memory deficits is methodologically more complex than a similar examination in amnesic patients (Albert and Moss, 1984).

In designing experiments to assess memory dysfunctions in DAT patients, it is important to be aware of the possibility that other cognitive deficits may be confounded by or interact with memory factors. If the task instructions are too complicated, poor performance may be the result of not understanding what to do rather than being due to memory deficits. For example, mildly to moderately impaired DAT patients usually display difficulty with naming. Testing memory with tasks that require verbatim responses may be confounded by those naming problems. Tests that use reaction time as the dependent variable may also give cause for confusion. Name-finding problems and a general slowing of responses are relatively common among the healthy elderly.

This issue also attests to the intricacy of finding a proper control group. First, there is the problem of the variation in competence. Within the elderly population this variation is extremely large and tends to increase with aging (Benton and Sivan, 1984). In addition, overlap in performance between a population of supposedly normal elderly people and a population of DAT patients might be due to the inclusion in the former group of subjects that will later prove to be at an early, not yet diagnosed, stage of Alzheimer's disease. All these factors that result in a vague borderline between normal aging and DAT, should be taken into account. One way to avoid heterogeneity in control groups or the healthy elderly is to exclude all people who in the past have suffered from any form of psychiatric disease, trauma, prior surgery, etc. It will be obvious that such a group will not be very representative of the elderly population. In such cases, it will be more likely that differences are found between patients and healthy elderly people. On the other hand, not using such exclusion criteria may mask the boundaries between morbidity and normality. For example, subjects with chronic conditions such as hypertension or minor cardiovascular disease tend to perform less well than subjects with excellent health condition (Benton and Sivan, 1984). The proper solution, then, is to strive towards a delicate balance between conditions that can be accepted as falling within the limits of normality and the conditions that interfere too much with the purposes of the study.

A second difficulty in research on dementia is the presence of floor and ceiling effects. When the tasks are too easy, ceiling effects can be expected for the control group and their motivation might wane. Conversely, when the tasks are too difficult, floor effects for the DAT group may arise and, as the patients might be aware of their poor performance, especially in the early phase of the disease, unnecessary anxiety may ensue. This can be avoided by equalizing base-line performance of both groups prior to testing (e.g. by manipulating the study time).

And third, there is the problem of interpreting the results. Because of the diffuse nature of the brain deterioration in DAT, deficits in the overall performance are always to be expected. Differences in the pattern of performance across groups of patients and controls might result from quantitative differences in the level of performance and not from qualitative differences. In other words, a selective deficit in one or another stage of memory will manifest itself in qualitative performance differences, but these may be hard to discern among the many quantitative differences. Yet these qualitative differences are what is most important in reference to the above-mentioned purposes of the neuropsychological assessment of dementia.

Although we have painted a somewhat gloomy picture of the research on dementia, we do believe that careful description of the experimental and control groups and of the tasks that are employed, and an agreement with respect to the terminology that is used will eventually lead to a better insight into the specific deficits of dementia.

With this perspective in mind, we will discuss in the next section some traditional views on learning and memory and its relation to dementia. These traditional concepts include the distinction between short-term memory (STM) and long-term memory (LTM), recall and recognition and acquisition, storage and retrieval. Standard psychometric batteries, that are mostly used by clinicians, are largely based on these traditional concepts. We will discuss some of the research employing these concepts in relation to aging and dementia. It will be argued that the traditional concepts may be useful for initial screening purposes but that they are too global to contribute to the differential diagnosis (or, as the case might be, for the evaluation of performance changes or the analysis of individual patterns of performance deficits).

This will be followed by a description of some more recent developments based on contemporary theories of memory. Here a distinction can be made between models that relate to (a) the kind of information that is to be stored in or retrieved from memory (e.g. the episodic/semantic dichotomy) and (b) the different kinds of memory processes involved (automatic vs. controlled processing) and (c) different ways of testing memory (implicit vs. explicit memory tests). In the final section we will discuss some implications of the recent developments in the theories of learning and memory with respect to their use in clinical practice.

TRADITIONAL MEMORY TASKS

Most of the currently used clinical tests for memory disturbances are derived from traditional memory tasks such as recognition, recall, short-term memory, etc. Erickson and Scott (1977) have provided a detailed review of the available clinical tests of memory. They conclude that there is no really satisfactory test of memory for clinical usage. There are several reasons for this unfortunate state of affairs.

The first main factor is that performance on these tests is influenced by a number of factors other than the memory ability *per se*. One of these is the motivational state. Subjects who find the test difficult can often still recognize this and realize that they are making very little progress (Miller, 1984). For example, learning a list of words is not an easy task. Depressed subjects in whom motivational state is very important for good performance, are afraid to fail the test, suffer from anxiety and thus perform often as badly as demented subjects, though from another cause. Furthermore, the instructions and responses required by many memory tasks are quite complex. This complexity alone may prevent a DAT patient who already has problems inhibiting irrelevant responses and focusing on the relevant dimensions of the task, from accurately revealing his or her memory ability (Albert and Moss, 1984).

Another problem in testing older subjects has to do with the fact that some tests rely on speed of responding. As mentioned by Benton and Sivan (1984), the drop in performance level is likely to be particularly marked on tasks in which the speed of responding is a component of the performance level or which make heavy demands on short-term memory. For example, verbal associative fluency, as measured by the Thurstone word fluency test, shows a relatively early onset of decline with advancing age. This test requires the subject to write as many words beginning with a certain letter in a 5-minute period. However, oral-fluency tests do not show a decline before the age of 75.

Much of the research has been based on the familiar multi-stage model of memory (Atkinson and Shiffrin, 1968). In this model, the information processing is divided in three stages: sensory memory, short-term memory

(STM) and long-term memory (LTM). Sensory memory refers to the initial registration of information by one of the senses (the so-called sensory registers). The information is next transferred to short-term memory, also called working memory. This memory store is concerned with the processing of information, as required by the task in hand. As a result of the processing in short-term memory, information is transferred to long-term memory, the permanent repository of information. One of the most important characteristics of short-term memory is its limited capacity: there is a clear limit to the amount of information that can be held simultaneously in working memory.

We will now describe some of these results in order to see what light they shed on the memory deficits of Alzheimer patients. It should be emphasized from the outset that although certain functions are almost universally impaired in the early stages of the disorder, there is considerable heterogeneity among patients with respect to the degree and pattern of dysfunction on certain tasks as it manifests itself as the disorder progresses.

Not much research has been conducted on sensory memory processing in demented patients. Miller (1981) mentions one experiment in which an array of six letters was briefly presented followed by a masking stimulus. It was observed that demented patients were much less able to report the letters than controls. There is some evidence that the peripheral aspects of iconic memory (the visual sensory memory) are preserved and that the impairment is located in the more central aspects of visual processing (see Morris and Kopelman, 1986).

More studies have been conducted with short-term or primary memory tasks. A rather mixed set of results has been obtained. Thus, digit span (a typical measure of STM based on the number of digits that a person can recall immediately after first presentation) is reported by some investigators to be normal in mild to moderate DATs and by others to be impaired (Huppert and Tym, 1986). In general it may be said that DATs show deficits on a variety of primary memory tests. These include the recency component of free recall (the better recall of the final items on a list, a measure of short-term memory), memory span (immediate serial recall of digits, letters and words, and the Corsi block span test) and the Brown–Peterson test (considered to be a measure of short-term forgetting). Morris and Baddeley (1988) present a review of studies using primary and working memory tasks. In most cases, moderate impairments have been observed.

A more severe impairment is generally observed in the performance of DAT patients on long-term memory tests. Deficits have been reported for a wide variety of tasks (see Morris and Kopelman, 1986), including free recall (recall of a list of unrelated items), paired-associate learning (learning associations between pairs of items) and recognition memory (judging whether a given item was presented on a list).

Several attempts have been made to pinpoint the exact nature of the long-term memory deficits in Alzheimer patients. These attempts have not been very successful, however. For example, Miller (1981) describes a number of experiments that were designed to test whether the deficit of DAT patients is caused by an inability to inhibit incorrect responses. The data provided no support for this hypothesis.

Summarizing, DAT patients show an almost universal impairment on traditional measures of memory functioning. This should not be taken to imply, however, that such measures are useful for diagnostic purposes. The problem is that most other memory disorders (Korsakoff's syndrome, pseudodementia) involve similar 'global' deficits on traditional memory tasks. This means that such measures may be helpful for screening purposes and for monitoring purposes but that they are not useful for differential diagnosis or research on drug treatment for dementia. What would be useful is a way of measuring aspects of memory required for everyday functioning. In the next section we will discuss some recent research on so-called implicit tests of memory that could be useful for such purposes.

RECENT DEVELOPMENTS

In recent years there have been a number of new developments in the analysis of the memory deficits of amnesic patients. The distinguishing characteristic of these studies is that a much more detailed approach to memory functioning is taken. We believe that such an approach will also prove to be useful in the case of DAT patients.

For example, Weingartner et al. (1983) observed no difference between Korsakoff patients and Alzheimer patients in the early stages of the disorder with respect to the performance on the Wechsler memory scale and a number of other conventional memory tasks. However, in other tasks, aimed specifically at aspects of semantic memory, there was a substantial deficit in the performance of the DAT group while there was no significant difference between the Korsakoff patients and normal controls.

This result is one among many that indicate that the distinction between episodic memory (the memory for personal experiences) and semantic memory (the general knowledge including the knowledge about concepts and the rules of language) may be important for the differentiation between various types of memory disorders. According to a number of investigators (e.g. Kinsbourne and Wood, 1975; 1982) patients suffering from the amnesic syndrome show a deficit in episodic memory but not in semantic memory. Alzheimer patients, on the other hand, do suffer from a deficit in semantic memory (Weingartner et al., 1982; 1983).

A similar conclusion has been advocated by Martin and Fedio (1983). They hypothesized that DAT patients suffer from an impairment in the organization of semantic knowledge. Such a conclusion is in agreement with the observation that DAT patients are particularly impaired in 'naming' and 'fluency' tasks.

A second distinction that should be mentioned is that between so-called automatic and controlled processing (Shiffrin and Schneider, 1977). Briefly, automatic processes make no demands on processing capacity, that is, they do not have to be consciously monitored; controlled processes, on the other hand, have to be monitored and are thus subject to capacity limitations but are more easily influenced by strategies. This distinction might prove valuable for the differentiation between Alzheimer patients and depressed elderly persons. It might be assumed that the depressed will show deficits on tasks that involve controlled processing but not on tasks that may be executed automatically. A similar hypothesis has been advanced by Weingartner and his associates (Weingartner et al., 1982; 1983). They assume that depressed patients will show deficits on those tasks that require sustained attention or effort, but that deficits are less likely on tasks that only require automatic processing. The reason for this is that their deficits are caused by motivational problems rather than being due to memory factors per se. Demented patients would also show clear deficits on passive or automatic tasks.

Not all results reported in the literature fit such a hypothesis. For example, it does not explain the discrepancies between the results obtained by Nebes et al. (1984) and those obtained by Ober and Shenaut (1988). Nebes et al. observed no significant difference between DAT patients and controls with respect to the priming effect in a naming task. The priming effect refers to the facilitation observed when a word is preceded by a semantically related word. Ober and Shenaut, on the other hand, observed that DAT patients did not show the expected positive priming effect in lexical decision tasks (i.e. deciding as quickly as possible whether an item is a word or a non-word). Instead, a negative priming effect was obtained. In other words, DATs were slower to decide whether a target was a word when it was related to the prime than when it was not related. According to Ober and Shenaut this difference is due to the fact that the lexical decision task requires more elaborate semantic processing. It is not clear, however, whether the results of Nebes et al. can be replicated. A definite conclusion should probably be postponed until this experiment has been replicated.

Tariot and Weingartner (1986) have presented an intriguing hypothesis that ties the automatic/controlled distinction together with the semantic/ episodic distinction. They assume that DAT patients, in contrast to other memory disorders, suffer from a deficit in the use of semantic memory. This deficit also affects their performance on episodic memory tasks because effective encoding of an episode requires access to semantic information. The more the task requires semantic processing, the more clearly this shows up. Therefore, the extent to which episodic memory is impaired in patients with DAT, is directly related to impairments of semantic memory. Tasks that require relatively little semantic processing (such as most priming tasks) will not show significant deficits.

Finally, there has been a recent flurry of research on various types of implicit or unaware forms of memory testing. In such tasks, memory is tested indirectly, that is, through its effects in ostensibly non-memory tasks. This usually involves some sort of repetition priming, e.g. the facilitation obtained in naming words that are repeated in a test session. Such effects may be obtained even though the subject is unaware of the repetition. This distinction between implicit and explicit forms of memory testing has been shown to be quite useful in the analysis of the memory deficits of amnesic patients (see Graf *et al.*, 1984; Jacoby and Witherspoon, 1982).

A natural question to ask is whether Alzheimer patients also show normal performance on implicit memory tasks. Moscovitch (1982) observed a normal repetition priming effect in DAT patients even though they showed severe deficits in normal recognition memory. Similarly, Nebes *et al.* (1984) obtained an equivalent semantic priming effect in Alzheimer patients. Similar results have been reported by Miller (1975) and Morris *et al.* (1983) using a word-stem completion task. That is, the patients were more likely to complete a word when given the first three letters, if that word had been previously presented.

Such results indicate that some basic aspects of memory processing may in fact be spared in Alzheimer patients. To what extent this holds up for other forms of implicit memory remains to be seen. In any event, such sparing will be important for understanding the exact nature of the memory deficits of Alzheimer patients.

EVALUATION AND DISCUSSION

In this review, we have placed a strong emphasis on the issue of differential diagnosis. As we have explained, early diagnosis is important even though no treatment for Alzheimer's disease is yet available. First, diagnostic tools may be used to differentiate between dementia and pseudo-dementia. Second, early diagnosis may avoid family problems due to a lack of understanding of what is wrong. Third, it may lead to the introduction of potential pharmacological treatments at a stage when they are most likely to prove effective.

There are also other reasons why a proper understanding of the memory problems of these patients is important. Decisions about the proper management regime have to be based on some form of evaluation or assessment of the patient. For this purpose it is important to know which abilities are still more or less intact in different subtypes of dementia. The extent of the memory problems has consequences for such decisions as to whether it is advisable to let the patient continue to live in the home environment (possibly alone and with minimal support from relatives or neighbours) or whether some form of sheltered accommodation is necessary. In addition, it is important to monitor the course of the disease since this may have consequences for the optimal type of management regime.

Finally, a proper understanding of the nature of the disease is important for those that are involved in the care-giving of these patients. This includes not only the family members but also the nursing staff if the patient resides in a geriatric hospital. Both groups may become frustrated over the lack of response to their efforts at trying to improve the patient's condition.

In fact, one of the biggest tragedies of Alzheimer's disease is the often physically gruelling and emotionally exhausting task that it imposes on the care-giver. As the disease progresses, the patient may no longer recognize the spouse (or other family members). In a sense, the spouse has already lost his or her partner even though she/he is still living. In addition, the care-giver has to invest so much time that he/she becomes socially isolated and cut off from the world at large, yet receives little recognition for these efforts. Perhaps, the best advice that can be given is to seek professional help as soon as possible and to join one of the existing associations of family members of Alzheimer patients.

REFERENCES

Albert, M. and Moss, M. (1984) 'The assessment of memory disorders in patients with Alzheimer disease', in L.R. Squire and N. Butters (eds) *The Neuropsychology of Memory*, New York: The Guilford Press.

Atkinson, R.C. and Shiffrin, R.M. (1968) 'Human memory: a proposed system and its control processes', in K.W. Spence and J.T. Spence (eds) *The Psychology of Learning and Motivation: Advances in Research and Theory*. vol. 2, New York: Academic Press.

Benton, A.L. and Sivan, A.B. (1984) 'Problems and conceptual issues in neuropsychological research in aging and dementia', *Journal of Clinical Neuropsychology* 6: 57–63.

Erickson, R.C. and Scott, M.L. (1977) 'Clinical memory testing: a review', *Psychological Bulletin* 84: 1130–49.

Estes, W.K. (1975) 'The state of the field: General problems and issues of theory and metatheory', in W.K. Estes (ed.) *Handbook of Learning and Cognitive Processes, Vol. 1: Introduction to Concepts and Issues*, Hillsdale, N.J.: Erlbaum.

Graf, P., Squire, L.R. and Mandler, G. (1984) 'The information that amnesic patients do not forget', *Journal of Experimental Psychology: Learning, Memory, and Cognition* 9: 164–78.

Heckler, M.M. (1985) 'The fight against Alzheimer's disease', *American Psychologist* 40: 1240–4.

Huppert, F.A. and Tym, E. (1986) 'Clinical and neuropsychological assessment of dementia', *British Medical Bulletin* 42: 11–18.

Jacoby, L.L. and Witherspoon, D. (1982) 'Remembering without awareness', *Canadian Journal of Psychology* 36: 300–24.

Kinsbourne, M. and Wood, F. (1975) 'Short-term memory processes and the amnesic syndrome', in D. Deutsch and A.J. Deutsch (eds) *Short-term Memory*, New York: Academic Press.

Kinsbourne, M. and Wood, F. (1982) 'Theoretical considerations regarding the episodic-semantic memory distinction', in L. Cermak (ed.) *Human Memory and Amnesia*, Hillsdale, N.J.: Erlbaum.

Martin, A. and Fedio, P. (1983) 'Word production and comprehension in Alzheimer's disease: the breakdown of semantic knowledge', *Brain and Language* 19: 124–41.

Miller, E. (1975) 'Impaired recall and the memory disturbance in presenile dementia', *Psychological Medicine* 3: 221–4.

—— (1981) 'The nature of the cognitive deficit in senile dementia', in N.E. Miller and G.D. Cohen (eds) *Clinical Aspects of Alzheimer's Disease and Senile Dementia*, New York: Raven Press.

—— (1984) 'Neuropsychological assessment', in D.W. Kay and G.D. Burrows (eds) *Handbook of Studies on Psychiatry and Old Age*, Amsterdam: Elseviers Science Publishers.

Morris, R.G. and Baddeley, A.D. (1988) 'Primary and working memory functioning in Alzheimer-type dementia', *Journal of Clinical and Experimental Neuropsychology* 10: 279–96.

—— and Kopelman, M.D. (1986) 'The memory deficits in Alzheimer-type dementia: a review', *The Quarterly Journal of Experimental Psychology* 38A: 575–602.

——, Wheatley, J. and Britton (1983) 'Retrieval from long-term memory in senile dementia: cued recall revisited', *British Journal of Clinical Psychology* 22: 141–2.

Moscovitch, M. (1982) 'A neuropsychological approach to perception and memory in normal and pathological aging', in F.I.M. Craik and S. Trehub (eds) *Aging and Cognitive Processes*, New York: Plenum Press.

Nebes, R.D., Martin, D.C. and Horn, L.C. (1984) 'Sparing of semantic memory in Alzheimer's disease', *Journal of Abnormal Psychology* 93: 321–30.

Ober, B.A. and Shenaut, G.K. (1988) 'Lexical decision and priming in Alzheimer's disease', *Neuropsychologia* 26: 273–86.

Shiffrin, R.M. and Schneider, W. (1977) 'Controlled and automatic human information processing: II. Perceptual learning, automatic attending and a general theory', *Psychological Review* 84: 127–90.

Tariot, P.N. and Weingartner, H. (1986) 'A psychobiologic analysis of cognitive failures', *Archives of General Psychiatry* 43: 1183–8.

Weingartner, H., Grafman, J., Boutelle, W., Kaye, W. and Martin, P.R. (1983) 'Forms of memory failure', *Science* 221: 380–2.

——, Kaye, W., Smallberg, S., Cohen, R., Ebert, M.H., Gillin, J.C. and Gold, P. (1982) 'Determinants of memory failures in dementia', in S.H. Corkin, K.L. Davis, J.H. Growdon, E. Usdin and R.J. Wurtman (eds) *Alzheimer's Disease: A Report of Progress in Research* (*Aging*, vol. 19), New York: Raven Press.

Chapter 4

Attachment theory and dementia

Bère Miesen

SUMMARY

Sooner or later, most elderly demented patients think that their deceased parents are still alive. In the study reported here, this is called 'parent-fixation' (PF). This phenomenon can be considered within several theoretical frameworks, but Bowlby's attachment theory is the most useful. A standard visiting procedure (SVP) was developed so that attachment behaviour of demented elderly persons towards their family could be videotaped and studied in detail.

The research results show that feeling unsafe and insecure is a common feature of the dementing process. The way in which these feelings manifest themselves depends mostly on the stage of dementia. Concrete attachment behaviour is strongest in early stages of dementia and is gradually replaced by PF as the disease progresses. PF is illustrated by a number of case examples and can be readily understood as a form of attachment behaviour.

INTRODUCTION

How demented elderly persons experience memories of their parents (the phenomenon of PF)

Patients with Alzheimer's dementia, or senile dementia of the Alzheimer type (SDAT), that is, the form generally occurring after the age of 65, are afflicted with functional, cognitive and behavioural disturbances. This means that their contact with persons and literally their whole environment is affected, and that they are dependent on assistance to some degree, depending on the stage of the disease, in performing activities of daily living.

From clinical observations of elderly demented persons, it appears that memories of their parents are an important component of their realm of existence (their inner reality) (Miesen, 1985). Sooner or later, elderly demented persons think that their long-since deceased parents are still alive, and they ask, for example, to 'go home' or 'where their parents are'. The following is a list of typical behaviours exhibited by persons with SDAT which will help to focus the reader on PF:

- trying or wanting to go home
- trying or wanting to go to their parent(s)
- expressing the need for parental attention
- expressing concern about the well-being of their parent(s)
- imagining themselves back in the parental family
- behaving according to certain parental expectations
- being threatened by parental authority
- asking where their parent(s) is/are
- asking how their parent(s) is/are keeping.

The clinical evidence for these behaviours and their persistence in clinical settings are contrasted by the observation that they have received little attention in the research literature on dementia. Within psychiatric literature (Levy and Post, 1982; Charazac, 1985; Lishman, 1987) such behaviours are subsumed under confabulation (Kopelman, 1987), delusions (Reisberg et al., 1984) and hallucinations (Bacherikov and Elizerov, 1982). Usually, however, this behaviour is treated as being a consequence of 'living in the past', and is accepted as fitting within the constellation of memory-loss patterns in dementia.

This lack of attention is not particularly surprising because research about dementia is directed primarily towards neurobiological (Fliers, 1985; Katzman, 1986), medical (Miller, 1977; Mayeux and Rosen, 1983) and cognitive (Diesfeldt, 1983; Woods and Britton, 1985) aspects of this disorder. With regard to this latter aspect, recent research literature indicates that demented persons seem to have a certain awareness of their waning cognitive abilities (Woods and Britton, 1985; Solomon, 1985; Hausman, 1985; Hagberg, 1987). Just as the emotional awareness of terminally ill patients about their condition has been acknowledged (Glaser and Strauss, 1965), so too, the possibility of an emotional awareness related to the bereavement or loss process in demented patients is now being considered. It appears that even demented persons experience and feel threatening losses, and it seems that the process of dementia creates an environment which fosters feelings of uncertainty and the lack of safety. This could mean that demented persons are struggling with emotional problems, which have been hitherto underestimated. Their insistence that their parents are still alive, is possibly a critical response to the fear evoked by the dementing process. Their perpetual requests for their parents could therefore be more readily interpreted as a cry of distress, as a cry for security, than as a muted memory from the faded past.

So far, what has been said might sound reasonable, but how does one go about investigating such ideas? This must be done within strict research frameworks and both through qualitative and quantitative explorative observations. The following paragraphs show how this was done.

For purposes of this study, the term 'parent-fixation' will be applied to behaviours relating to elderly demented persons maintaining that their parents are still living. This definition assumes that: one or both of the parents is thought to be alive, whilst one or both of them have actually been dead many years. In the preceding discussion, it was suggested that PF could have a deeper meaning than merely being a result of memory deficit. Several aspects of the reality experienced by demented persons crystallize around the theme of 'parents'.

Research into the meaning of PF can lead to a further understanding of this phenomenon as experienced by demented persons. Their behaviour can be better understood and guided by this understanding.

A number of interesting questions arise from the phenomenon of PF and these questions lead us to several theoretical niches (approaches) which are not particularly specific to dementia. Such questions are: Is PF related to memory loss, and to intact memories of early experiences? Does PF indicate a (strong) need to have one's parents close at hand? Is PF related to reminiscing, and what role do concrete memories of parents have to PF? Do unresolved conflicts with parents have any relationship to PF, and/or are they related to a (strong) longing for what elderly persons symbolize? These questions will be simplified in the form of four more specific questions that arise from studying the typical example of Mrs Vos.

The example of Mrs Vos

Mrs Vos was a 90-year-old, married lady who spoke to the author during several interviews. She had been diagnosed as having SDAT several years earlier and had been placed in a nursing home when her husband was hospitalized. During this conversation, and others, it became clear that, overall, in spite of a few lucid moments, she assumed that her parents were still alive (PF) and she acted accordingly.

Mrs Vos initially said to me 'My parents are well.' Thereafter she went on to say, 'My mother has been dead for some time. My father is also dead. He died first.' In reply to my question, 'So your father died before your mother?', she answered, 'No, father is still alive and mother too for that matter.'

Later in the conversation she said, 'My parents are both dead.' I enquired whether she thought of them often. 'Oh yes, certainly I think of them often. Not necessarily every day, you understand, but I always feel close to them. I mean I want to keep them alive, hold them tight. I miss them.'

At the end of the conversation Mrs Vos added: 'So, I'll be getting home now. My parents are expecting me.' 'Your parents are still alive?' I asked cautiously. 'Oh yes! father and mother are still alive.'

Four interpretations of PF arise from this example of Mrs Vos.

1   Is it retrograde amnesia when Mrs Vos thinks that her parents are still alive? Does she have a good memory for the distant past when she realized that they are dead? If PF is associated with a good memory for the distant past, then such behaviour cannot be corrected as it were, since all efforts to convince Mrs Vos of the reality of her parents' death (for example, trying to impress upon her her own age) will fail. She will remain resolute about her intention of going home. If her memory dysfunction is of a changing nature, (that her disorientation is interspersed with lucid moments) then the only intervention is to wait for her awareness of their death to return.

2   Mrs Vos clearly longs for her parents; this is possibly an extension of her feeling that her parents are strongly present in the world (or inner reality) that she experiences. If PF reflects a strong need to have one's parents close at hand, then in theory, the behaviour could be corrected. The question arises whether it is wise to do so. Maybe Mrs Vos misses them, but by telling her that her parents are dead, she will feel the pain of their loss again, and her need for them may be intensified. In this conception of PF, the belief that the parents are still alive is functional for the demented person because it helps to create feelings of safety. It is preferable to talk to Mrs Vos about how she feels when she is talking about her parents as if they were alive, talk to her about general memories of her parents, not referring to whether they are alive or dead. This view is supported by the validation method of Feil (1982).

3   What part do Mrs Vos' memories of her parents play in PF and is reminiscing helpful in such instances? If remembering the parents is regarded as a part of memories of times gone by, then PF is less significant. When elderly persons appear to be thinking of former times and their parents, it could be regarded as normal for their time of life. Perhaps Mrs Vos keeps very happy memories of her parents available because thinking of them gives her a pleasant feeling. What remains then, is the question why and how her parents became a living reality in her memory. When she makes a lucid, startling announcement that her parents have long since died, a care-giver should always encourage her to review her life, and to talk to her about her parents.

4   What part do unresolved experiences or conflicts with her parents play in PF for Mrs Vos? Or could she be experiencing a general (primitive, according to Jung) longing for parents or parental figures which does not only apply to Mrs Vos but to everyone? When PF is connected with unresolved or undigested experiences with parents, the question arises to what extent waning cognitive abilities are responsible for

this. Perhaps, besides happy memories, Mrs Vos also has unhappy memories which compel her to go home quickly because otherwise she might be punished. In such a situation there are arguments for, as well as against stimulating memories of parents. If undigested experiences with parents are involved, it is perhaps most useful to make every possible attempt to reassure the demented person that everything is in the past and that the parents have long since died. But it is also possible that concrete experiences with parents do not play any significant part at all in dementia. Perhaps demented persons are just longing for all of the positive memories from their life which made them feel secure and safe, and this might be symbolized by good parental figures.

BRIEF SUMMARY OF FOUR THEORIES USED TO EXAMINE PF

In connection with the four points made above, four theoretical frameworks were examined in this study: the search of associative memory theory (Raaijmakers and Shiffrin, 1980; 1981), Bowlby's attachment theory (1969; 1973; 1980), theories about the retrieval and the spontaneous surfacing of memories, i.e. reminiscence (Merriam, 1980; Molinari and Reichlin, 1984–5; Coleman, 1986), and analytical psychology (Jung, 1934, 1938a, 1938b). A brief review of these theoretical frameworks follows.

The search of associative memory theory

Within the literature on memory (e.g. Baddely, 1986; Squire, 1987; Bayles and Kaszniak, 1987), the search of associative memory theory (Raaijmakers and Shiffrin, 1980; 1981) is unusual because it avoids detailed assumptions about how information is represented in long-term storage. In this theory about memory, a distinction is made between long- and short-term storage of information. Both are treated as two different states of one memory. The capacity of short-term store is limited. The intake of information into long-term store depends on which information in short-term store is rehearsed. The greater the correspondence between internal and external 'retrieval cues' on the one hand, and the early information in long-term store on the other hand, the greater the chance that information can be retrieved from long-term store (Raaijmakers, 1984).

Bowlby's attachment theory

Within Bowlby's attachment theory (Bowlby, 1969; 1973; 1980), attachment behaviour is defined as all behaviour which has the goal of obtaining and/or retaining the proximity of another person. Attachment behaviour is activated under particular circumstances, e.g. in unfamiliar situations and in the presence of fear, especially when one is alone. Some forms of attachment behaviour remain potentially active throughout the lifespan. On the one hand this theory demonstrates how the individual, by nature, is driven to form emotional ties with special persons; with parents but also with others. The other side of attachment theory provides insight into the manner in which an individual reacts to (threatened) loss of particular affective bonds.

Reminiscing theories

The importance of theories about reminiscing, and the retrieval and spontaneous surfacing of memories, is self-evident (e.g. Merriam, 1980; Molinari and Reichlin, 1984–5; Coleman, 1986). On the one hand, because not having, or no longer having parents forms a part of the past of every person, and because the memories of parents are a special type of memory; on the other hand, because reminiscing is an active process which takes place only in present time. Reminiscing is in fact an actual process occurring in everyone's life, and it is natural that in old age, memories also surface spontaneously.

Jung's analytical psychology

In his analytical psychology (e.g. Jung, 1934; 1938a, 1938b), Jung differentiates between consciousness (the ego), the personal unconscious and the collective unconscious. A removable consciousness is paired with the spontaneous surfacing of the contents of the personal unconscious, e.g. unresolved conflicts. According to Jung, many psychological situations exist wherein, under certain conditions, the contents of the collective unconscious surface, e.g. the archetypes of the parents.

EXPLANATIONS OF THE CONCEPT OF PARENT-FIXATION

With the help of these theoretical frameworks, some answers to the preceding questions can be formulated to four specific questions about the phenomenon of PF in demented elderly persons namely: How can the theme of 'parents' in demented elderly persons be understood? When does PF occur? How can PF be explained? What is the relationship between PF and the process of dementia?

In fact, PF can be translated into each theoretical framework. In the following schematic these 'translations' of PF are stated for each particular theory (see Table 4.1).

Table 4.1 Schematic of the 'translation' of the four questions about parent-fixation for each theoretical framework

	The four questions about parent-fixation in dementia			
Theoretical framework:	How can the theme of parents be understood?	When does parent-fixation occur?	How can parent-fixation be explained?	What is the relationship between parent-fixation and the process of dementia?
Search of associative memory theory	As episodic information in long-term store	When there is overlap between internal contextual episodic information in long-term store and 'recognized' information serving as 'retrieval cue'	As a result of activation of episodic information in long-term store	With dementia, instantaneous perception of internal and external information activates (emotional) contextual retrieval cues
Bowlby's attachment theory	As attachment figures	When there is no other available attachment figure around	As a form of attachment behaviour	Dementia implicates an unusual condition that activates attachment behaviour and/or results in experiences of (threatening) permanent loss.

Theories of reminiscence	As part of the content of the natural process of reminiscing	When 'parents' begin to fall under the category of new information	As content of the actualization of new information rather than as the content of the reproduction of episodic information	Dementia implies a permanent actual problematic situation wherein the decreased ability to experience oneself as a continuity, activates the process of reminiscing
Jung's analytical psychology	Early on as a manifestation of the personal unconscious; in the later phase, as part of the collective unconscious	When transfer is no longer possible in interactions with the outside world	As parent-complexes in the early phase, and as parent-archetypes in later phases of dementia	Dementia is coupled with loss of ego (awareness) whereby the borderline between the inner and outer world slowly fades

THE STUDY OF PARENT-FIXATION AND ATTACHMENT BEHAVIOUR

Introduction

The central statement of the problem posed in our research asks whether the phenomenon of PF in the demented elderly is an expression of the need for safety and security?

Of the theoretical frameworks mentioned, the search for associative memory theory and Bowlby's attachment theory appear to have most relevance for the study of PF. Bowlby's attachment theory is the most useful of these two. The search for associative memory theory is applicable because memory impairments which occur in general cognitive dysfunctioning, are taken to be the key symptoms of dementia.

Methods and population

Methods

Both of the theories selected for use in this research, give rise to a number of tangential questions. PF, attachment behaviour and the level of cognitive functioning (including memory dysfunctions) comprise the most important variables; forming as it were, the cornerstones for this research which examines the meaning of the theme of 'parents', that is, the phenomenon of PF in the inner-world of demented old persons.

The assessment of the level of cognitive functioning helped to determine the extent of the dementing process. The schematic in Table 4.2 provides a brief summary of the methods used in this research.

Population

The subjects were patients who were admitted to a psychogeriatric nursing home (Mariënhaven/Warmond) between the end of 1986 to October 1987. According to the medical diagnosis, almost all subjects had a probable diagnosis of (pre)senile dementia, comparable with senile dementia of the Alzheimer type (SDAT). Each subject's behavioural problems were readily identifiable as those typical to dementia.

The research group consisted of 40 persons – 27 women and 13 men. The oldest person was 90 years, and the youngest was aged 64. More than half were older than 80 years. Almost 40 per cent, especially males, were still married. Half of the group, mostly women, were still married.

This subject group is a representative sample of first-time psychogeriatric admissions in the Netherlands during 1987, and reasonably representative for all admitted psychogeriatric patients in the Netherlands in 1987.

Table 4.2 Schematic of the research methods used in this study

Parent-fixation	The replies to six questions were scored by two independent raters on a 5-point scale
Level of cognitive functioning:	
Medical classification	Medical status before and/or after admission, according to the ICD-09-CM classification made by the resident physician
Behaviour rating scale for elderly patients (BOP)	The 'Dependency' and 'Orientation and Communication' scales were rated by care-giving staff on the ward
Mini-mental state examination	Test administered and scored by researcher
Memory problems	Tests administered by the researcher and research assistant
Attachment behaviour on the ward	An observation questionnaire of 60 items on a 3-point scale, completed by two of the care-giving staff, independent of each other. Distinctions are made between total scores and attachment behaviour scores in different situations: general, morning care, eating, during visits, and at bedtime.

Preliminary results which led to the development of the standard visiting procedure

PF occurred in two-thirds of demented persons examined, and was related to their level of cognitive functioning. PF occurred primarily in demented elderly with a low level of cognitive functioning (inclusive of severe memory disturbances). (See Table 4.3.)

Table 4.4 shows that PF is also related to attachment behaviour on the ward, particularly to attachment behaviour during family visits and at bedtime. Especially demented elderly who exhibit little attachment behaviour, manifest PF.

Other research findings not reported in this chapter (see Miesen, 1990) indicate that attachment behaviour in addition to PF exhibited during family visits, also showed a strong correlation (Kendall's tau $r = 0.37$; $p \leqslant 0.01$) with cognitive functioning. Demented elderly persons with a low level of cognitive functioning demonstrate less attachment behaviour than those persons with a high level of cognitive functioning. The schematic in Figure 4.1 shows a summary of these results in picture form.

Tabie 4.3 Parent-fixation and the level of cognitive functioning

	Level of cognitive dysfunctioning:		
Parent-fixation	*low (MMSE $\leqslant$ 11)*	*high (MMSE $>$ 11)*	*Total*
Fully present	9	2	11
Almost present	3	1	4
Fluctuatingly present	7	2	9
Absent	1	15	16
Total	20	20	40

Note: Chi^2 = 20.48; p $\leqslant$ 0.0001.

Table 4.4 Parent-fixation and attachment behaviour during family visits and at bedtime

	Attachment behaviour				
	Visit			*Bedtime*	
Parent-fixation	<9	$\geqslant 9$	*Total*	<7	$\geqslant 7$
Present	12	3	15	12	3
Fluctuatingly present	4	5	9	4	5
Absent	4	12	16	7	9
Total	20	20	40	23	17

Note: Chi^2 = 9.51 (p $\leqslant$ 0.01)   Chi^2 = 4.97 (p $\leqslant$ 0.05)

THE STANDARD VISITING PROCEDURE (SVP)

Experimental visits (referred to henceforth as the standard visiting procedure (SVP)) enabled analysis of the more subtle details of attachment behaviour and facilitated exploration of some of the conditions in which there are variations in attachment behaviour in demented elderly people.

The SVP is based in part on clinical observations of demented persons' behaviour which occurs during visits, on the ward, and in part on Ainsworth's 'strange situation'; an experimental research setting with young children (Ainsworth *et al.*, 1978). The SVP utilizes a friendly, specially constructed, living room (see Figure 4.2), wherein subjects remain for about 15 minutes. There are five distinguishable parts to the SVP. The demented person is alone twice, alternatively with the researcher and with a

Figure 4.1 Schematic summary of early results

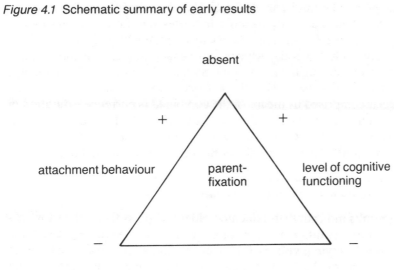

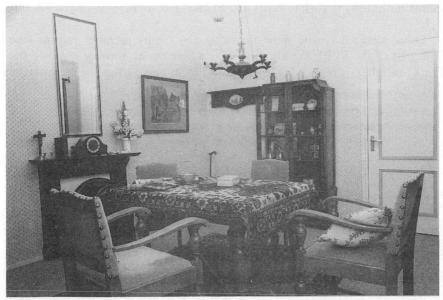

Figure 4.2 The living room of the standard visiting procedure

Picture by Aad Kralt

family member. The third part of the SVP is the critical one. It focuses on the moment when the family member indicates that he or she must leave and suddenly ends the visit. This creates a potentially 'threatening' moment for the person with dementia. Attachment behaviour (e.g. touching, calling after) is recorded during the parts of the SVP in which the family member is with the demented person. The ultimate score for the various attachment behaviours is comprised by means of the combined occurrence – duration of each behaviour within the five distinct parts of the SVP. The scoring was done by two independent observers who rated video recordings of the visit. See Miesen (1990) for more details of the procedure and method.

Results of the standard visiting procedure

Research results indicate that demented elderly express themselves towards their family through different forms of attachment behaviour, e.g. touching, turning towards, crying, visually following, calling after, which are more or less independent of the level of cognitive functioning. It is apparent that demented persons with a high level of cognitive functioning use different or longer-lasting forms of attachment behaviour than persons with a low level of cognitive functioning. This is largely dependent on whether family members are arriving or departing.

Table 4.5 shows that low-level demented elderly people are especially prone to touching after unexpected arrival of family members. The sudden departure of family members is often the trigger for the high-level demented elderly to turn towards and to call after them. See Tables 4.6 and 4.7.

Other research results show that after the family member returns (the fifth part of the SVP), the duration of the time spent 'turning towards' the family member, is reduced. The transition from one part to the next part of

Table 4.5 Attachment behaviour in the second part of the SVP (the family is arriving) according to the level of cognitive functioning

Level of cognitive functioning:	Mean attachment behaviour scores		
	Touching	Turning towards	Crying
low (MMSE $\leqslant$ 11)	40.9	89.7	1.7
high (MMSE $>$ 11)	17.9	93.9	1.8
t-values	2.71*	−0.85	−0.10

Note: * = p $\leqslant$ 0.01.

Table 4.6 Attachment behaviour in the third part of the SVP (the family is departing) according to the level of cognitive functioning

	Mean attachment behaviour scores		
Level of cognitive functioning	Touching	Turning towards	Crying
low (MMSE ≤11)	21.7	81.7	0.6
high (MMSE >11)	19.7	94.9	7.8
t-values	0.46	−2.37*	−1.80

Note: * = p ≤0.05.

Table 4.7 Attachment behaviour in the third part of the SVP (the family has departed) according to the level of cognitive functioning

	Mean attachment behaviour scores		
Level of cognitive functioning	Watching after	Walking after	Calling after
low (MMSE ≤11)	17.6	12	27.7
high (MMSE >11)	19.7	4.4	45.6
t-values	−0.47	1.49	−2.95*

Note: * = p ≤0.01.

the SVP, gives rise to apparent differences, namely in the duration of 'touching'. Immediately after the abrupt message from family members that they will be leaving, demented elderly persons with a high level of cognitive functioning touch them longer than before.

Demented elderly persons with a low level of cognitive functioning are not at all affected by this abrupt message; they keep touching them just as much or just as little as before.

The relationship in the SVP between these concrete forms of attachment behaviour and the level of cognitive functioning with PF, confirms the preliminary results. Demented elderly persons without PF exhibit more attachment behaviour than demented persons with PF. A clear exception, in fact the reverse result, occurs in the case of touching when demented persons unexpectedly meet their family member. Here it is the demented elderly with PF who touch more than demented elderly people without PF. Because it is demented elderly with a low level of cognitive functioning who react thus, it would appear that PF serves the same function for them as touching, namely, a form of attachment behaviour.

Individual differences

The research results reported here are based (mainly) upon statistically significant differences between subgroups of high (MMSE > 11) and low (MMSE ≤ 11) levels of cognitive functioning. In this analysis, an important feature of both subgroups disappears, namely the individual differences within the groups. This is particularly true for the attachment behaviours but also for PF.

More detailed analysis indicated that in the high-level cognitive subgroup, there were three persons who exhibited PF, which led to the following questions. Is the relationship between PF and attachment behaviour different in a person with a high level of cognitive functioning than in a person with a low level? Does PF mean something different for the person with a high level of cognitive functioning than for the demented person with the low level?

The first person was a widow who exhibited strong attachment behaviour on the ward. In the SVP, she continuously touched herself in spite of the presence of her daughter. In her case, PF could mean permanent accessibility to her parents. The second person was a widower who also exhibited strong attachment behaviour on the ward. In the SVP he manifested this clearly, even in the presence of his son. He did not seem to have the ability to come to grips with the problems arising from his waning physical strength. In his case, PF meant the constant support of his mother. The third person was a married lady who, both on the ward and during the SVP with her son, exhibited very 'clinging' attachment behaviour. Because of her minimal memory impairments, she had a strong awareness of her problems, and of the fact that her husband tried to deny them. Her PF could mean the continual availability of the protection of her parents.

Interpretation and discussion of the results

PF in demented elderly people is possibly an expression of their need for safety and security. The research results can be interpreted as follows: dementia activates attachment behaviour, and dementia itself apparently functions as a type of 'retrieval cue'. These interpretations answer some of the questions formulated at the end of the paragraph on pp. 41–2.

Dementia activates attachment behaviour

The process of dementia for the persons affected, can be more or less understood as a 'strange situation' which gradually becomes permanent. The more dangerous this situation feels, the more attachment behaviour is exhibited in consequence. If the bond with the outside world disappears through memory dysfunction, then the demented person will search for some kind of a 'hold'. But it is precisely these memory dysfunctions which erode feelings of safety and security, because durable affective bonds are not obtainable. This means that the demented elderly person is caught up in a situation that is comparable to a bereavement process which can never be resolved. A vicious circle begins. The exposed needs for safety and security can never be fulfilled. Dementia activates attachment behaviour but, at the same time ensures that old and new attachment figures will not remain present in the social environment of the demented person.

Dementia itself functions as a type of 'retrieval cue'

In the first stage of dementia, the increasingly frequent experience of feeling 'unsafe and insecure' functions as a 'retrieval cue', which activates attachment behaviours in the form of e.g. touching, turning towards and calling after. Basically, PF does not occur in this stage, because the safety and security provided by attachment figures outside of the demented person, are temporarily useful. If PF occurs in the first stage of dementia, it can be explained as so-called unreciprocated attachment behaviour, as demonstrated in the three previous examples. This early stage of dementia is accompanied by an awareness of the disabilities which fuels additional feelings of unsafety and insecurity.

In the next stage of dementia, the 'strange situation' remains constantly present, and the experience of feeling unsafe becomes permanent. The continuous care-requiring circumstances of the demented persons function as a 'retrieval cue'. Less of the explicit attachment behaviour of the early stage is manifested, but PF and touching are particularly evident. In this stage, PF no longer means unreciprocated attachment behaviour. PF becomes attachment behaviour which reciprocates the need for safety from within the person him/herself.

In the end stage of dementia only speculation about the meaning of PF is possible. It appears that PF itself has become a 'retrieval cue', and that parents symbolize the archetypal attachment of man.

THEORETICAL SUPPORT FOR THE VALIDATION APPROACH

The research study reported in this chapter and described in detail elsewhere (Miesen, 1990 and 1993) seems to confirm Feil's qualitative observations that reference to parents in an early stage of dementia arises because of the need to find safety in an increasingly unsafe environment. Our study confirms also the usefulness of speaking and interacting in terms of 'universal symbols' in a later stage of dementia. Another interesting result is the empirical support for the demented elderly person's need to have a validation worker around because validation workers seem to function as attachment figures.

CONCLUDING REMARKS

In spite of the current emphasis on neurobiological research on dementia, we are still in the dusk; the aetiology of dementia is still unknown, and no therapies exist to treat or cure it once assessed. It is important to give independent attention to the experiential world of the demented elderly person; to understand the meaning of dementia for the sufferers themselves. Our research has attempted to address that issue. It appears that the phenomenon of PF is a key to the experiential world of demented elderly people, wherein, more-or-less permanent feelings of a lack of safety and security trigger attachment behaviours.

Throughout the duration of this research we gradually achieved some insight into the manner in which demented elderly people (can) interpret their situation, and a means of understanding their behaviour. Aside from the awareness of their disabilities, demented elderly people do not have an easy time of it. They appear to wrestle with the emotional problems which are more typical of people in general, than specific to persons with dementia. It has become clear how a number of their behaviours can be perceived and understood, namely as attachment behaviours in a situation that is experienced as strange and being unsafe.

This shift in understanding has important implications for care-giving because it allows us to relate to demented elderly people with more satisfaction and hence less frustration. The demented elderly person can only be blessed by this.

ACKNOWLEDGEMENT

The author gratefully wishes to thank Joep Munnichs, Henk van der Ploeg, Gemma Jones (who also translated this chapter) and Anne-Marie van Dam for their support, comments and advice.

REFERENCES

Ainsworth, M.D.S., Blehar, M.C., Waters, E. and Wall, S. (1978) *Patterns of Attachment: Assessed in the Strange Situation and at Home*, Hillsdale NJ: Lawrence Erlbaum.

Bacherikov, N.E. and Elizerov, Y.A. (1982) 'Adaptational disturbances of the auditory, visual and motor analyzers in atherosclerotic and presenile psychoses', *Zhurnal Nevropatalogii i Psikhiatrii* 82 (4): 547–51.

Baddely, A.D. (1986) *Working Memory*, Oxford: Oxford Science Publications.

Bayles, K.A. and Kaszniak, A.W. (1987) *Communication and Cognition in Normal Aging and Dementia*, Boston: Little, Brown & Co.

Bowlby, J. (1969) *Attachment and Loss, Volume 1: Attachment*, London: Hogarth Press.

—— (1973) *Attachment and Loss, Volume 2: Separation: Anxiety and Anger*, London: Hogarth Press.

—— (1980) *Attachment and Loss, Volume 3: Loss: Sadness and Depression*, London: Hogarth Press/New York: Basic Books.

Charazac, P. (1985) 'L'angoisse du vieillard dement. De la clinique a la theorie', *Evolution Psychiatrique*, 50 (3): 707–14.

Coleman, P.G. (1986) *Ageing and Reminiscence Processes. Social and Clinical Implications*, Chichester: J. Wiley.

Diesfeldt, H.F.A. (1983) *De draad kwijt. Over organisatie van het geheugen bij dementie*, Proefschrift, Deventer: Van Loghum Slaterus.

Feil, N. (1982) *Validation. The Feil Method. How to Help Disoriented Old–Old*, Cleveland: Edwards Feil Productions.

Fliers, E. (1985) *Hypothalamic Changes in Aging and Alzheimer's Disease*, Proefschrift: Amsterdam.

Glaser, B.G. and Strauss, A.L. (1965) *Awareness of Dying*, Chicago: Aldine Publishing Company.

Hagberg, B. (1987) 'Coping with dementia. The interaction between primary and secondary symptoms with functional level of the brain', paper presented at the Conference of European Regions of the International Association of Gerontology, Brighton.

Hausman, C.P. (1985) 'Dynamic psychotherapy with Alzheimer's disease patients', paper presented at the thirteenth International Congress of Gerontology, New York.

Jung, C. (1934) *Ueber die Archetypen des kollektiven Unbewussten*, Zurich: Eranos-Jahrbuch, Rhein-Verlag.

—— (1938a) *Die Beziehungen zwischen Ich und den Unbewussten*, Zurich: Rascher Verlag.

—— (1938b) *Die psychologische Aspekte des Mutterarchetypus*, Zurich: Eranos-Jahrbuch, Rhein-Verlag.

Katzman, R. (1986) 'Medical progress: Alzheimer's disease', *New England Journal of Medicine* 314 (15): 964–73.

Kopelman, M.D. (1987) 'Two types of confabulation', *Journal of Neurology, Neurosurgery and Psychiatry* 50 (11): 1482–7.

Levy, R. and Post, F. (1982) *The Psychiatry of Late Life*, Oxford: Blackwell Scientific Publications.

Lishman, W.A. (1987) *Organic Psychiatry. The Psychological Consequences of Cerebral Disorder*, 2nd edn, Oxford: Blackwell Scientific Publications.

Mayeux, R. and Rosen, W.G. (eds) (1983) *The Dementias. (Advances in Neurology*, vol. 38), New York: Raven Press.

Merriam, S.B. (1980) 'The concept and function of reminiscence: a review of the research', *Gerontologist* 20 (5): 604–9.

Miesen, B. (1985) 'Meaning and function of the remembered parents in normal and abnormal old age', paper presented at the thirteenth International Congress of Gerontology, New York.

—— (1990) *Gehechtheid en dementie. Ouders in de beleving van dementerende ouderen (Attachment and Dementia. How Demented Elderly Persons Experience Their Parents)*, Almere: Versluys.

—— (1993) 'Alzheimer's disease, the phenomenon of parent-fixation and Bowlby's attachment theory', *International Journal of Geriatric Psychiatry* 8(2): 147–53.

Miller, E. (1977) *Abnormal Ageing*, London: Wiley.

Molinari, V. and Reichlin, R.E. (1984–5) 'Life review reminiscence in the elderly: a review of the literature', *International Journal of Aging and Human Development* 20 (2): 81–92.

Raaijmakers, J.G.W. (1984) *Psychologie van het geheugen*, Deventer: Van Loghum Slaterus.

—— and Shiffrin R.M. (1980) 'SAM: A theory of probalistic search of associative memory', in G.H. Bower (ed.) *The Psychology of Learning a Motivation: Advances in Research and Theory*, vol. 14, New York: Academic Press.

—— and Shiffrin, R.M. (1981) 'Search of associative memory', *Psychological Review* 88: 93–134.

Reisberg, B., Ferris, S., Anand, R., De Leon, M. and Buttinger, C. (1984) 'Functional staging of dementia of the Alzheimer type', *Annals of the New York Academy of Science*, 435: 481–3.

Solomon, K. (1985) 'The subjective experience of the patient with Alzheimer's disease', paper presented at the thirteenth International Congress of Gerontology, New York.

Squire, L.R. (1987) *Memory and Brain*, New York: Oxford University Press.

Woods, R.T. and Britton, G.G. (1985) *Clinical Psychology with the Elderly*, London: Croom Helm.

Chapter 5

Reminiscing disorientation theory

Gemma Jones and Alistair Burns

SUMMARY

Reminiscing disorientation theory (RDT) developed from our frustration with seeing many moderately demented persons unhelpfully labelled 'confused' and 'psychotic', whilst their behaviours were clearly different from other adults exhibiting psychotic behaviour. This chapter suggests that the causes and manifestations of psychotic behaviour accompanying dementia may be sufficiently different from psychotic behaviours in other populations to warrant a new label and description. The application of the traditional label 'psychotic' to the patient with dementia has serious consequences, both in terms of the medication prescribed and the care provided by nursing staff.

RDT is an explanation of some of the behaviours exhibited by moderately demented persons who have been labelled 'psychotic', so that these behaviours can be understood in a context specific to dementia and so that new care-giving approaches can be generated from this new conceptualization. RDT describes particular 'misrepresentational, psychotic' behaviour in terms of an inability to control shifts between the 'state of intense reminiscing' and the 'state of being oriented to reality'. The decreased sensory perception and social stimulation often accompanying normal aging, combined with the decriments in sensory, attentional and mnemonic information-processing accompanying dementia are thought to be responsible for the loss of the ability to move voluntarily and quickly between states. Resultant interventions suggested by this theory include:

1   active reminiscing (both planned and spontaneous),
2   the use of special therapies and approaches which utilize reminiscing,
3   specific communication techniques for working with the disoriented elderly and,
4   more accurate charting of 'confused' behaviour so that interventions can be individualized and incorporated as part of the nursing care plan and interdisciplinary plan.

INTRODUCTION

Before introducing RDT, four examples will be given to illustrate the kinds of behaviours that have led to development of this theory. These four examples came from amongst the 75 residents of a geriatric hospital, where the mean age of the residents was 83.4. These examples do not attempt to cover all aspects of behaviour but they have been chosen either because they are typical or particularly illustrative.

Example one

Mrs H is 87 and has been residing in a geriatric hospital for 3 years. Her eyesight and hearing are poor and she is physically very fragile. She has no family and few visitors. She has been diagnosed as 'probable' dementia of the Alzhiemer type (DAT). Her short-term memory is poor, she has difficulty using specific nouns in speech. She can still speak in sentences although the content of her communications is limited and she loses the 'thread' easily. She spends most of the day sitting in a geriatric chair in one of the dimly lit hospital corridors. Within the past 6 months, when people pass by, particularly visitors wearing coats and the kitchen staff pushing the meal trolleys, she has started to become agitated and to call out to them 'Has the train to London gone yet?' 'Is there still time to buy a ticket?' 'I hope it comes on time.' Is this lady psychotic? She was labelled as such and given not only mild doses of antipsychotic medication, but vigorous doses of reality orientation (RO): 'You're not waiting for the train, you're in a hospital for old persons where they go when they can't look after themselves anymore.' The medications and RO did not appear to help because the vocalizations and agitation continued, and Mrs H became increasingly desperate to have answers to her questions and began to hold onto people's arms until they gave her an answer instead of ignoring her or trying to orient her. She was often lied to, to keep her quiet, and told such things as 'We'll buy your ticket for you and call you when the train comes so stop shouting now.'

It turned out that Mrs H had taken the train to London to get to work for many years. If you acknowledged the content of Mrs H's conversation and spoke of it as part of her past, she responded well and was happy to continue reminiscing although she could not use the past tense continuously in her conversation. Her agitation settled quickly, though temporarily, with even a few minutes of conversation that was directly relevant to her. Examining the situation objectively: Mrs H had a poor memory, poor eyesight and hearing and could not remain oriented to reality for any length of time. Sitting in a dim corridor with lots of people in different types of clothing rushing past, some with trolleys and carts, none of whom spoke to her, must have been giving her cues very similar to that of sitting waiting for a train.

Example two

Miss T is 93 years old and moderately demented. She practised nursing for over 45 years. In the evenings, unlike most of the other residents, she doesn't want to go to bed until after 11.00 p.m. She prefers to sit alone at a table in the darkened dining area in front of the nursing station. She talks to herself, and seems to be drawing and counting on the empty surface of the table, just as if she is working with real paperwork. If she is interrupted to be helped to bed while engaged in this activity, she becomes irate and very aggressive. It is routinely charted that she is 'psychotic: hallucinating again'. If, instead of trying to force her to bed, you ask her how the day has gone and if she has worked hard, the reaction is quite different. She'll say things like,

> The girls are nearly ready to change shifts and I thought I'd stay up long enough to help them with the drug count. I've drawn up the charts. It's been a busy shift. You've interrupted my count dear, but if you come back later I'll be finished and then we can talk.

Is Miss T's interpretation of events in her world so distorted, given her dementia? She is listening to nurses talking about work; shift change, drug counts, patient anecdotes. It is very likely that this conversation reminds her of experiences during her own years of nursing. Disoriented, unaware of her fragile memory and yet wanting to be useful, is her behaviour so much out of line with the sensory and perceptual information available to her? Could anti-pychotic medications or sedatives possibly help her in any way?

Example three

Mrs R is 84 years old and has started to become quite disoriented and disinhibited in the past year. She has begun to swear, and to make racist remarks to the coloured staff. She is often left in her private room for the entire day, even to eat her meals. If you were to go into her room to visit with her she would say things like:

> Did anybody see you sneak in here? Aren't you afraid to be caught with me? They'll punish you too, you'll get locked up in your room too. I was getting very lonely though, and I sure am glad to see a friend.

Once again, this lady has been labelled psychotic and hallucinatory. On examining her life history you will discover that she spent many years, unhappily, in a boarding school, and was frequently punished by being locked up alone in her room. Is it surprising that with a frail recent memory, poor eyesight, only an occasional visitor, and left in a little room with only a bed, wardrobe, chair and sink, she mistakes this environment for a boarding school of the past? Antipsychotic medications and RO did not improve this lady's behaviours, her memory or her frequent feelings of loneliness.

Example four

Mrs G, 81 years old, is sitting in front of the window in her room. She is getting cataracts and her hearing is deteriorating such that she often mistakes the consonants of words. She has been napping on and off throughout the afternoon. You come into the room and notice that she is looking out of the window at the children who have just come out of school and are walking along the sidewalk in front of her room. Mrs G stands up and begins to shout at them 'I told you a hundred times that you should button up your coats and wear your hats and scarves in this weather. Why will you never listen to your Mother?' Is this lady psychotic?

What are our goals in giving such persons antipsychotic medications and either using RO-type communications, ignoring them or telling them overt lies? If their behaviours are associated with the progressive brain damage of dementia and failing sensory functioning, currently available drugs will not reverse this; at best they will only be temporarily silenced and isolated. Let our goals instead be directed towards utilizing the memories and abilities that persons with dementia still have, to make them as content as possible in spite of their enormous handicaps.

Psychotic on experiencing reminiscing disorientation?

Psychiatrists would argue that the label 'psychotic' is technically appropriately applied to each of the above examples because of the following features: they are indicative of a severe form of mental illness in which the patient lacks insight and is unable to distinguish abnormal experiences (such as hallucinations or delusions) from reality. In dementias in general, and in Alzheimer's disease in particular, the difficulty arises when these symptoms occur in addition to the organic brain disease. Some authors regard them as 'psychotic symptoms associated with Alzheimer's disease' but little is known about their exact relationship to DAT.

Clearly, such behaviours are not grossly out of touch with reality or overtly 'crazy' if one takes into account the failing memories, senses, lack of stimulation and the environmental cues available to such residents with DAT. Their behaviours are not newly generated fantasies or thoughts that have no basis in reality. In fact, in each example the interpretation of the present environment accurately reflects the limited amount of informational input received, and in most is related to events that have actually occurred in their lives. Each of these instances shows a desire to place a 'meaningful' interpretation on a world which must be experienced as increasingly chaotic and alienating as dementia progresses.

We prefer to consider the problems associated with such 'misidentifications' as being the result of a person having (1) extremely impoverished sources of stimulation or information, and (2) a severely damaged information processing system to deal with this limited information. It therefore seems possible that persons in moderate stages of dementia, who cannot remain oriented, probably experience their environment as somewhat of a 'collective reality', a melange of the memories and sensory cues that are still available to them, rather than as 'objective reality' or even 'chronological reality' which can be selectively retrieved, examined and restored at will by careful control of mental 'states'.

This concept of state functioning is not exclusive to RDT. Several information-processing models have recommended that cognitive functioning be examined in terms of 'states' (Warburton, 1986; West, 1962; Horowitz, 1975) but these models have not yet permeated through to practice in clinical settings.

As if the term 'psychotic' were not complicated enough to consider on its own, the term 'confusion' must also be addressed. The term 'confused' is found in patient charts even more frequently than 'psychotic' and 'hallucinating'. In gerontology the term confusion is often used synonymously with disorientation and dementia (Wolanin and Phillips, 1981). In geriatric psychiatry, researchers are beginning to make distinctions between 'misperceptions, delusions, hallucinations, reduplications, and substitutions', but these terms are not generally used in the clinical settings nor are they explained by any current model. The term confusion is used both as a behavioural descriptor as well as a medical diagnosis. 'Confused' behaviour observed in an individual may be due to a multiplicity of factors including post-surgical trauma, head injury and systemic infection. Confusion is used to describe so many conditions and states in geriatrics, psychiatry and general medicine, that it has become an unhelpful word for the purpose of directing personalized nursing care. The lack of consistency and specificity in the use of the term 'confusion' as applied to dementia, complicates the development and implementation of effective assessment and useful care plans in the same way that the word 'psychotic' does. Our reasons for choosing the word 'disorientation' rather than 'confusion' will become apparent later in this chapter.

REMINISCING DISORIENTATION THEORY (RDT)

Identification of the population

This theory applies to elderly persons with dementia who are:

1 generally over 75 years of age,
2 handicapped by decreased sensory perception, particularly vision and hearing,

3   experiencing the cognitive impairments associated with dementia, such
     as reduced short-term memory, and attention and information-
     processing ability,
4   in stages 2, 3 and 4 of the Hughes dementia rating scale (Hughes *et al.*,
     1982),
5   experiencing multiple losses and decreased stimulation, arising from
     having a dementia, institutionalization and/or limited social, family
     and supportive interactions, and,
6   making errors in interpreting their environment and relationship by
     mistaking present reality for similar situations that have occurred in the
     past.

Background and definitions

Before proceeding, some terms and concepts used throughout this theory
need to be described and defined.

Sensory impairments in old age and dementia

Let us begin by clarifying the prevalence of visual and hearing impairments
in elderly people. Weale (1963) found that using a standard white-light
source, only one-third of the light enters the retina of a normal, healthy 60-
year-old, compared to that of an average 20-year-old. If this is so, then
what additional impairments must accompany eye pathology and visual
processing deficits?

Corbin and Eastwood (1986) in reviewing the literature on sensory
deficits in old age, report that visual acuity poorer than 20/50 in the better
eye was found in about 10 per cent of persons aged 60–69, 30 per cent of
persons aged 70–79 and in 35 per cent of those over 80 years. They remind
us of the common presbyopic changes due to thickening and yellowing of
the lens and the reduced speed and adaptation to the dark; additional
commonly occurring eye pathologies in old age are macular degeneration,
cataracts, glaucoma and diabetic retinopathy. White (1980) has described
the occurrence of complex visual hallucinations which accompany partial
blindness due to eye disease.

Profound bilateral hearing loss ('deafness') is relatively rare although
bilateral or unilateral losses sufficient to interfere with communication are
not uncommon. Estimates of hearing loss in persons over the age of 65,
based on questionnaires, are between 30 and 40 per cent, whereas surveys
which used audiometric assessment indicate that about 60 per cent of those
living at home or in homes for the aged, and up to 80 or 90 per cent of
elderly people in chronic care facilities have significant hearing loss (Corbin
and Eastwood, 1986). Unlike sensory deficits, there is little evidence to
indicate that the incidence of most mental disorders increases with age

(Corbin and Eastwood, 1986). Little research has been performed regarding the coexistence of sensory deficits and mental disorder in old age. Some researchers have described what appears to be an excess of sensory deficits in old-age psychiatry populations (Eastwood *et al.*, 1985). Post (1966) and Mayer-Gross *et al.* (1969) described paraphrenics and persons with organic brain syndrome (or dementia) as exhibiting vision and hearing loss more often than could be accounted for by advanced age alone. Gilhome-Herbst and Humphrey (1980) investigated the association between sensory deficits and psychiatric symptoms in persons over 70 years old, and found high correlations between the degree of hearing loss and evidence of depression or cognitive impairment. Corbin and Eastwood (1986) make an important statement about the difficulty of conducting research on sensory deficits and dementia. Of their sample of 102 patients in a home for the aged the sample was reduced to 40 with dementia. This sample was further reduced by the time sensory deficits were sought, and person with multiple complications eliminated, leaving them with a population that was not large enough for meaningful statistical analysis.

Berrios and Brook (1984) assessed 150 successive referrals to a psycho-geriatrician, for visual hallucination. Over 29 per cent reported visual perceptual disturbances. No age, sex, psychiatric status or cognitive-score differences were found between 'hallucinators' and 'non-hallucinators'. A highly significant correlation was found between the presence of 'hallucinations' and eye pathology and delusions. They conclude by saying that visual hallucinations can contribute to other psychiatric symptoms in elderly people and may contribute to their dysphoria and poor orientation and may result in psychosocial incompetance. Perceptual interference (through hallucinations) of the external reference systems for place and time can lead to false orientation. Both Berrios and Brook (1984) and Post (1965) report that neuroleptic medication is of little benefit in controlling visual perceptual disturbances in this group. Alroe and McIntyre (1983) query the role of visual pathology with the Charles Bonnet syndrome as well.

Visual pathology in DAT

Relatively little has been written about visual and perceptual attentional deficits in DAT specifically. The first study on visual perceptual performance in DAT was by Williams (1956), who concluded that 'it is not so much that [the person with dementia] is unable to receive information through his senses, but that he is unable to select or abstract from all of the information, that which is relevant'. Alexander (1973) studied attention in DAT using a non-computerized continuous-vigilance task, in which subjects had to identify one letter on its own, or a pair, from amongst a string of letters presented individually. He reported that persons with dementia were able to perform the single-letter search at a level appropriate to their age. They showed decreased accuracy and increased false alarms when they had to detect the pair of letters. This led him to postulate that DAT might be associated with a disturbance in selective attention. Jones (1990) has shown that DAT patients, even in early stages of the illness exhibit attentional deficits. Control populations of similar age did not make similar attentional errors. It seems reasonable to suppose that if pathology occurs throughout the visual system, from the point of stimulation, through to the processing centres, then we must expect to find aberrations throughout the visual system, from perception, attention, to visual-information processing. This pathology has now been substantiated. Hinton et al. (1986) showed that there is a significant reduction in the number of ganglion cells and in the thickness of the nerve-fibre layer of DAT patients. In addition, widespread axonal degeneration in the optic nerves of 80 per cent of the DAT patient sample was found, though the characteristic plaques and tangles were not. Many research teams have shown that the occipital regions, particularly region C-17, responsible for higher levels of visual processing, have large numbers of plaques and tangles when examined post mortem. Hutton et al. (1981) and Hutton et al. (1984) have shown that eye-tracking dysfunction is significantly worse in Alzheimer's disease patients than in persons with pseudodementia or elderly normal controls, and furthermore, that the severity of the visual tracking abnormality correlates highly with the severity of dementia.

How common are such behaviours?

The types of behaviours described in the four examples are not uncommon. Burns et al. (1990) found that of the 178 of patients with Alzheimer's disease in their study (mean age 80.4; range 56–99), over 30 per cent exhibited 'misidentifications'. Table 5.1 describes other psychiatric symptoms present in this group.

Table 5.1 Psychiatric symptoms and behaviours exhibited by Alzheimer's disease patients in the Burns et al. (1990) study

Symptom/behaviour	% affected
Delusions	16
Hallucinations	17
Misidentifications	30
Reduplications (doubles)	0.5
Substitutions	0.5
Aggression	20
Wandering	19
Sexual disinhibition	7

They found that complicated delusions were associated with calcification in the basal ganglia. Aggression was associated with temporal-lobe atrophy and wandering was associated with atrophy in the Sylvian fissure region as seen in computed tomography (CT) scans.

1   *Delusion* refers to a false and unshakeable belief developed by a person which is out of keeping with their social and cultural background. Common delusions by DAT patients include believing that property has been stolen and that a spouse is being unfaithful.

2   *Hallucination* refers to a perception without an object, i.e. something is perceived (e.g. a voice or vision) which occurs without any stimulation. This makes a hallucination different from an illusion, which is seeing a face or a pattern in a fire. Hallucinations can be auditory (voices or sounds), visual (visions), tactile (feeling things) or olfactory (smells) (Cline *et al.*, 1980; Siegel and West, 1975).

3   *Misidentifications* fall under four categories. Misidentification of other people occurs where the person fails to recognize others, most obviously family or close friends. They may say that a daughter is a mother or that a brother is a son. In the extreme case, a patient may believe that a loved one has been replaced by another person (substitution), or that there are two of them (delusion of doubles; Capgras syndrome) and that the present one is an impostor. Some persons experience misidentification of television images; in this category the patient believes that events on the television are taking place in real, 3-dimensional space, and these events are experienced as real. Mirror images can also be misidentified as being another person; this 'other person' can elicit friendly or violent reactions. Last, the belief that there are other persons in the house, is included under misidentifications, although it may also be classified as a delusion. The patient often cannot describe this other person but may set an extra place at mealtimes.

4   *Reminiscing* in the aged is defined as being the activity of recalling events and experiences in one's life. It is part of the normal life review process brought about by both the conscious and unconscious realization that one is near the end of one's life and approaching death (Butler, 1963).

5   *Intense reminiscing* is distinguished from the common understanding of reminiscing (i.e. the act of relating an experience) in that eidetic imagery (or seeing with the mind's eye as in daydreams, dreams or hypnogogic states) occurs concurrently with the reminiscence (Jones and Zeiss, 1985).

6   *Reality* is defined as being a state of awareness of, and an ability to respond knowingly to the four dimensions of (a) person, (b) place, (c) time and (d) situational context. (Merckelbach (1989) emphasizes how complex time perception is.)

7   *Orientation* is defined as being the uninterrupted transit or movement
    (voluntary or spontaneous) between the states of reality and other
    states such as sleep, daydreaming, hypnotic and meditative states,
    hypnogogia, hypnapagogia and intense reminiscing. This transit or
    movement occurs without the loss of control necessary for independent
    and safe functioning.
8   *Disorientation* is defined as being an interrupted transit between the
    state of reality and other states, resulting in an impaired ability to
    return to the state of reality voluntarily. Consequently, a disoriented
    person cannot function in reality fully, safely or independently.
9   *Reminiscing disorientation* is a specific type of disorientation occurring
    when a person cannot return to a state of reality from the state of
    intense reminiscing. For moderately demented persons this occurs in
    the presence of decreased sensory perception (primarily vision),
    sensory stimulation and cognitive abilities. Reminiscences are super-
    imposed onto the present environment (reality) such that present time,
    people and surroundings are mistaken for situations or persons from
    past reality.

Assumptions and related research

RDT incorporates several assumptions. The first is that all behaviour has
meaning. This assumption implies that the health care worker must attempt
to identify and understand the meaning and patterns of behaviours and
communications observed in demented, disoriented elderly persons. The
second assumption is that reminiscing is a normal activity occurring
throughout the lifespan, which becomes increasingly important in our older
years (Butler, 1963; 1974; 1980–1; Lewis and Butler, 1974; Jordon,
1988; McMahon and Rhudick, 1964). Reminiscing is seen to be essential
for the attainment of the developmental goals of resolution and self-
acceptance as postulated by Erikson, 1963; Butler, 1963; Feil, 1982. The
next assumption stems from the former, and holds that meaningful
communication with disoriented elderly people is possible utilizing a
number of current verbal and non-verbal approaches and therapies, and
that these approaches must continue to improve and evolve as our
understanding of the psychopathology increases. These approaches include
validation therapy (Feil, 1982), remotivation therapy (Hoskins Smith,
1973), reminiscing (Coleman, 1986) and life-review therapy
(Taylor *et al.*, 1983). The next assumption is that loss theory (Crate,
1965; Schmidt and Hatton, 1972), maturational development theory
(Erikson, 1963) and the concept of chronic illness (Perdue, 1981), help
our understanding of what happens as persons age, and how they may
react to foreseen and unforeseen losses or changes in their life before the
advent of dementia. Without a preliminary conceptualization of the diffi-

culties associated with normal aging, additional difficulties posed by having a dementing illness cannot be fully appreciated by care-givers. The last assumption involves the belief that the attainment of the developmental goals of resolution and acceptance are not restricted to oriented elderly people, but are also possible for disoriented elderly people (Butler, 1960; Lewis, 1971; Feil, 1982; Jones and Zeiss, 1985; van Amelsvoort Jones, 1985).

RDT is based on the following facts and research findings.

The activities of reminiscing and life review have beneficial effects on the behaviour and mood of elderly people (Butler, 1963; 1974; Havighurst and Glasser, 1971; Lewis, 1971; McMahon and Rhudick, 1974; Pincus, 1970). but as yet, little formal attention has been given to incorporating 'one-to-one' and group reminiscing in clinical settings, or to prescribing these activities in nursing-care plans.

Multiple factors contribute to disorientation. Some may be reversible, some not. Research indicates that with specific planning and intervention, stabilization or, occasionally, the partial reversal of disorientation may be possible in some persons. These findings need to be tested thoroughly on a variety of populations of patients, and with a variety of techniques and protocols, but it gives us hope that the decline seen in dementia does not always have to be a rapid, progressive slope downwards, and that inter-personal interventions may have a role to play in ameliorating some of the negative variables secondary to dementia which, no doubt, contribute to the isolation and alienation of demented persons. (Figure 5.1 suggests how interpersonal intervention might work.)

Finally, research has shown that communicating with disoriented elderly persons is not only possible and essential, but is beneficial to the quality of their everyday life. This is evidenced by increased verbal and non-verbal expressions of contentment and happiness (Feil, 1982; Jones and Zeiss 1985).

Remember that these various lines of research form but a platform upon which RDT is based. They must be developed in their own right as part of the literature for care-giving in dementia. The value of RDT as a teaching and research tool must also be tested in the future.

Postulates for the concepts of disorientation and orientation in RDT

RDT will be described here in the traditional way for describing theories, as a set of eight postulates.

1   RDT maintains that participating in the state of reality encompasses the 'recognition of one's temporal, spatial, personal relationships, and environment' (Stedman, 1982). This participation in reality thus involves the abilities to function, cognizant of person, place, time and

Figure 5.1 How interventions are thought to work

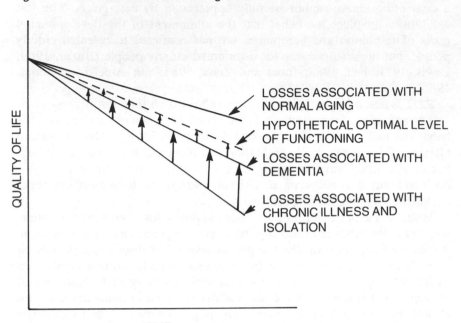

Note: Interpersonal and environmental interventions are thought to compensate for some of the losses and impairments associated with having dementia, the additional negative variables associated with social isolation, and a chronic illness. The overall goal is to help a person with dementia achieve the highest level of enjoyment of life and functioning possible, given their individual limitations and the severity of the dementia.

situational context. In order for an elderly person to be assessed as participating in a state of reality (what is commonly thought of as being oriented), he or she must be able to function cognizant of person, time, place and situational context, recognizing temporal, spatial, personal and environmental relationships.

2   RDT enlarges upon the traditional concept of orientation as described in the first postulate, by holding that all persons normally participate in states other than reality, daily, although we are not used to thinking about or labelling these states. These states make up a part of the daily activities of all healthy persons and include:

(a) hypnogogia: the traditional state preceeding the oncoming of sleep (Stedman, 1982).

(b) hypnapagogia: the transitional state through which the mind passes in coming out of sleep and the delusions experienced at such times (Stedman, 1982).

(c) daydreaming: the state in which the individual lets his or her mind wander aimlessly through gratifying images.

(d) dreaming; those sensations, thoughts and emotions experienced in sleep.

(e) meditative and hypnotic states; an artificially sleep-like or contemplative (though conscious) state in which recollection of events and reflection on one's perceptions and emotions occur (Hilgard and Hilgard, 1975; Schuman, 1980).

(f) intense reminiscing; is the state of being absorbed in the process of reflecting on the occurrences and events of one's life, to the extent that eidetic images of the events being reviewed are seen.

Both reminiscing, and intense reminiscing are normal for all persons, particularly the elderly.

3   RDT maintains that healthy persons can voluntarily or spontaneously transit between reality and other states (particularly between reality and intense reminiscing). When no difficulty is experienced in transiting between these states, we perceive persons as being 'oriented'. In the case of a person with dementia not being able to make this transition voluntarily, spontaneously or quickly, the person is considered to be disoriented. This damaged transit ability is understood to be related to the multiple types of damage that occur to cognitive functioning in dementia.

4   In RDT, orientation is the process and behaviour which indicates that there has been a successful transit between reality and other states such that no difficulty or interruption was experienced when return to the state of reality was necessary. Disorientation is the process and behaviours which occur when this transition between states does not occur without interruption (i.e. quickly and smoothly). This is evidenced by the inability of a person to participate in reality consistently and voluntarily. In the case of dementia, we perceive a person to be 'disoriented' on those occasions during which elderly persons superimpose their reminiscences on objective reality such that they mistake present for similar situations in the past.

5   This theory holds that a variety of factors or negative variables influence the transit or movement between the state of reality and other states. Some of these factors are reversible or can be manipulated, others cannot. These include: (a) organic disturbances or imbalances associated with the progress of dementia, (b) decreased sensory functioning (primarily vision and hearing), (c) decreased personal and environmental stimulation, arising from accumulated losses and decreased roles and responsibilities, such that the person is experiencing psychosocial deprivation or impoverishment and (d) decreased control over manipulating the environment.

7   RDT maintains that reversible and irreversible factors interact over time in such a manner as to cause increasingly complicated 'cycling' of

a person's participation in reality and other states. Many care-givers have reported this in terms of seeing even very demented persons having occasional 'lucid' moments.

8   RDT maintains that there are other kinds of compromised behaviours associated with the inability to transit freely between states, in conditions of sleep deprivation, psychiatric pathology and the use of particular drugs. (This chapter confines itself to RDT experienced by elderly demented persons.) Figures 5.2 to 5.4 illustrate RDT.

Implications

This theory directs care-givers to utilize interventions directed towards decreasing the effects of the factors or negative variables which influence disorientation in dementia, such that voluntary transit between the state of reality and other states is improved or regained, even temporarily.

Assessment

Sample questions that can be used to explore behaviours that appear to be involved with reminiscences and disorientation include:

1 What/whom were you thinking of just then?
2 Do you miss ——— ?
3 Did you have good times with ——— ?
4 Can you tell me about (event) ——— ?
5 Do I remind you of ——— ?
6 It's hard when you miss people and can't have them here with you.

Figure 5.2 Reminiscing disorientation theory

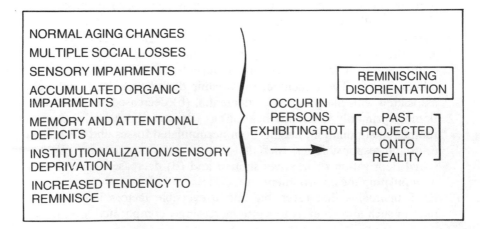

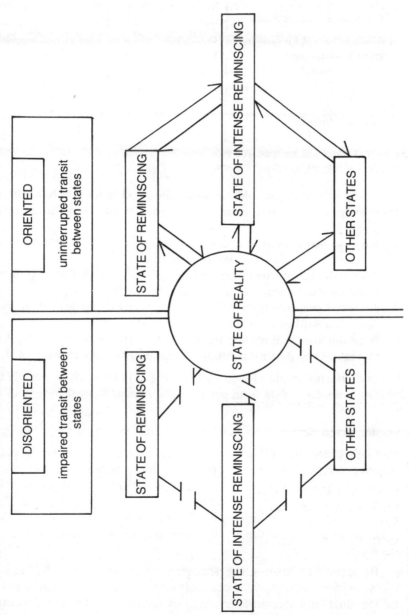

Figure 5.3 Schematic of reminiscing disorientation theory. The symbol ⇌ represents normal, unimpaired transit between states, and for access to the state of reality; ⊥⊢ represents impaired transit between states and irregular access to the state of reality

Figure 5.4 Intervention and goals

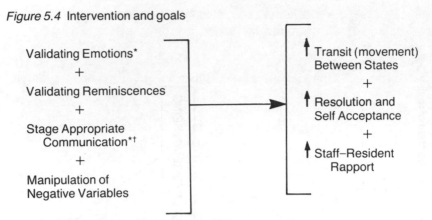

Note: *Feil, 1982; van Amelsvoort Jones, 1985.
         †Feil's four stages of disorientation.

Would it help if you told me about the good times you had with them when you are missing them? Could you tell me about some of those times?

7 What do you miss most about ——— ?
8 Do you like to talk about your memories?
9 Does it make you feel better when you talk about them? (when you sing, when we're together in a group like this?)
10 Do you have enough good memories to make up for all of the sad times and hard times you had in your life?
11 What did your parents and friends do to help you when you felt badly? Maybe we can do some of those things here for you or with you?

The mini life-review developed by Feil (1982) is also helpful for obtaining baseline assessment data from persons who appear to be disoriented.

Nursing diagnoses

Although there are numerous diagnoses that could be formulated for persons exhibiting disoriented behaviours, the following 'skeleton form' can be tailored specifically to any resident's behaviour. The characteristics of the disorientation should be observed and documented while various communication and reminiscing interventions are tried.

The skeleton form of the nursing diagnosis is composed of parts a, b and c as follows:

a   Resident X is experiencing disorientation or reminiscing disorientation:
b   *As evidenced by*: (give specific observations with as much detail as to the time and circumstances and recurrence of these behaviours as possible). For example, mistaking female staff for her mother every morning when being assisted with care; or, expressing a desire to go

home and feed her children often, usually at dinner time; or, referring to the environment around her with labels from her time spent at a boarding school.

c   *Due to*:

1   decreased short-term memory functioning, attention, or other cognitive changes,

2   decreased personal stimulation,

3   decreased control over the environment (state specific situations in which lack of power or decision making is experienced, if appropriate or helpful to the understanding of a particular behaviour).

4   decreased number of roles and responsibilities with/for significant persons (by choice, involuntarily? Who/What has been lost, substituted and maintained?),

5   decreased sensory–perceptual functioning (be very specific as to the losses and the effect that they have in limiting function and interaction with the environment),

6   other physiological imbalances (infections, dehydration),

7   feelings of loss (collecting notes about the feelings that a person expresses when they are disoriented, and a list of their favourite activities (or things that make them 'feel better') can be helpful in planning care interventions. (See Chapter 7 on nursing care model by Jones, this volume).

Interventions

Interventions directed towards decreasing the effects of these negative variables may help an elderly demented person to improve mobility or transit between the state of reality and the state of intense reminiscing, or they may just help a person to feel better in spite of the lonelinesses and fear which must be present with disorientation and isolation.

The most desirable goal is for an elderly person to continue experiencing normal reminiscing while maintaining the ability to return and participate in reality voluntarily. If continuous participation in reality is not possible, the next priority is to assist the person to reminisce liberally; help them follow the thread of the communication and place their comments into a chronological or historical time context for them if that is meaningful, otherwise, just reminisce. (I.e. Mrs Gibson is telling you about the horses they had at the farm when they were little. She suddenly wants to take you outside to show them to you. You might comment 'How nice that you grew up with horses, and saw how everyone started using cars later on.' 'Many children today have never even seen a live horse, tell me about some of your memories of horses.') Arrange for the person to participate in group reminiscence activities as well as encouraging reminiscence on a one-to-one basis.

In our experience, the intervention of validating a disoriented person's reminiscences and feelings (Feil, 1982) may often facilitate their reorientation even though this was not necessarily a goal of the intervention.

The importance of adapting the environment so as to minimize sensory deficits (Bolin, 1974) cannot be overemphasized. In addition, life review, remotivation therapy, validation therapy and sensory stimulation can be used simultaneously as interventions to help a person reminisce with the goal of maximizing the current abilities of persons to function socially, and to be appreciated in spite of their cognitive limitations.

It is essential that all staff members use a similar approach. Families can also be encouraged to understand misrepresentations, psychotic or confused behaviour in terms of RDT. This is a more humane vision to give them than that of the notion of 'craziness' associated with psychosis. This theory also provides us with a framework within which to study nursing and psychological interventions for disorientation.

ACKNOWLEDGEMENT

Ellen Zeiss is thanked for her contributions to the original ideas about RDT as presented at the 13th International Congress on Gerontology, New York, 1985.

REFERENCES

Alexander, D. (1973) 'Attention dysfunction in senile dementia', *Psychology Reports* 32: 229–30.

Alroe, C.J. and McIntyre, J.N.M. (1983) 'Visual hallucinations: the Charles Bonnet syndrome and bereavement', *Medical Journal of Australia* 2: 674–5.

Berrios, G.E. and Brook, P. (1984) 'Visual hallucinations and sensory delusions in the elderly', *British Journal of Psychiatry* 144: 662–4.

Bolin, R.H. (1974) 'Sensory deprivation: an overview', *Nursing Forum* 23 (3): 240–59.

Burns, A., Jacoby, R. and Levy, R. (1990) 'CT scan correlates of behaviours commonly exhibited in moderate and severe dementia of the Alzheimer type' (submitted).

Butler, R.N. (1960) 'Intensive psychotherapy for the hospitalized aged', *Geriatrics* 15 (9): 644–53.

—— (1963) 'The life review: an interpretation of reminiscence in the aged', *Psychiatry* 26 (1): 65–76.

—— (1974) 'Successful aging and the role of the life review', *American Geriatrics Society* 22 (12): 529–35.

—— (1980–81) 'The life review: an unrecognized bonanza', *International Journal of Aging and Human Development* 12 (1): 35–8.

Cline, D., Hofstetter, H.W. and Griffin, J.R. (1980) *Dictionary of Visual Science*, 3rd edn, Kadnor, Penn.: Chilton Book Co.

Coleman, P.G. (1986) *Ageing and Reminiscence Processes.* Chichester: J. Wiley & Sons.

Corbin, S.L. and Eastwood, M.R. (1986) 'Sensory deficits and mental disorders of old age: causal or coincidental associations?' *Psychological Medicine* 16: 251–6.

Crate, M.A. (1965) 'Nursing functions in adaptation to chronic illness', *American Journal of Nursing* 65 (10): 72–6.

Eastwood, M.R., Corbin, S.L., Reed, M., Nobbs, H. and Kedward, H.B. (1985) 'Acquired hearing loss and psychiatric illness; an estimate of prevalence and co-morbidity in a geriatric setting', *British Journal of Psychiatry* 147: 552–6.

Erikson, E.H. (1963) *Childhood and Society* 2nd edn, New York: W.W. Norton.

Feil, N. (1982) *V/F Validation: the Feil Method: How to Help the Disoriented Old-Old*, Cleveland: Edward Feil Productions.

Gilhome-Herbst, K. and Humphrey, C. (1980) 'Hearing impairment and mental state in the elderly living at home', *British Medical Journal* 281: 903–5.

Havighurst, R.J. and Glasser, R. (1971) 'An exploratory study of reminiscence', *Journal of Gerontology* 27: 245–53.

Hilgard, E.R. and Hilgard, J.R. (1975) *Hypnosis in the Relief of Pain*, Los Altos, California: William Kaugmann.

Hinton, D., Sadun, A., Blanks, J. and Miller, C. (1986) 'Optic nerve degeneration in Alzheimer's disease', *New England Journal of Medicine* 315(8): 485–7.

Horowitz, M.J. (1975) 'Hallucinations: an information processing approach', in R. Siegel and L.J. West (eds) *Hallucinations*, London: J. Wiley & Sons.

Hoskins Smith, D. (1973) 'Remotivation therapy', in G.K. Barns, A. Sack and H. Shore (eds) *Guidelines to Treatment Approaches*, Round table abstract in *Gerontologist* 13: 513–27.

Hughes, C., Berg, L., Dnziger, W., Cohen, L. and Martin, R. (1982) 'A new clinical scale for the staging of dementia', *British Journal of Psychiatry* 140: 566–72.

Hutton, J.T., Nagel, J.A. and Loewenson, R.B. (1984) 'Eye tracking dysfunction in Alzheimer-type dementia', *Neurology* 34: 99–102.

——, Shapiro, J., Loewenson, R.B., Christians, B.L. and Nagel, J.A. (1981) 'Abnormal eye movements in dementia and aging', *Transcript of the American Neurological Association* 106: 320–3.

Jones G.M. (1990) 'The cholinergic hypothesis of dementia: the effects of lecithin and nicotine on human memory and attention', PhD thesis, University of London.

—— and Zeiss, E. (1985) 'Reminiscing disorientation theory', 13th International Congress of Gerontology, New York, July 12–17 (Abstract).

Jordon, B. (1988) 'Preserved learning of novel information in amnesia: evidence for multiple memory systems', *Brain and Cognition* 7: 257–82.

Lewis, C. (1971) 'Reminiscing and self-concept in old age', *Journal of Gerontology* 26: 240–3.

Lewis, M.I. and Butler, R.N. (1974) 'Life-review therapy: putting memories to work in individual and group psychotherapy', *Geriatrics* 29(11): 165–75.

McMahon, A.W. and Rhudick, P.J. (1964) 'Reminiscing', *Archives of General Psychiatry* 10(3): 292–8.

Mayer-Gross, W., Slater, E. and Roth, M. (1969) *Clinical Psychiatry*, London: Bailliere, Tindall & Cassell.

Merckelbach, H. (1989) 'Tijdwaarneming als psychologische functie', *De Psycholoog* 545–9, November.

Perdue, B.J. (1981) *Chronic Care Nursing*, New York: Springer.

Pincus, A. (1970) 'Reminiscence in aging and its implication for social work practice', *Social Work* 15: 47–53.

Post, F. (1965) *The Clinical Psychiatry of Late Life*, Oxford: Pergamon.

—— (1966) *Persistent Persecutory States of the Elderly*, London: Pergamon.

Schmidt, L. and Hatton, C.L. (1972) 'The concept of loss', in I. Smith (ed.) *Five Years of Cooperation to Improve Curricula*, Colorado: Western Interstate Commission for Higher Education (WICHE).

Schuman, M. (1980) 'The psychophysiological model of meditation and altered states of consciousness: a critical review', in J.M. Davidson and R.J. Davidson (eds) *The Psychobiology of Consciousness*, New York: Plenum Press, pp. 333–78.

Siegel, R. and West, L.J. (eds) (1975) *Hallucinations*, New York: J. Wiley & Sons.

Stedman, T.L. (1982) *Illustrated Stedman's Medical Dictionary*, 24th edn, Cincinnati: Anderson.

Taylor, S., van Amelsvoort Jones, G.M. and Zeiss, E. (1983) 'Collecting and conducting life reviews', proceedings of the 1st National Conference on Gerontological Nursing (vol. 2), Victoria, B.C., Canada, 7–10 June.

van Amelsvoort Jones, G.M. (1985) 'Validation therapy, a companion to reality orientation', *Canadian Nurse*, pp. 22–6, March.

Warburton, D. (1986) 'A State model for mental effort', in G.R. Hockey, A.W. Gaillard and M.G. Coles (eds) *Energetics of Human Information Processing* Dordrecht, Netherlands: Martinus Mijhof.

Weale, C. (1963) 'On the Eye', in C.C. Welford and J.E. Birren (eds) *Behavior, Aging and the Nervous System* Springfield, Ill.: Charles, C. Thomas, pp. 307–25.

West, L.J. (1962) 'A general theory of hallucinations and dreams', in R. Siegel and L.J. West (eds) *Hallucinations*, London: J. Wiley & Sons.

White, N.J. (1980) 'Complex visual hallucinations in partial blindness due to eye disease', *British Journal of Psychiatry* 136: 284–6.

Williams, M. (1956) 'Studies of perception in senile dementia: cue selection has a function of intelligence', *British Journal of Medical Psychology* 29: 270–87.

Wolanin, M.P. and Phillips, L.R. (181) *Confusion: Prevention and Care*, St Louis: Mosby.

Chapter 6

A communication model for dementia

Gemma Jones

SUMMARY

The rules for communicating with normal healthy people must be completely readapted when one is working with persons with dementia of the Alzheimer type (DAT). The rules for normal communication demand a fairly equal exchange between two communicating parties; in working with persons with dementia the exchange cannot be equal and a care-giver must make a decision to provide extra energy and input into the communication, if it is to be a meaningful one. Although there is a general pattern of language change in DAT, there are large variations between persons. If health care professionals believe that it is important to communicate with their patients, they must compensate for the barriers to communication as much as possible and choose a method of interacting with them, even when the factual content is not clear, correct or based in reality. There are four main options: correct all conversation that is not factual or based in reality; try to distract the person from the topic at hand onto one that is easier to talk about (including lying); speak to the person about social pleasantries; or last, try to find out what the person is talking about, what topics are still meaningful to them and help them to say whatever they still can. This chapter presents three studies about communication with institutionalized elderly persons with dementia. A model for conceptualizing communication processing and response is presented to show how and where barriers to communication can accumulate. Finally, specific guidelines for communicating optimally with persons in different stages of dementia are given.

GENERAL INTRODUCTION

The increasing awareness of the importance of communicating can be seen readily when one looks in the self-help, business and psychology sections of book shops. This increasing awareness has also been occurring in nursing as reflected by the many nursing studies which focus on communication between nurse and patient. Studies have been reported for the acute care setting where therapy and support are identified closely to nursing function (Skipper *et al.*, 1963; Petrollo, 1976; Macilwane, 1978a, b; MacIntosh, 1979; Faulkner, 1979; Mercer, 1980; Forrest, 1983), and also for specific settings such as psychiatry, oncology, hospice care, paediatrics and maternity (Paton and Stirling, 1974; Blacker, 1976; Moores and Grant, 1976; 1977; March, 1979; Bond, 1983.)

It can therefore be seen that nurses are very conscious of the importance of communication in the delivery of nursing care. However, it is equally obvious that the process of communication is not all 'plain sailing'. There are many barriers to good communication in healthy people, and even more so in persons who are acutely or chronically ill. The number of barriers to good communication escalates even further for persons who have dementia and complicated physiological problems in addition to the normal sensory deficits accompanying old age. (Jones and Burns discuss these sensory deficits further in Chapter 5, this volume)

In this chapter, three studies will be presented about communicating and interacting with persons with dementia. The first study is descriptive, and compares the total amount of communication exchanged between nursing staff and residents, and residents and nursing staff during 2 hours of the day. Four groups of aged residents with different communication abilities were compared in a geriatric hospital setting.

The second study is a survey of the nursing staff in the same hospital, describing: the subjective criteria that staff use to select their favourite and least favourite residents; which residents they see as most demanding to communicate with; and what information staff would like to have in order to do their work optimally. The final study is a case study, showing the results of a structured attempt by nursing staff to communicate more with one such 'least favourite' resident in the moderate stage of dementia.

The last part of this chapter is a model which shows how communication deficits and barriers can accumulate. It can be used to problem-solve difficulties with individual residents, to optimize communication with them. The literature on the specific types of language change in dementias is very specialized and will not be covered here. Gewirth *et al.* (1984) and Miller and Hague (1975) provide a good introduction.

STUDY ONE: COMMUNICATION BETWEEN NURSING STAFF AND THREE GROUPS OF RESIDENTS IN A GERIATRIC HOSPITAL

Introduction

Faulkner's (1979) study of communication between nurses and patients showed: that interaction between nurses and patients was mostly initiated by nurses; that nurses employed avoidance behaviours when a patient enquired about their clinical condition; and that communication and interaction between nurses and patients was mainly task orientated. If this is how normal interaction occurs in acute care settings then the question arises: How do nursing staff interact with residents in 'extended or chronic care' settings, where persons often remain for many years, with no prospect of returning to their home or participating in the community again? Bakdash (1977) has shown the positive outcome of paying careful attention to verbal communication with the frail elderly, and Fox (1976), Griffin and Gerber (1980), Hardiman *et al.* (1979), Harrington (1975), Parkinson (1979) and Bartol (1979) have shown the importance of non-verbal communication techniques with this group and with persons who have special neurological barriers. Smith *et al.* (1980) in assessing nurses' perception of self-care in geriatric patients, showed that whereas the primary emphasis of nurses was on physical care, this was not reflected by the priorities of patients, who, in fact perceived the need for teaching activities as being the most important. Lipman *et al.* (1979) noted that nurses saw the most important verbal communication interactions as those encompassing physical tasks and not the provision of affective, supportive communication.

Given the plethora of studies on communication interactions in such a diversity of nursing settings, it is rather surprising to find that there has been little, if any, attention given to the qualitative and quantitative structural analysis of communication patterns between nursing staff and patients in geriatric and extended care settings. This gap in our knowledge led to the following study being conducted. The main question of this study is: what are the communication patterns between nursing staff and residents in a geriatric hospital? Are there differences in the total amount spoken to normal elderly residents versus those with dementia? (A partial version of this study was reported by Jones and Jones (1985).)

Methods

Description of the facility

This study was conducted in a 77-bed geriatric hospital in Vancouver, Canada, which provided care for persons in the intermediate to extended-care levels of the care classification system used in the province of British Columbia. This care facility had two wings, containing a total of fifteen private rooms, seventeen two-bed rooms, and seven ward rooms of four beds each. There was a nursing station and a combined dining/activity room on each wing. Nursing staff were of a number of ethnic origins, but all had a functional command of the English language.

Group selection

Four groups of residents were chosen for comparison in this study. Twelve persons (six male and six female) who were Canadian-born, and frail, but not having a dementia, were allocated to group 1. Twelve persons (six male and six female) who were immigrants from non-Commonwealth countries (including Russia, Sweden, Poland, Denmark, Greece, China, Italy, Norway, Romania and Germany), and who were also frail, but not demented, were allocated to group 2. Six persons (three male and three female), who were in Hughes *et al.* (1982) stages 2 and 3 of dementia, were allocated to group 3. Three residents who were very hard of hearing, but not completely deaf (two females and one male), were allocated to group 4. Persons in single-bed rooms, and those who had private nurses in addition to the care provided by hospital staff were eliminated from the patient selection.

Ethical permission to conduct this study was obtained from the hospital administration, the residents, family of the residents and/or their legal guardians, and physicians of the residents. Four meetings were held with all of the staff at the hospital, including laundry and housekeeping, to explain the nature of the study, and its duration. Staff were told both that tape recordings would be made, and that observations would be made during morning care, lunch times and evening care. Anyone who felt uncomfortable about being taped or included in the study was encouraged not to participate, but virtually every staff member registered their desire to participate. The total nursing staff in this facility consisted of eight registered nurses, five non-registered nurses who had completed their training but not completed their examination and twenty-six patient-care aids and licenced practical nurses.

Tape recordings and data collection

Staff and patients were unaware of when their interactions were being recorded. Tape recordings were collected during the 2 hours of the day, in which there was maximal contact between residents and nursing staff in the resident's rooms, namely during morning care (from 7 to 8 a.m.), and during evening care (from 6 to 7 p.m.). Tape recordings were made by carefully hiding microtape recorders, with 1-hour tapes, in inconspicuous locations in the resident's rooms just before the two time periods specified. Tapes were transcribed, and specific observations were recorded on two forms: one for 'communication by nursing staff to residents', the other for 'communication by residents to nursing staff'. Each form contained the following category headings: 'total number of words spoken', 'number of commands', 'number of statements', 'number of questions asked' and 'number of questions answered'.

Commands were defined as being statements made without a subject, whereas statements referred to either sentences or phrases which did have a subject. Questions were considered to be either proper questions, or statements that were asked with an interrogative intonation.

Thereafter the data were tabulated for each group, for the combined 2 hours during which the tape recordings were made. Student's T-tests were performed to compare the normal elderly resident in group 1, with the residents with dementia in group 3. Statistical analysis was not done on group 4 because there were only three people in this group. However, the measurements taken, are useful for comparative, illustrative purposes.

Results

The data from this study represent the results of a two-way communication flow; from the nursing staff to the resident, and from the resident back to the nursing staff.

The total number of words spoken between nurses and residents is shown in Figure 6.1. This is not high for any of the groups, but there is a

Figure 6.1 Total number of words spoken by nursing staff to residents, and residents to nursing staff

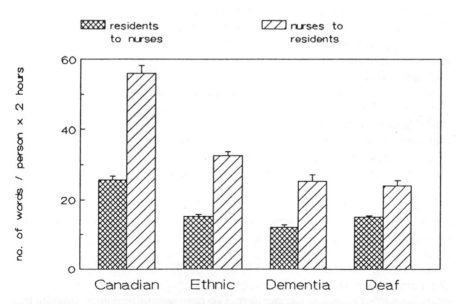

Note: Histogram bars represent standard errors. Recall that the Canadian group represents the group with the least communication impairments in contrast to the other three groups. Nursing staff spoke significantly more to the Canadian group than the dementia group (T = 6.5; p < 0.005).

significant difference (T=6.5; p < 0.005) between the amount spoken to the Canadian-born elderly group (representing persons with the least communication problems) and the three groups which have definite types of communicational barriers. Nursing staff almost always initiated conversation, and it is apparent that residents in all groups communicate less to nursing staff, than nursing staff do to them. This is deceptive though, because as you will see later on, many of the sentences residents use to initiate 'social conversation' with the nursing staff, and many of the questions the residents ask of nurses, are not answered or used to generate conversation.

Before showing the results for the different types of speech, i.e. statements, commands and questions, two sample conversations that occurred during morning care, between nurses and residents with dementia will be presented. These demonstrate typical examples of communication interaction with residents.

Two sample conversations with residents with dementia

Example one

Nursing staff: (Has come into the room and started washing Mrs G. No conversation has taken place yet)
Resident: I haven't got a towel to wipe my face.
Nursing staff: You want to use a towel?
Resident: (screams) Ahhhhhhh! Ahhhhhhh!
Nursing staff: Do you want to go to the toilet?
Resident: Yes.
Nursing staff: Stand up dear. Stand up please. Pee in the toilet.
Resident: I have to talk to you.
Nursing staff: Finished?
Resident: Yes.
Nursing staff: Good. (Nurse leaves room)

Example two

(Mrs H. was helped to get washed and dressed earlier than usual. She was dressed and sitting in a chair in her room)
Resident: What? Am I to go?
Nursing staff: Go there.
Resident: Go there?
Nursing staff: Come here, come here. (To another staff member passing by, nurse says 'Follow her to the lounge.')
Resident: Damn!
Nursing staff: Don't talk like that. (Nurse goes on to another room)

Commands

Commands are the most common form of communication between nursing staff and all types of residents, and commands are directed proportionately more frequently to residents with dementia and hearing problems than other forms of communication. This contrasts with commands being the least frequent form of communication used by residents to the care-givers. Figure 6.2 shows the number of commands made to and by each of the four groups. Recall that the Canadian group represents the group best able to communicate.

Statements

During the 2 hours measured, an average of only two statements were made by nursing staff to residents with dementia, as opposed to 5.1 to the Canadian elderly group (representing those best able to communicate). This difference is significant ($T=2.26$; $p < 0.05$). The number of statements that residents in all groups made to the nursing staff were nearly the same amount as the amount addressed to them.

Figure 6.3 shows the number of statements made to and by each of the four groups of residents.

Figure 6.2 Total number of commands addressed by nursing staff to residents, and residents to nursing staff

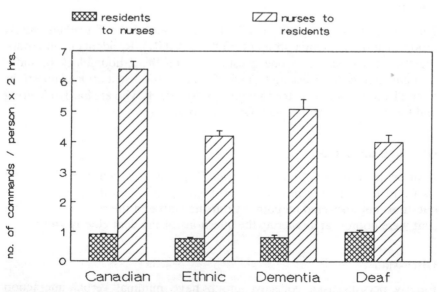

Note: Histogram bars represent standard errors. Commands are the most frequent form of communication used by nursing staff to address all groups of residents.

Figure 6.3 Total number of statements addressed by nursing staff to residents, and residents to nursing staff

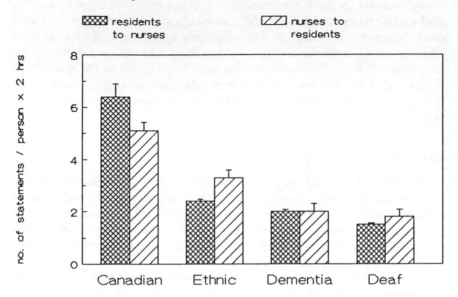

Note: Histogram bars represent standard errors. There are significantly more statements made by nurses to the Canadian group (those best able to communicate) than to the dementia group (T = 2.26; p < 0.05).

Questions

Nursing staff asked significantly more questions of the Canadian elderly group than the dementia group (T=3.88; p<0.01). Residents in all groups together, asked less than one question during the 2-hour block of staff–resident interactions measured. Figure 6.4 shows the distribution of questions to and by the residents in the four groups. Residents who are hard of hearing and those with dementia, again fare the worst.

Questions answered

A surprising number of questions, over 50 per cent, asked by both nursing staff and residents are not answered. Figure 6.5 shows the percentage of questions not answered by both the nursing staff and the residents. Nursing staff were poorest at answering the questions of the deaf elderly group.

Discussion

Elderly persons as a collective group have minimal verbal interaction directed towards them during morning and evening care, but this paucity of

Figure 6.4 Total number of questions asked of residents by nursing staff, and of nursing staff by residents

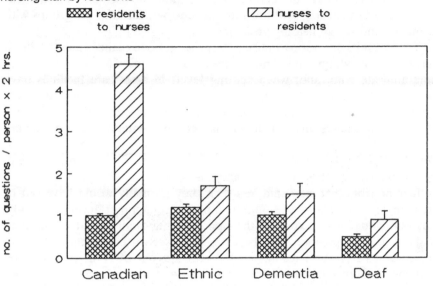

Note: Histogram bars represent standard errors. There are significantly more questions asked of the Canadian group (those best able to communicate) than the dementia group (T = 3.88; p < 0.01).

Figure 6.5 Total percentage of questions answered: questions asked of residents by nursing staff, and of nursing staff by residents

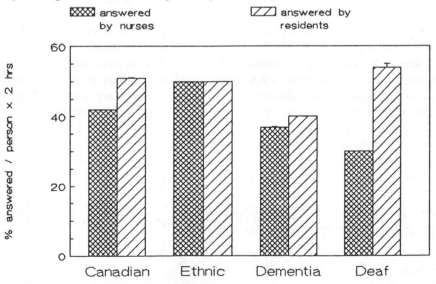

Note: The deaf group has the least number of questions answered. Overall, only about 50 per cent of questions asked by residents are answered.

communication is most evident in the groups of elderly people who, for a variety of reasons have difficulty communicating themselves. Communication directed by nursing staff towards residents was least for the groups with dementia and severe hearing problems.

These results are not particularly surprising if one realizes that it takes a great deal of energy and time to speak to persons who are difficult to communicate with, and, when staffing levels in most care facilities have been pared down to a minimum, staff feel pressured to become task oriented rather than communication oriented. These orientations unfortunately are still seen as distinct rather than complimentary. These results are worrying if one tries to imagine what the contents of a communication could be with an average of less than 15 words during time of peak personal contact between nurses and patients.

It is possible that staff said less than they normally would have out of shyness, knowing that they would be taped at some point during the study, but one would have expected the opposite, that staff would try hard to make a good impression, and be extra attentive to the residents. Even if these results have underestimated the real amount of communication by half, one cannot imagine that residents can actually thrive in an environment in which they are spoken to so little, and in which the primary form of communication takes place as 'commands'.

Distinctly absent from the communication interactions were 'introductions'. Nursing staff rarely told residents who they were and what sort of help they were going to be given. This would be considered to be an especially important orientation technique for those residents with dementia, aside from considerations of social and professional courtesy.

Tape recordings cannot pick up on non-verbal communication, and it is possible that much of what was not said with words was indeed carefully related with non-verbal interaction. However, if a person with dementia does not hear their name spoken several times a day, if staff do not encourage them to use their waning speech and if they are not stimulated generally to express themselves at the level which they still can, by how much and how quickly are they deteriorating unnecessarily? The literature on sensory deprivation in acute care settings suggests that deterioration can occur quickly; how much more so then for persons who have dementia and are permanently confined to care facilities?

STUDY NUMBER TWO: NURSING STAFF PERCEPTIONS OF THE RESIDENTS THEY CARE FOR

Introduction

The results of the first study were so incongruent with the dedication that the majority of nursing staff members reported feeling for their work, that I wanted to interview staff, and find out more about what was contributing to the very limited communication profile seen in study one.

Methods

Four meetings were held with nursing staff. The results of the first study were not disclosed to them, instead, staff were asked a series of questions: (1) Which patients do you speak to most, and least? (2) What makes someone your 'favourite'? (3) Who is most difficult to speak to and why? (4) Are male residents harder to speak to than female residents? and (5) What specific kinds of information do you wish you had been taught about caring for older people, before you started work here?

Results

The following were typical answers to the first question: 'To whom do you speak most and least?'

'I enjoy residents with a sense of humour, who remember who you are and what your name is.' 'Residents who can speak well, and who are polite are the easiest to work with.' 'Some of these people are really nice, they smile a lot, they love to tell you about their grandchildren, and they don't complain.'

The residents whom staff least liked to work with were described by the following statements:

'Some of them just give you such a hard time, they are not nice people to be with.' 'I find it hardest to speak to the ones who are lost, I just don't know what to say to them, or, if saying anything to them does any good.' 'I need feedback when I'm doing heavy, hard work with these people all day long; if they have strokes and things, I just don't get anything from them.' 'The ones who are deaf are the ones who drive me crazy; I started trying to say everything in a loud voice, and to keep repeating it, but it just takes too much time.' 'We have many persons here from other countries and they do not speak English; I don't have the time to learn Polish or Chinese ... I feel sorry for them, but there's nothing I can do about it.'

When nursing staff were asked for specific examples of their favourite and least favourite residents, some nurses maintained initially, that they had no favourites and that they treated everyone the same. Other staff members immediately accused them of hiding behind an ideal, yet acknowledged that in reality some persons really irritated them and others readily become 'favourites'. We made a list of residents who were the favourites and least favourites. There was a large degree of agreement as to which residents were placed in what categories. Then, two more categories were identified: those persons to whom one felt 'neutral', and those who were 'unusual favourites' for special personal reasons; not because they generally fit into the category of being 'everybody's favourite'. Specific examples of these four categories were very interesting and a few examples follow.

Category 1: everybody's favourite resident

Mrs R: 'She is so lovely. She has a calendar on which she marks staff birthdays, and even some of the staff's children's birthdays. She doesn't have much money, but she always has a chocolate or a candy in her room to give you. She knows everything about everyone and never complains that she can't walk anymore.'

Mr M: 'He has had such an interesting life. He always tells the most amazing stories. He's very polite, and loves to tell jokes.' 'When I have a coffee break I sometimes go to sit with him because he is so nice to be with, and really appreciates the time you spend with him.'

Category 2: those least favoured residents

Mrs W: 'Always complains about everything. She doesn't like the food, her room mates, she says the care isn't good, and that she hates this place. She is always accusing Mrs C of stealing her clothes and she hides everything in the cupboards, even old food.'

Mrs S: 'She is so confused. She doesn't apply reason to anything. Her behaviour is so variable and unpredictable. She doesn't let you wash her perineal area. Sometimes she yells just like a rooster "cock-a-doodle-doo". She threw the basin of wash water over me last week.'

Mrs B: 'She repeats everything you say to her, and fights you when you try to undress her for bed, and calls for the police. She messes everything up and wants to keep folding things and playing with them. She is very uncooperative and wanders into everybody's room. Sometimes she just yells for help all afternoon, unnecessarily. She just makes more work for everybody.'

Mr E: 'He comes from another country, and he doesn't know what you are saying to him. He likes to fight a lot with the other men and sometimes the nurses. He's big and stubborn; I always get out of his room as fast as I can.'

Category 3: neutral residents

Mrs K: 'She just seems O.K. She doesn't give you a hard time, but she's not particularly friendly. She likes to sit quietly in her room. Only when her family visits does she seem to be really happy.'

Mr V: 'He's very difficult to dress because his bones and joints always are sore, but he does his best. He is quiet and polite.'

Category 4: personal favourites

Mrs S: 'She is completely blind now, and has been in bed for a few months. She has a lot of bed sores and is in a lot of pain, but never complains. She's a very tiny lady with long, white hair, and somehow she reminds me of my mother. I sneak in to spend a few minutes with her every day, even though she's not one of my patients.'

Mrs O: 'She doesn't have any family and is just beginning to become confused. She has been here for so many years and she always liked to sing. Every year I helped to decorate her room at Christmas time, and I bring in some of the desserts she really likes, but which they don't serve here.'

Mrs C: 'She just wants to die now. She won't eat. Not everyone likes her, so I do.'

Although the allocation of residents to three of the four categories was expected, the existence of the 'personal favourite' category was surprising. When a list had been compiled of those residents fitting into the above four categories, the 'neutral' and 'least favourite' categories were examined together. It was evident that most of the persons from ethnic origins, who did not speak the language well, but who otherwise did not show 'crazy', 'rude' behaviour had been placed in the neutral category, whereas the majority of the persons with dementia and deafness had been placed in the 'least favourite' category. These were precisely the persons whom the staff did not understand, and felt powerless to help. It was apparent from the content of the communications in study one that staff often resorted to speaking to these 'least favoured' residents like children, and otherwise minimized their interactions with them. This certainly helps to explain the paucity of communication addressed to this group that was seen in the first study.

Male versus female residents

Only a few of the staff members had real preferences for working with males or females in particular. Some of the pros and cons of working with men were stated as follows:

'The men don't seem to complain as much as the women, and I find them easy to talk to.' 'Men are more work because they are generally bigger and heavier than the women. You can't just move the men into a wheelchair, it always takes at least two people.'

What staff would like to have known

None of the nursing staff had had any specialized training in geriatrics either during their initial or postgraduate training. The following is a list of things that staff members expressed a desire to have known about before they started working in a geriatric setting, and which they wished to know for their present work.

1   'When these people are so confused and demented, what is happening to the brain? I just don't see how their behaviour can fluctutate so much?'

2   'I would like to know the theory behind what happens to people as they get old, and to have the practical knowledge how best to help them. I try my best, but I just don't know what to do for a lot of them.'

3   'What programmes are there that we could use in this hospital to make people a little livelier? They all just sit there, and most of them don't even try to talk to each other. I heard about another hospital trying to use pets with older people, and another hospital that tried to start a programme where school children visited older people in a nursing home every week, but there must be other possibilities.'

4   'So many people have no visitors. We just don't have the time to be a nurse, and a friend to everyone. I would like to find out how to get more volunteers in here, just to be nice to people, and to take them outside for walks and do the things that we don't have time to do.'

5   'So many things we have to try to discover ourselves! No-one has ever taught us how to lift people, how to position them in wheelchairs, how best to feed people who have dificulty swallowing, what to say to the ones who are wandering all day long and really confused. I wish I knew more about these practical things.'

6   'Some of these people have such crazy behaviours (i.e. smearing and eating bowel movements; thinking they are in their own homes; biting you when you are trying to wash them; rude sexual behaviour; their mouths constantly twitching; and some of them not even recognizing their own children anymore). No-one has ever explained why these things happen, and if I knew, I think that I would not be so afraid of these people, and would not dislike working with some of them so much.'

7   'Family members of residents can be so difficult. How are you supposed to deal with family members who feel guilty that they can't look after their parent or spouse themselves, but who never have a kind word or a compliment for staff but constantly criticize all aspects of care?'

Discussion

It seems clear that nursing staff often feel bewildered and helpless before a number of problems that arise in having to interact with residents, particularly those with dementia. Staff derive some sort of support from residents who are cheerful and interact sociably with them, and tend to avoid those persons who they do not understand, and with whom they do not know how to interact.

Many staff members expressed the desire for concrete information about what was wrong with persons with dementia, and for intervention techniques that would help to interact with them. Many stated that if they understood what was happening to the brain, they could be more sympathetic to the residents and would not have to think of them in the simplistic terms of 'being difficult and crazy'.

In addition to the four categories of resident described (i.e. favourite, least favourite, neutral and special), two broader categories could be identified – 'complainers' and 'non-complainers'. This distinction arose frequently in the descriptions staff gave of residents. Staff were extremely conscious of trying to do their best, but not being able to make everyone happy. Those residents who emphasized that staff's 'best' was not good enough, and who made them aware of their limitations, were subsequently labelled as complainers, relegated to the 'least favourite' category, and avoided wherever possible, presumably as a form of self-defence.

An important question that arose from this study was: Is the staff's avoidance behaviour of certain residents, particularly those with dementia, really a form of self-defence, and helplessness? More specifically: If the staff were given specific knowledge about the type of brain damage involved in dementia, were informed of relevant details about residents' lives that are related to their 'difficult' behaviour, and were taught specific intervention techniques for working with the difficult behaviours of particular residents in question, would staff-interaction patterns change positively? This was the objective of the third study.

STUDY THREE: PLANNED INTERVENTION FOR A 'LEAST FAVOURED' RESIDENT WITH DEMENTIA

Introduction

From discussions with staff in the second study, it appeared that one female resident with dementia was particularly unpopular. Her medical history and life history were studied and discussed in detail in staff in-service education sessions and thereafter interventions for particular behaviours were planned. This study was designed to see if staff interactions with Mrs S would change if specific, relevant information about dementia and her life history were provided.

Methods

Four additional discussions were held, with the same groups of nursing staff as in the second study. The discussion for the meeting was divided into four parts: (1) a description of progression, brain pathology and sensory and cognitive deficits in dementia of the Alzheimer type, (2) a review of Mrs S's medical and life history, (3) a discussion of the major behaviours which staff found difficult to cope with and (4) the design of a nursing care plan for Mrs S.

Unannounced visits to the hospital were made six times during the next 3 months to assess: whether staff behaviour towards Mrs S had changed and to ask staff if planning specific interventions had changed their attitude towards her, how they spoke to her and the amount of time they spent with her.

Mrs S was born on a reserve among one of the tribes of Canadian West Coast Indians, of a Caucasian father and an Indian mother. She had very distinctive Indian features, and when as a young girl, she moved away from the reserve to a small, white community, she was often teased about her appearance. Later she went to a boarding school, often felt alone, and was apparently frequently punished by having to stay in her room. She felt very close to her godmother, and a part-time domestic helper called Sarah. Later, Mrs S became a teacher, married and had several children. The marriage was not a happy one, and during the depression, the husband left home for good, leaving her with the worries of providing for the children.

By all accounts Mrs S was a very proper 'lady' throughout her life. She continued to study and work, enjoyed the company of her friends and participated in community life until her eyesight deteriorated and she started showing signs of dementia in her late seventies. She was placed in the care facility when she could no longer live safely alone.

Several behaviours which staff found most troublesome will be described. The first behaviour, which was particularly annoying to staff members who came from other ethnic origins themselves, was that Mrs S tended to refer to them all (whether they were from the Caribbean, the Philippines or of Chinese extraction), as 'Darkie' or 'Sarah', depending on whether she was in a bad or good mood, respectively. These terms were either accompanied by swearing, or demands for attention and affection.

Because of her native Indian features, Mrs S had been called 'Darkie' herself, as a child by other school children. With the general disinhibition occurring in moderate stages of dementia, when Mrs S was upset, she passed this racial slur onto other people; something she had never done when she was healthy. Conversely, when Mrs S called staff 'Sarah', it was meant as a term of endearment. With the cognitive and memory impairments in dementia, she could no longer retain staff member's names, and when she felt close to them she used the name Sarah (someone who she had loved and trusted) for all of them.

Another behaviour which staff found disconcerting was that Mrs S often said 'crazy things and hallucinated'. Consequently, she was often left in her room throughout the day by staff, even for meals. She did not have a radio or television set in her room, and there were no photographs or personal memorabilia to help keep her oriented. When you stepped into her room, she would often make comments like: 'Do they know you snuck in here to visit me?' 'You better not stay too long or they'll punish you too.' 'I never thought I'd see you today.' 'Do you think Mr S will let me out tomorrow?' 'Where's Helen, I haven't seen her in ages, and I do love her so.'

After her life history was discussed, it was not hard for staff to realize that Mrs S's private room in this hospital must have had a lot in common with a room in a boarding school. Given that persons in the moderate stage of dementia exhibit disorientation to person, time and situational context, it was not hard to imagine that without much normal conversation and stimulation, all of Mrs S's environmental clues were ones of being locked up in her room and punished at boarding school.

Planned interventions

The following list of suggestions was generated and put into practice by staff.

1   Not to 'take it personally' when Mrs S called them names, but to realize that somehow situations from the present triggered unpleasant and pleasant memories from her childhood, and that she could no longer identify them as memories from the past because of her dementia.
2   To try to find out what things Mrs S liked, and to help decorate her room with some personal items. (One staff member found out that gold-coloured velvet was her favourite material, another staff member had a remnant of gold velvet at home and a third staff member sewed a pillow for Mrs S.) Mrs S was also fond of Canadian wild animals, and everyone began to save pictures of deer, bears, racoons, chipmunks, skunks and porcupines, etc. to put up in her room.
3   Staff were asked to introduce themselves to her when they went into her room, and to explain what they were going to be doing. If she called them 'Sarah' they were to say, 'I'm not Sarah, I'm X, but do I remind you of Sarah? Tell me about Sarah.' If she called them 'Darkie', staff were to say, 'I can see that you're upset, does my skin look dark to you?'
4   Staff were also asked to encourage Mrs S to sit in the lounge, to have

her meals in the dining room, to make sure she was present at weekly singsongs for the residents, and to encourage her to play the piano (which she had done when she was well).

5   Staff were also asked to encourage Mrs S to reminisce about her childhood, and particularly her school years. Some of the recommended questions were: 'Did you enjoy school?' 'Tell me something about your friends and teachers?' 'Did you learn any songs at school, can you remember any of them?'

Results

After 3 months, staff reported that Mrs S was much easier to work with, and that they were actually beginning to understand her better. She was being included in the hospital activities more frequently, was rarely in her room, had actually started picking some tunes out on the piano and did not say 'crazy' things as often as before. When she was in her room, Mrs S often had her new gold velvet pillow on her lap and stroked it gently. Pictures of animals covered the wall just next to her chair.

Staff related that they understood her behaviour better and that they were spending more time talking to her. Indeed, I found staff members talking to Mrs S in her room on two of the six unannounced follow-up visits, and Mrs S sitting behind the piano on another occasion. Mrs S's bad moods had decreased in frequency from all accounts, and staff were pleased with the success of the nursing care interventions.

A MODEL FOR COMMUNICATING WITH RESIDENTS WITH DEMENTIA

Residents with dementia can be thought of as having been sentenced to solitary confinement without trial. The only chance they have at communicating and sharing fragments of normal life, is through the efforts of those staff members who do not pass judgement on their behaviours, but try to remove as many of the barriers to communication as possible, even if it is for just a short while.

Figure 6.6 is a generalized schematic of what is involved in being able to perceive a message, and to respond to it. It is not intended as a psychological model of information processing, but rather, as a practical model to help care-givers understand why communicating with persons with dementia can be so difficult; that they have deficits at almost all levels and stages of processing a message; and therefore that they cannot be expected to initiate or sustain conversation, unassisted. The objective of this model is to help care-givers understand why they must provide the majority of the input into communicating with persons with dementia, and why

Figure 6.6 Communication processing and response schematic

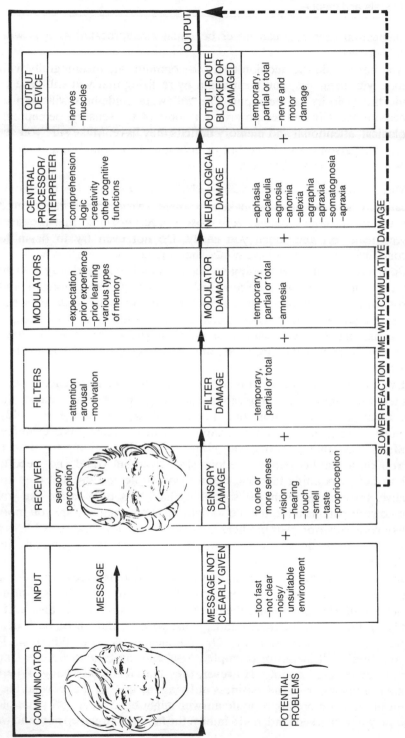

Note: Schematic diagram showing a conceptualization of the communication processing and response process in addition to where potential problems can occur for persons with dementia.

communication exchange can never be equally reciprocated as it is with healthy persons.

If you have made the decision to try to communicate meaningfully with someone with dementia, you must begin by realizing that you will have to provide the majority of the input. The following guidelines will help to compensate partially and temporarily for some of the sensory–perceptual, neurological, attentional and memory deficits they have. Make sure you get a sense of a person's overall level of orientation/disorientation, and assess how well their senses are functioning.

1   Make sure that you have optimized the environment for communicating. Check the lighting, make sure there isn't too much background noise and position yourself very close to the person so that they can see, hear, feel and touch you easily. Do not even try to begin to communicate until you have established eye contact.

2   Body contact, such as holding someone's hand is a good way to help them realize that you are there, even when their eyes, thoughts and concentration wander. It will help them to focus on your presence because you are providing continual sensory stimulation. If you keep a distance between you, you expose their weaknesses because they have to remember that you are there, and keep trying to find you in their visual field.

3   Even if a person loses the train of a conversation, or a sentence, or gets their facts mixed up, you can acknowledge the feeling behind the content of their communication. (This is called validation (Feil, 1982), and is described in detail in Chapter 12, this volume.) For example, Mrs S was talking about going home to visit her parents for dinner. You know that her parents are long since dead but you do not need to hurt her by pointing that out, neither do you lie and say that they are alive. Instead you might say something like: 'It sounds to me like you miss your parents a lot, tell me something about them . . . are you more like your father or your mother? Was your mother a good cook? When you miss them, does it help to think about the nice times you had with them?'

4   Re-orient a person as required, that is; when there is a reason for doing so, or if they ask you to. For example, if you must end a visit and bring them to the dining room for their next meal, it is appropriate to say, 'It's nearly 12.00, lunch is ready and I must go now, but I'll be back next week on Wednesday morning.' Or, if someone asks you 'Where am I', you should tell them, for example, 'You're in the Extended Care Unit in Camberwell, London.' However, they may really be asking 'Where am I in my life or in this business of living my life?' If that is what they mean, then a more appropriate answer might be 'You are 85 years old now, you've worked hard, had a family, the family is grown up now and we

are all proud of you that you have done so well. In spite of all the hard times, you always did the very best that you could and we respect you for that.'

5   Give people lots of time to respond, reaction times in moderate dementia can be reduced by more than five times that of normal elderly persons (Jones, 1990). Repeat yourself if necessary. Don't be embarassed by long pauses.

6   Follow the 'thread' of the conversation. Help the person with dementia to maintain the thread when their memory is too weak to do so, or when there are distractions. For example, 'You were just telling me about ...'

7   Reminisce liberally, and help persons to put things into the context of their own unique 'life story'.

8   Choose themes and topics of conversation that are relevant to the person's interest, life work and hobbies. Current events are no longer meaningful for persons in moderate stages of dementia.

9   Use props or 'triggers' to stimulate and prompt memory recall. Encourage family to bring in photos, personal possessions and memorabilia. These can be used to orientate a person, start conversation and reminisce throughout the day.

10 Be aware that intense reminiscing often evokes strong 'eidetic images', similar to those in dreaming and daydreaming states (see Chapter 5, this volume). When eyesight is decreased, a person may superimpose those 'inner images' from the past onto a poorly perceived present environment. This misperception in dementia is not the same as hallucinations occurring in other forms of mental illness, so do not be perturbed by it. These images often relate to memories of parents and children (see Miesen, Chapter 4; Jones and Burns, Chapter 5; Feil, Chapter 12, this volume).

CONCLUSIONS

The material presented in this chapter has shown that nursing staff find it difficult to work with persons with dementia, and that they say less than half to residents with dementia, than to non-demented elderly residents who can still communicate well. Persons who come from other ethnic origins and who are deaf, also have less communication directed towards them than elderly residents who can still communicate well.

If we believe that communication is an integral part of nursing care, then we must assess the reasons for the paucity of communication some residents receive. These include frustration and helplessness at not understanding the cause of behaviour changes in dementia, and not knowing how to intervene positively. Most staff, instead of focusing on communication, avoid it, and concentrate on custodial activities instead. There is evidence that staff will readily change their interaction patterns with persons with dementia if they are given the information they need to understand anomalous behaviours, and if the whole nursing or multidisciplinary team is involved in planning appropriate care interventions for residents.

Nursing staff continually express concerns that they need special education; care-giving does not 'come naturally' and must be learned. Communication with persons with dementia must also be learned. (The need for special multidisciplinary education for all health care professionals working in the field of old age psychiatry is discussed in Chapter 24, this volume.)

REFERENCES

Bakdash, D.P. (1977) 'Communicating with the aged patient: a systems view', *Journal of Gerontological Nursing* 3 (5): 29–32.

Bartol, M.A. (1979) 'Dialogue with dementia; nonverbal communication in patients with Alzheimer's disease', *Journal of Gerontological Nursing* 5 (5): 21–31.

Blacker, H. (1976) 'Talking to patients', *Nursing Times* pp. 1212–14, August.

Bond, S. (1983) 'Nurses communication with cancer patients', in J. Wilson-Barnett (ed.) *Nursing Research: Development in Nursing Research*, vol. 2, New York: John Wiley & Sons.

Faulkner, A. (1979) 'Monitoring nurse–patient conversations on a ward', *Nursing Times* 75: 95–6.

Feil, N. (1982) *V/F Validation: the Feil Method: How to Help the Disoriented Old-Old*, Cleveland: Edward Feil Productions.

Forrest, D. (1983) 'Analysis of nurses' verbal communication with patients', *Nursing Papers* 15 (3): 48–56.

Fox, M. (1976) 'Patients with receptive aphasia; they really don't understand', *American Journal of Nursing* 76: 1596–8.

Gewirth, L., Shindler, A.G. and Hier, D. (1984) 'Altered patterns of word associations in dementia and aphasia', *Brain and Language* 21: 307–17.

Griffin, H.D. and Gerber, P.J. (1980) 'Non-verbal communication alternative for handicapped individuals', *Journal of Rehabilitation* 46 (4): 36–9.

Hardiman, C.J., Halbrook, A. and Hedrick, D.L. (1979) Non-verbal communication systems for the severely handicapped geriatric patient', *Gerontologist* 19 (1): 96–101.

Harrington, R. (1975) 'Communication for the aphasic stroke patient: assessment and therapy, *American Geriatric Journal* 23 (6): 254–7.

Hughes, C.P., Berg, L., Danziger, W.L., Coben, L.A. and Martin, R.L. (1982) 'A new clinical scale for the staging of dementia', *British Journal of Psychiatry* 140: 566–72.

Jones, G.M.M. (1990) 'The cholinergic hypothesis of dementia: the effects of lecithin and nicotine on human memory and attention', PhD thesis, University of London.

Jones, D.C. and Jones, G.M.M. (1985) 'Communication patterns; ethnic elderly and nursing staff in a long term care facility', *Perspectives* 9 (3): 12–16.

Lipman, A., Slater, R. and Harris, H. (1979) 'The quality of verbal interaction in homes for old people', *Gerontology* 25 (5): 75–84.

Macilwaine, H. (1978a) 'Communication in the nurse–patient relationship', *Nursing Mirror* 146 (7): 32–4.

—— (1978b) 'Breaking through the communication barrier: liaison nursing', *Nursing Mirror* 147 (12): 19–21.

MacIntosh, T.B. (1979) 'The nurse–patient relationship', *Nursing Mirror* 148 (4): 1–11.

March, N. (1979) 'The patient needs to talk', *Nursing Mirror* pp. 16–18, June.

Mercer, L. (1980) 'Pseudocommunication with patients', *Nursing* 10 (2): 19–22.

Miller, E. and Hague, F. (1975) 'Some characteristics of verbal behaviour in presenile dementia', *Psychology in Medicine* 5: 255–9.

Moores, B. and Grant, G. (1976) 'On the nature and incidence of interactions in hospitals for the mentally handicapped', *International Journal of Nursing Studies* 13 (2): 69–81.

—— and —— (1977) 'The "avoidance" syndrome in hospitals for the mentally handicapped', *International Journal of Nursing Studies* 14 (2): 91–5.

Parkinson, T.L. (1979) 'The way back to simple pleasures for a withdrawn patient', *Nursing Times* 20 (27): 2213–14.

Paton, X. and Stirling, E. (1974) 'Frequency and type of dyadic nurse–patient verbal interactions in a mental subnormality hospital', *International Journal of Nursing Studies* 11: 135–45.

Petrollo, J. (1976) 'Your patients hear you, but do they understand?', *Registered Nurse* 39: 37–9.

Skipper, J., Mauksh, H. and Tagliacozzo, D. (1963) 'Some barriers to communication between patients and hospital functionaries' *Nursing Forum* 2 (1): 15–23.

Smith, C.E., Buch, S., Colligan, E., Kerndt, P. and Sollie, T. (1980) 'Clients and staff view nursing activities', *American Journal of Nursing* 272 (2): 79–88.

Chapter 7

A nursing model for the care of the elderly

Gemma Jones

SUMMARY

This model arose out of specific concerns that elderly persons who are difficult to communicate with, and those who are seen by staff as requiring 'special' attention, are often thought of as exceptions, and even nuisances. These elderly include the ethnic elderly, those with dementia and persons with severe hearing loss and deafness. In an attempt to relate all patient needs to universal, rather than exceptional needs, a nursing care model was devised to show how any given patient need relates back to Maslow's universal needs hierarchy via a graded series of intermediate steps. This system incorporates the use of a philosophy, family contract, patient contract, interdisciplinary care plan, a life history, material needs record, 'likes and dislikes' record and an avocational assessment. It is designed to be used by everyone in the care-giving network, especially 'nurse aides' and 'patient care aides'; the very persons who do the majority of the hands-on care with the elderly.

INTRODUCTION

The studies on communication and conducting life histories in Chapters 6 and 9, this volume, show that certain groups of elderly residents, particularly those with dementia, are difficult to communicate with and that special techniques are required to do so. And yet communication is only one aspect of care. Is there a way in which to combine a 'philosophy of care' with a 'nursing care plan' in such a way that it remains obvious that the needs of certain groups of elderly are universal needs, not special, exceptional, a nuisance and only extra work? Nursing is not the only profession to face this problem; Challis and Chesterman (1985) state that the problem of developing adequate recording systems has been a concern of social services departments since their development. Existing recording systems have been criticized for their lack of comparability, inaccessibility, variability and vagueness . . . indeed though a client record may resemble a long novel, this detail may still provide inadequate information to monitor activity.

The system suggested in this chapter is an attempt to keep the basic or 'universal' needs rather than merely the physiological needs (Maslow, 1954) of elderly persons foremost in mind when providing long-term or chronic care.

This model arose out of three particular types of experience in working with elderly persons in long-term care settings. The first involved seeing that there was no special system, or means of co-ordinating nursing, or interdisciplinary care for persons with communication problems, even though there were options for intervention. The results of the communication studies (described in Chapter 6) had shown that staff genuinely did not know how to speak to persons with dementia, and hence this group of elderly were deprived of significant amounts of meaningful interaction. Persons who were hard of hearing, and persons who complained, were also often ignored.

(There were voluntary translation services to assist with persons from non-English-speaking backgrounds, but staff did not know about them and hence they were not used. Several residents had lost all the English they had learned, and could only speak in their original language (loss of second language is discussed by Riegel, 1966). Of this group of residents, several without family or friends who lived nearby, had not had anyone speak to them in their language in over 6 months.)

The second type of experience that led to the development of this model, involved doing intensive one-to one work with persons who were moderately-to-severely demented, to see what their best level of functioning could be with intensive stimulation. It was very difficult to start any type of work with them often because there simply was no information available about their likes, dislikes, special avocations, life history or the circumstances that had led to their permanent institutionalization, and, as verbal abilities and comprehension diminish, it becomes difficult to collect such information from residents themselves. For example, when playing music for someone, it took a long time to discover their favourite songs, melodies and types of music because this sort of information was not collected in the traditional medical notes. Another example: if a person had been politically active during their life, it would please them more to watch the national elections on television than cartoons. If a lady had enjoyed being mother of a large family, it would make more sense to take her to a park for an outing, where she could watch children and families interacting, than to a cafe which mostly young adults attended. But such practical information was scarce. In discussing this problem with nursing staff it was surprising to see how much 'unofficial' information a collective group of care-givers had collected about a person, but none of which was available, as a unit on paper, to any given individual care-giver. It seems to have escaped the notice of many health care teams that the information collected in the type of medical notes used in acute care settings is of very limited practical use to staff who work in chronic care settings. Is it unreasonable to have as a goal, simply that you want to make a person as happy and comfortable as possible until they die? If not, then we need practical information about what makes individuals happy and comfortable in order to plan meaningful care for them.

The third type of experience which led to the development of this model, involved working in a support group for families of demented residents. There seemed to be so much unnecessary grief and misunderstanding because families did not know what they were and were not allowed to do for their family member. (In fact, there was very little they would not have been allowed to do; nursing staff would have been relieved to see more planned involvement and input from families.) One such misunderstanding arose from a change in institution policy, which, next of kin who did not visit frequently, were inadvertently not informed of. Due to economic restraints, skin lotion and talcum powder were no longer being supplied out of the institution budget. If this was not supplied by family or friends, residents did not have any available for personal care.

Two complaints were particularly frequently expressed by family members. 'I don't know what to do when I visit', and, 'What's the point of visiting, my (mother/spouse) doesn't know my name, has a poor memory and hence can't be benefiting from my visits?'

Both of these complaints led to irregular visiting patterns on the part of many family members, because they felt helpless and unappreciated. Nursing staff on the other hand spent much time trying to persuade residents to join in activities, or to come out of their rooms, but they would not, out of fear that they might miss a visit. The more irregular visiting patterns were, the more difficult it was to include residents in activities.

Nursing staff were not used to speaking to family members about how to visit, or remembering to tell family members about the small positive signs indicating that their visit had been appreciated (which usually occurred after the visit was over), or suggesting the types of activities that might be most appreciated or successful, or how important, short, but regular visits were. Neither did they feel comfortable telling some family members not to wear themselves out by visiting for many hours, every single day, at the expense of their own health. Interaction with family was unnecessarily frustrating because they were not included in practical planning although everyone paid lip service to their inclusion in the interdisciplinary team.

In addition to seeing a great need for a comprehensive model for care came the realization that although traditional, acute-care medical notes were not very useful for planning care, neither were existing nursing care models which have generally been developed for use in acute care settings. Long discussions with the nursing staff at the geriatric hospital described in Chapter 6, this volume, confirmed the observation that some sort of *needs framework* (Kraegel *et al.*, 1972) rather than a *problem-oriented* framework would be more appropriate for planning care for elderly residents who would be living out the rest of their lives in chronic care settings.

Staff concluded that working with the concept of 'needs' rather than 'problems' would be a more positive way of approaching care planning and interventions and one nurse gave the example of a Chinese resident, Mrs L, who wanted to eat rice with each meal and to eat with chopsticks rather than cutlery. Mealtimes were busy enough without having to order special food and remember that Mrs L preferred chopsticks. Only if staff had the time and/or the inclination did they get them for her. These requests had not been incorporated into Mrs L's care plan and were regarded as a nuisance. Only after Mrs L's family complained about her weight loss; when they explained that she had emigrated in her sixties and had never in her life used a knife or fork, and that she had never eaten bread or potatoes, did staff begin to take her requests seriously. Eventually, a small pouch was attached to Mrs L's wheelchair with velcro. It was agreed that she keep her chopsticks in the pouch so that she would always have them handy for meals, and that she was responsible for washing them up in her bedroom. Family agreed to provide rice cakes, and the kitchen staff agreed to cook a pan of rice for Mrs L in time for her lunch and evening meal. This is a good example of how a request can change appearances when it is viewed as a need rather than a problem.

STARTING ASSUMPTIONS AND CRITERIA FOR A 'NEEDS' MODEL

When examining the prerequisites and goals for a new model, it was apparent that there had to be four underlying assumptions. The first was that persons in chronic care settings may have needs related to lifelong routines and traditions that are not met by existing nursing care models or charting methods; the second was that any framework developed would have to incorporate the concept of basic (or universal) needs so that all aspects of care and interventions could always be related directly back to these needs. The third assumption involved the necessity for developing special tools so that relevant, personal, life-history information could be collected, charted and used in planning care. The last assumption was that nursing staff had to find a way to make family and friends feel welcome, and as involved in care as they could or wanted to be. There had to be a way to contractually agree, before a person was taken into care, what needs care facility staff could realistically meet, and which needs exceeded their responsibility and ability, and would have to be met by others.

These four assumptions led to the generation of a list of tools that should be developed or borrowed from existing systems, and collated into a new package, a new model specifically designed to meet the needs of the chronically institutionalized elderly. The model also had to be general enough so that it allowed one to work with a person who started off physically frail, and who proceeded to become mentally frail and pass through all of the stages of dementia. This is the list that was generated:

1   A statement of philosophy of chronic care provision so residents, family and staff would know what the overall aims of care provision were.
2   A family contract form so that family and staff could be clear about who was providing for which needs, and so that volunteer services could be directed particularly to persons without families, or whose families lived far away.
3   An avocational interest inventory, so that staff could get an idea of activities that would be most likely to please a resident, given their previous interests.
4   A life history form, (see also Chapter 9 this volume) so that particular highlights, and the sense of a persons 'life story' could be assimilated in a concise way.
5   A list of a person's favourite and least favourite things (or dislikes), so that an account of their preferences could be met wherever possible.
6   A personal property and clothing inventory of personal possessions, special treats, the minimum clothing and toiletry items needed, with instructions 'how' and 'by whom' they are to be supplied when new or additional items are needed.
7   A care plan form which would allow for nursing and interdisciplinary interventions to be generated directly from a listing of the basic or universal human needs. This form had to be simple enough so that it could be of immediate, practical use by all care staff, without much additional preparation or special education.

MASLOW AS THE STARTING POINT FOR THE UNIVERSAL NEEDS FRAMEWORK

No-one has described basic, universal human needs more simply and intuitively convincingly than Maslow (1954; 1968). Hence his framework was used as the cornerstone on which to build a new model for nursing care for the eldery in chronic care facilities. His work is popular and generally well covered in most nursing curricula. It will not be reviewed here, other than the listing given on the care plan. In reviewing existing nursing care models, it was found that Johnson et al. (1970) had already adapted Maslow's needs hierarchy to design a system of care for acute care settings. (Their work is a valuable resource for anyone wanting to study the applications of Maslow's hierarchy from the acute-care point of view.) This was further adapted to meet the criteria just described for the current model.

Tables 7.1 to 7.5 and Figures 7.1 and 7.2 show the instruments developed.

Table 7.1 Philosophy of chronic care statement

(a) Health care staff in this institution believe that all persons have physical, mental, spiritual and social needs. When elderly persons require long-term, or chronic care, outside of a home environment, these needs continue to be experienced.

(b) We believe that the term 'family' is meant in the widest possible sense of the word, and that this includes extended family, very close friends and pets.

(c) We believe that not all of a person's needs can be fully met by the health care staff and volunteers employed in this institution, and that family, friends and special services must be utilized collaboratively so as to design a system of care that optimally meets the needs of a given individual.

(d) The care planning involved in meeting these needs should be routinely reviewed every 6 months (and more frequently if necessitated by rapidly changing conditions or circumstances) at interdisciplinary team meetings, together with the resident and their family members.

(e) Each health care professional working in this institution adheres to this philosophy statement of beliefs about the provision of care in long-term, or chronic care settings. In addition, each profession has its own philosophy statement and care-objectives statement, as well as an interdisciplinary philosophy and care-objective statement (see Chapter 24, this volume, for samples of these).

(f) We believe in supporting the independence of a person, and their right to freedom of choice, and will encourage these abilities as long as possible. But, when cognitive and memory abilities become fragile, we will not insist on a 'reality-based' approach to care. We support the use of a range of activities which encourage a person to reminisce, and enjoy physical and social stimulation, with the sole goals of making them comfortable and happy, and functioning to the best of their capability, for as long as possible.

(g) We recognize that the move to an institution is not only a difficult transition for the older person, but also for their family. Therefore we ask the family to make a regular commitment (not necessarily frequent) to visit, so we can help remind, plan, prepare, and help their relative look forward to their visit.

(h) In addition to including family members in interdisciplinary care conferences and planning sessions, we also encourage their participation in monthly family support meetings where we undertake to provide (1) social contact with other families, (2) extra support for special problems or circumstances that arise, (3) general education about conditions in the elderly, research into these conditions, and information about other programmes.

CONCLUSIONS

Each of the individual parts of this model have gone through preliminary testing successfully in nursing homes in Canada, the Netherlands and England but this package has never been used together, as a unit, by all the members of nursing staff in a care facility.

Table 7.2 Sample contract of care facility with families

Dear _____ (*family member(s)*)

Although this is not a legal document, we do take this signed agreement as a serious sign of your desire to negotiate for and provide the best possible care for _____ (*name of resident family member*).

This agreement will be re-negotiated at your request, as often as necessary, or if the condition of your family member changes rapidly.

We strive to meet as many of the physical, mental, spiritual and social needs of _____ (*your family member/guardian*) as possible; however, because we cannot replace family and friends and previous social contacts, and because we do not know the details of their life as well as you do, we ask for your co-operation and collaboration in arranging the following:

Clothing (specify)
Toiletries (specify)
Sundries
Favourite foods
Christmas present
Birthday present
Radio
Television
Memorabilia (photos, items of furniture, knick-knacks)
Hobby supplies
Writing paper and cards
Holiday outings
List of phone numbers of close friends and special people

Did your family member participate in any religious group or church activities, receive visits from a particular member of the clergy or church society? If your family member wishes to continue receiving these, or similar visits, we may need your help to organize this.

We realize that circumstances may change rapidly and hope that you will inform us of such changes as often as necessary so that we can try to arrange for optimal continuity of care in meeting your family member's needs.

(*Specify agreements reached*)
(*Signatures and date*)

This model needs to be tested and further refined, but because it was generated from the experience and requests of nursing staff working in long-term care settings, it seems to be a more appropriate and practical system to pursue than nursing models designed for use in acute care settings. Hopefully this model will be seen as a starting point, and a challenge to persons in practice to develop it further, or to design better methods based on similar assumptions.

Table 7.3 Avocational interest inventory

Please rate each activity according to how much it appeals to you, even if you have not tried it yet, on a scale from 0 to 5. If you really like it write 5, if you dislike it, write 0, and if your feelings fall in between, choose a number in between that represents your level of enthusiasm for this activity.

Have you ever done this activity?	Rating	Specific activity
Art appreciation		
————————	———	Going to an art, sculpture or crafts exhibit
————————	———	Reading about the lives or painting methods of artists
————————	———	Watching a TV programme on art history
Politics		
————————	———	Discussing politics, campaigning, circulating petitions
————————	———	Doing committee work
————————	———	Attending community meetings
Arts and crafts activities		
————————	———	Making things
		models
		needlework, knitting
		sewing
		pottery
		leatherwork
		drawing, painting
		cutting/pasting/collages
Literature		
————————	———	writing letters, stories, poems
————————	———	reading
		novels, science fiction, plays, travelogues, biography, mysteries
————————	———	watching a documentary, play, live, or on television
Music		
————————	———	Playing an instrument (which?)
————————	———	singing
————————	———	listening to records and tapes (what sort of music?)
————————	———	attending or watching concerts, recitals or musical events
Gardening		
————————	———	growing and caring for plants
————————	———	watching gardening programmes
————————	———	hearing radio gardening news

Table 7.3 continued

Nature appreciation

——————————— ———— enjoying animals, pets
——————————— ———— enjoying landscapes, scenery
——————————— ———— following nature TV programmes
——————————— ———— being outside in nice weather

Physical exercise

——————————— ———— walking, strolling
——————————— ———— dancing
——————————— ———— swimming
——————————— ———— group exercises, yoga

Science appreciation

——————————— ———— attending museums, planetariums
——————————— ———— watching science documentaries
——————————— ———— reading related articles

Social/community/volunteer work

——————————— ———— volunteer work with help agency
——————————— ———— helping informally
——————————— ———— church activities
——————————— ———— visiting neighbours and friends

Travel

——————————— ———— local sight-seeing, day outings
——————————— ———— formal holidays away
——————————— ———— watching travel shows

Miscellaneous

——————————— ————
——————————— ————
——————————— ————
——————————— ————

Source: adapted from Meyer, 1980.

Table 7.4 Life review: general information sheet

Name: _____

Maiden name: _____

Birthdate: _____

Birthplace: _____

Languages spoken: _____

Religion: _____

Marital status: _____

Last address: _____

Admitting date: _____

Admitting diagnosis: _____

_____

_____

History of illness: _____

Current medications: _____

_____

Physician: _____

Special information: _____

_____

Father: _____ born:_____ died:_____

Mother: _____ born:_____ died:_____

Siblings: _____ born:_____ died:_____

_____ born:_____ died:_____

_____ born:_____ died:_____

_____ born:_____ died:_____

Friends: _____

_____

Spouse: _____

Children: _____

_____

_____

_____

Close relations: _____

_____

_____

_____

_____

Table 7.4 continued

1 Childhood: _____	7 Memories of people: __	12 Other memories: ____
2 Adolescence: _____		
	8 Memories of places: __	
3 Marriage: _____		
	9 Memories of events and	_____
	pets: _____	
4 Children: _____		
	10 Favourite 'things': __	
5 Work/avocations: ____	11 Hardest times and	
	things that might have	
	happened differently: __	
6 Health: _____		

Note: See Chapter 9, life review section for the recommended recording tool and condensed questionnaire guideline form. Make room for a special life history section in the resident's chart or notes. The headings in the table fit the sections of the 'condensed questionnaire guideline' in Chapter 9, pp. 153–4, this volume.

Table 7.5 Favourite and least favourite things: inventory

	Favourite things	Least favourite things/dislikes
Colours: in general		
for clothes		
Music: for listening to		
going to concerts to hear		
for singing along with		
for playing		
style		
types of instrumentation		
Authors		
Politicians		
Actors/actresses		
Singers		
Sports		
Sports personalities		
Heroes		
Flowers/plants/trees		
Holiday spots/countries		
Seasons		
People (i.e. grandchildren)		
Animals (pets)		
Books/biblical texts		
Activities/hobbies		
Food:		
appetizers		
meat		
vegetables		
deserts		
snacks		
Holidays of the year (i.e. Christmas, Easter, Passover, Hallowe'en, Guy Fawkes, May Day)		
Drinks		
Jewellery		
Casual clothes		
Formal clothes		
Shoes		
Hairstyle/haircut, etc.		
Personal possessions from life at home		

Figure 7.1 Personal property and clothing: needs inventory

Attention – family, RNs and AIDES

Should you notice that _____*(Female)*_____ is missing any of these items, please tick them off. Arrangements will be made to replace them.

Item	Date requested	Date received	No. of pairs

Personal grooming

Item	Date requested	Date received	No. of pairs
Hairpins			
Elastics			
Comb			
Brush			
Toothpaste			
Mouthwash			
Powder			
Body lotion			
Perfume			
Polident			

Clothing

Item	Date requested	Date received	No. of pairs
Bras			
Slip			
Underpants			
Dresses (wheelchair)			
Sweaters			
Socks			
Shoes			
Slippers			
Warm outdoor clothes			

Miscellaneous

Item	Date requested	Date received	No. of pairs
Radio			
Writing paper			
Pens, pencils			
?Any other items??			

Attention – family, RNs and AIDES

Should you notice that _____(Male)_____ is missing any of these items, please tick them off. Arrangements will be made to replace them.

Item	Date requested	Date received	No. of pairs

Personal grooming

Item	Date requested	Date received	No. of pairs
Brush			
Comb			
Toothpaste			
Polident			
Toothbrush			
Mouthwash			
Powder			
Body lotion			

Clothing

Item	Date requested	Date received	No. of pairs
Underpants			
Undershirts			
Socks			
Shirts			
Pants			
Belt and/or suspenders			
Sweaters			
Socks			
Shoes			
Slippers			
Warm outdoor clothes			

Miscellaneous

Item	Date requested	Date received	No. of pairs
Radio			
Writing paper & pens			
?Any other items??			

Figure 7.2 Care plan for the elderly (universal needs)

Categories of needs (Maslow*)	Description of needs (Johnson et al.†)	Basic/Universal need:	Specific need:
1. Physiologic needs.	1. Comfort. 2. Activity (rest and exercise). 3. Correct body alignment and mechanical functioning. 4. Oxygenation (circulation and respiration). 5. Nutrition (protein, fat, carbohydrates, vitamins and minerals). 6. Elimination of wastes. 7. Fluid and electrolyte balance. 8. Regulatory function (hormonal balance). 9. Sensory and motor functioning.	1. To be comfortable. 2. To have a balance of activity and rest. 3. To remain optimally mobile. 4. To have adequate gas exchange. 5. To use foods that are familiar, enjoyable and sustaining. 6. To dispose of toxins and waste products. 7. To experience substance/solute balance. 8. To experience organ system balance. 9. To experience optimal sensory and motor stimulation.	5. i.e. to use familiar products for dry skin (herbal salve). i.e. to eat steamed white rice with all meals.
2. Safety needs.	1. Freedom from threat of injury – mechanical, chemical, thermal, bacteriological, psychological, social and economic.	1. To be safe and feel free from harm, discomfort or fear.	To feel accepted for who one is and what one's ancestry is.
3. Need to belong.	1. Security, love and affection. 2. Companionship. 3. Productive relationship with others. 4. Means of communication.	1. To be called by name. 2. To be with family and significant others. 3. To partake in meaningful exchange. 4. To be able to make one's needs known.	4. To communicate and sing in one's mother tongue. To use the word/picture board and signs to make needs known.

Need			
4. Need for recognition, esteem and affection.	1. Self-concept. 2. Self-identity (includes cultural and sexual). 3. Self-esteem and self-worth. 4. Recognition. 5. Awareness of individuality. 6. Dignity. 7. Respect.	1. To feel satisfied with oneself. 2. To express one's identity. 3. To feel worthwhile. 4. To be as oriented as possible. 5. To be aware of one's own 'story'. 6. To live and die in dignity. 7. To be respected for one's total self.	2. To wear jewellery from the 'old country'.
5. Creative needs.	1. Expression of self. 2. Feelings of usefulness. 3. Need to be productive, to contribute.	1. To be able to express oneself optimally. 2. To feel needed. 3. To experience feelings of achievement.	To speak about the past, especially the good and difficult times in the 'old country'.
6. Need to know and understand.	1. Need for knowledge, understanding, comprehension. 2. Need to control matters concerning self. 3. Need to master self and environment.	1. To have a reasonable appropriate explanation of what is happening. 2. To have input into decisions. 3. To function as independently as possible.	1. To have medical procedures and special assistance explained slowly, carefully, and translated if necessary.
7. Aesthetic needs.	1. Order. 2. Harmony. 3. Beauty. 4. Truth. 5. Privacy. 6. A pleasing environment. 7. Spiritual goals. 8. The opportunity to celebrate meaningful occasions and events.	1. To experience a comfortable routine. 2. To experience comfort and inner calm. 3. To perceive beauty. 4. To perceive truth/fulness. 5. To be given privacy as needed. 6. To have meaningful possessions nearby. 7. To attend to spiritual matters as customary, or alone. 8. To celebrate life in all its phases.	1. To make bed in the customary way. 5. To say prayers before washing and retiring for the evening. 6. To keep a plant of special significance in the bedroom.

Figure 7.2 continued

	Resident objectives:	Nursing actions:	Family participation:	Other parties involved:

1. Physiologic needs.	Resident is responsible for washing and bringing her own chopsticks to meals.	Make arrangements with dietician and kitchen to have rice included with all meals.	Family will bring in traditional foods as per agreement with director.
			  Favourite sweets.
			  Foods for traditional celebrations.
			Family will bring in salves and other items as needed.
				Dietary and kitchen.

2. Safety needs.		Turn on German radio programme every Wednesday at 2.00 p.m.	Encourage reminiscing and facilitate use of mother tongue.	
3. Need to belong.		Learn 10 key words in the resident's language, and become familiar with the use of the picture/letter board.	Write out key words for staff and negotiate structure, with family member, of word/picture board.	Activity aid will include person in music group. Volunteer (Greek speaking) will be arranged.
4. Need for recognition, esteem and affection.		Encourage resident to wear jewellery. Arrange opportunities for residents of same nationality to socialize together.	Family will visit, utilizing traditional, favourite pastimes to stimulate their parent. Family will help older persons to spend money on meaningful items.	

5. Creative needs.		Encourage reminiscing and life review activities.	Family will provide hospital with a mini-life history and appropriate cultural data.
6. Need to know and understand.		Utilize an interpreter for emergencies if family is not available.	Will explain routine, activities, and changes in regimen as necessary.	Use services of MOSAIC FOR EMERGENCIES, as needed. Translation. Counselling.
7. Aesthetic needs.	Will make bed in customary way each morning.	Include quiet time into evening routine so that resident can be alone in room to say prayers.	Family will bring in meaningful possessions and memorabilia. Will arrange to take resident to church, or have visitors come in from church.	If there is no family, link person with desired church.

Note *Abraham H. Maslow, *Motivation and Personality* (New York: Harper & Row, 1954)
†M. Johnson, M. Davei and M. Bilitch, *Problem-solving in Nursing Practice* (NY: William C. Brown, 1970), adapted by Gemma Jones, 1985

REFERENCES

Challis, D. and Chesterman, J. (1985) 'A system for monitoring social work activity with the frail elderly', *British Journal of Social Work* 15: 115–32.

Johnson, M.M., Davei, M.L. and Bilitch, M.J. (1970) *Problem Solving in Nursing Practise*, New York: WMC Brown, pp. 18–99.

Kraegel, J.M., Schmidt, V., Shukla, R. and Goldsmith, C.E. (1972) 'A system of patient care based on patient needs', *Nursing Outlook* 20 (4): 257–64.

Maslow, A.H. (1954) *Motivation and Personality*, New York: Harper & Row.

—— (1968) *Toward a Psychology of Being*, New York: Van Nostrand Reinhold.

Meyer, G.R. (1980) 'Avocational interest inventory', in *Non-Traditional Therapy and Counseling with the Aging*, New York: Springer.

Riegel, K.F. (1966) 'Development of language: suggestions for a verbal fallout model', *Human Development* 9: 97–120.

Part II

Interventions for persons with dementia in care facilities

What can be learned from studies on reality orientation?

Bob Woods

SUMMARY

Reality orientation (RO) is probably the most widely applied and empirically evaluated approach to the management of dementia. Undoubtedly, it is an approach with major limitations, and so this chapter describes the implications to be drawn from the extensive literature on RO for the development of more satisfactory approaches. Emphasis is given to the central part played by the attitudes, values and principles of staff and services in the actual implementation of any approach and to the importance of a broader perspective in the evaluation of the effectiveness of such methods. The feasibility of achieving limited learning in some people with dementia is demonstrated, and means are described of ensuring that any changes obtained are relevant to the person's actual needs and difficulties.

INTRODUCTION

The use of RO will first be placed in a historical context, before briefly describing its key features. Some of the major criticisms of RO will be set out, and the most important implications drawn from the accumulated knowledge base on the evaluation of RO in practice. Finally, an integrated approach to work with people with dementia, emphasizing communication and an individualized approach, will be described as a viable way forward for those day by day faced by the challenging task of providing humane, sensitive care for those people afflicted with a dementia.

HISTORICAL CONTEXT

The origins of RO can be traced back at least 30 years to various Veterans Administration facilities, where Dr James Folsom developed a programme for hospitalized elderly patients, involving all staff, including those without professional qualifications (Taulbee and Folsom, 1966; Folsom, 1967;

1968). Such a programme was a tremendous innovation, at a time when care for elderly people in such institutions was predominantly custodial, and typically little status or responsibility would be given to the unqualified staff. Elsewhere, there had been some efforts to offer more stimulation and activity to confused elderly people (e.g. Cosin *et al.*, 1958; Bower, 1967), but it was RO that mushroomed in popularity. In 1969 a booklet was published by the American Psychiatric Association entitled *Reality Orientation: A Technique to Rehabilitate Elderly and Brain-damaged Patients with a Moderate to Severe Degree of Disorientation* (edited by Louise Stephens), and this, together with a training programme at Tuscaloosa (one of the hospitals where Folsom had developed RO), where nurses and other staff from all over the USA came to learn the RO approach, helped to consolidate RO's position as the major approach in this field. RO with its emphasis on orientation seemed tailor-made for use with people with dementia, where disorientation appears almost universally. It is interesting to note that some of the early work was in fact carried out with people suffering from long-standing psychiatric disorders, and was not targeted solely at those suffering from dementia.

For all its popularity, it was some years before RO was subject to the test of a controlled evaluation. In the USA several anecdotal studies and uncontrolled trials were reported (e.g. Letcher *et al.*, 1974; Barnes, 1974). It was, however, the first report of its use in the UK that evaluated patients in the programme in relation to those in a control group (Brook *et al.*, 1975). The majority of the numerous further controlled evaluations appeared in the five subsequent years (1976–1981). Holden and Woods (1988) review these studies in detail. Over the years, also, a number of descriptive and 'how-to-do-it' articles have been published. The flow of these similarly has dwindled in the latter half of the 1980s. With a few exceptions, people with a dementia have become the clear target population for the programme. Although subject to criticism for many years (e.g. Schwenk, 1981; Powell Proctor and Miller, 1982), its use is taught widely to the variety of professional groups involved. Most homes, centres and wards with any claim to adopting a positive approach to work with people with dementia will incorporate at least some of the RO techniques into their programme. There is, then, a wealth of experience of its use (and possibly abuse) to guide us in developing the approaches which should lead practice into the next decade.

KEY FEATURES OF RO

RO, like other therapeutic approaches, can at times be difficult to pin down. Sometimes, people assume the name says it all, and that it consists entirely of orientating the person to reality, at all times, in every situation. Sometimes the definition of RO is so broad that, as Hanley (1984) comments, 'RO can be all things to all people'. Several manuals are available (e.g. Drummond *et al.*, 1978; Hanley, 1982; Rimmer, 1982). The description of some of the most important aspects that follows is derived from the comprehensive account of RO in Holden and Woods (1988).

Two main types of RO are usually distinguished. The first is 24-hour RO (also described as 'informal RO' or 'the basic approach'). This is a continual process, where each interaction with the person is seen as an opportunity to present current information and to involve the person in what is happening around them, through providing a commentary on what is happening and reinforcing the person's awareness of and interest in their environment. The second aspect consists of RO sessions (or 'formal RO' or 'RO classes'). These are small group sessions, with three to six patients meeting with one or two staff, for 30 minutes or so, ideally on a daily basis. Research has tended to focus on RO sessions, probably because implementing 24-hour RO satisfactorily is a considerably more difficult undertaking (see Holden and Woods, 1988: 70–3).

Whilst presenting current reality is at the heart of 24-hour RO, this entails some consideration as to how best engage the person in interaction, how best to elicit appropriate responses and so achieve a better level of two-way communication. The first step must be to reduce the impact of any barriers to communication; sensory deficits need to be corrected as far as possible, and members of staff need to learn to speak clearly and sensitively so as not to amplify the person's difficulties. Environmental barriers must also be removed. These might include: distracting background noise, furniture arranged so as to make an ordinary conversation nearly impossible, large numbers of people gathered together, lack of privacy and so on. Staff need to become aware of the impact of their own body language, when working with patients consigned by memory loss to a world where 'first impressions' are among the few indicators to what might be expected from an impending interaction. The patient has to make the decision as to 'friend or foe?' in a split second when approached by a staff member. Poor recent memory means the person is unlikely to be recognized, or even have their role correctly identified. The staff member's demeanour, tone of voice, facial expression, speed and direction of approach may make the difference between a warm, friendly interaction and an 'aggressive outburst'. Using eye contact and gentle touch, staff can hold the attention of a distractable patient for longer, and again achieve a higher-level interaction. Staff also need to learn to read the patient's non-verbal communication. Where the patient has difficulty expressing thoughts and emotions in appropriate words, staff sensitive to non-verbal communication may be better able to grasp the meaning of what the patient is trying to communicate.

Guidelines also arise from 24-hour RO as to the form and content of what the staff member says, as well as how it is said. Holden and Woods (1988) recommend the use of short, simple sentences and the encouragement of response and repetition from the patient. Using varied means of repeating the same theme or topic, perhaps calling into play several senses may prove useful. Having something tangible as a focus for the conversation, helps ensure both parties to the conversation are talking about the same thing, and are not at cross-purposes, as is so often the case. *Very often drawing on the person's past experiences can be a powerful way of opening up discussion leading up to the present day.* Tapping into the person's sense of humour (often amazingly intact), can make way for a more relaxed and rewarding interaction. Finally, guidelines are given for the difficult area of responding to the patient when he or she appears *out of touch with reality.* This issue will be discussed in a later section in some detail; the essential rule in RO is *never to agree with what the person says if it is clearly wrong,* but there are then a number of options for responding depending on the particular circumstances.

Twenty-four-hour RO is built around interaction with the patient; underlying it is a commitment to the importance of explaining to the person what is happening, as clearly and simply as is necessary. Silent care is seen as undesirable, and potentially dehumanizing. Wards and homes where staff say 'if only we had time to talk to the patients' are viewed as missing out on opportunities for interaction during care tasks. Where levels of staff–patient interaction are low, the question must be asked as to whether this is because staff give higher priority to activities not involving contact with the patients. Twenty-four-hour RO places good-quality staff–patient interaction at the top of the many competing demands on staff time, but emphasizes it is not in competition with the fulfilment of personal care tasks, which should be accompanied by such contact.

The most tangible aspect of 24-hour RO, and perhaps the most ubiquitously applied, is the use of signposting and information boards, providing a back-up to the information provided by staff. The person with dementia has an even greater need of memory aids than a person with unimpaired memory; for the person with dementia these aids, if they are to be useful and relied upon, must be clear, striking and above all accurate. Yet it is commonplace to visit wards or homes where the RO board has not been updated for days, or where the clocks all tell a different time! The proper implementation of 24-hour RO involves a commitment to ensuring information given is accurate, and that staff make use of the orientation aids in their interactions with patients, so that patients can begin to use the aids themselves as orienting cues.

RO sessions were originally intended to supplement 24-hour RO, not to replace it, as has too often been the case. They provide an opportunity to use many of the techniques already described more intensively, and to help patients communicate more with each other as well as with staff. The groups use a variety of activities as a focus; these need to be carefully selected to be simple enough to enable group members to enjoy feelings of success and achievement, but not so simple as to be viewed as boring or demeaning. Different groups of different ability levels will need activities suited to their needs. Holden and Woods (1988) describe three levels of activities ranging from basic sensory stimulation, to baking cakes, to outings. Variety is important for patients and staff; the greater the range of activities the greater the range of responses likely to be forthcoming. Although many RO sessions begin with completing and rehearsing the basic current information on the RO board, often used as a focus for the group, Holden and Woods show how this current information (day, date, weather, place, etc.) is only a small part of the current reality to which patients may be reintroduced.

These, then, are the key features of RO. A brief guide to these techniques for direct care-staff is provided by Woods (1989a; b; c).

THE CASE AGAINST RO

RO has attracted a great deal of criticism over the years. Many have pointed out the lack of a sound theoretical foundation to RO and that some of the evaluative research is flawed or inconclusive, so that its empirical basis is also subject to uncertainty. For example, Hussian (1981) argues that RO has taken the place of custodial care before the 1960s as 'a "treatment" approach of less than empirically supported efficacy'. Hussian is rightly keen to ensure that premature complacency does not prevent the development of more refined and more helpful approaches. Reisberg (1981) is more scathing; his view is that RO 'appears to be little more than a sensible, scientific sounding-ritual' and that 'challenging their fantasies or attempting to educate and continually re-educate dementing persons is probably of no value'.

More specific criticisms relate to the lack of generalization of changes from the specific material taught to other domains of behavioural function (e.g. Burton, 1982) and the problem of using the training material in the evaluation of the technique (Hussian, 1981) – a fear almost that all that is being achieved is some sort of rote learning, artefactual and not of clinical significance. Others have queried the targets of the intervention, in particular the emphasis on current orientation (e.g. Powell Proctor and Miller, 1982; Morton and Bleathman, 1988). Again, it is the clinical significance of the changes which is being questioned, recognizing that the statistical significance achieved in most of the published evaluative studies may not have any real impact on the patients' day-to-day lives. The final group of criticisms to be mentioned focus on potentially negative aspects of RO. Burton (1982) argues that RO lacks ecological validity, in not using sufficiently techniques, materials and methods drawn from what would be valued by and familiar to the normal population. Gubrium and Ksander (1975) have given now well-known examples of how RO sessions can be run in an inflexible, rigid manner, to the extent of denying any reality not consistent with that put on the RO board at the commencement of the session. For instance, they report a resident who was pressured into reading 'correctly' from the board that it was raining, even though she could see perfectly clearly through the window that the sun was now shining! MacDonald and Settin (1978) found that nursing home residents in their study viewed RO as boring and unstimulating – perhaps again because it was inflexibly applied at too low a level for the group in question.

These criticisms can certainly not be dismissed, and they raise a number of issues *relevant both to RO and other approaches* to working with people with dementia. The concern here is not to defend RO, but rather to encourage an incremental approach to developments in this field, to avoid the cycles of therapeutic fashion which seem to occur so often elsewhere.

THE PRIMACY OF ATTITUDES, VALUES AND PRINCIPLES

Over the years it has become clear from articles such as those mentioned above by Burton (1982), Gubrium and Ksander (1975) and others, such as Buckholdt and Gubrium (1983), as well as from clinical experience, that the techniques of RO can be used to demean, devalue and patronize the patient. This occurs when the techniques are used rigidly, unthinkingly, insensitively by staff whose attitudes to the patients with whom they work are far from positive. RO is not alone in this; *virtually any method can be abused and distorted in this way.* In the author's view, staff attitudes need to be carefully examined before embarking on a RO programme. Indeed, much can be achieved when the patient's individuality as an adult is recognized and respected; when he or she is helped to retain dignity, even when very personal care is being given; when he or she is offered real choices, commensurate with his or her decision-making ability; and when as much independence as possible is nurtured and encouraged. Woods (1989a) summarizes these attitudes as considering the patient 'first and foremost as a *person.* The resident is not to be regarded as an object, vegetable, doll, a list of problems or a child'. It is recognized that these principles are by no means easy to achieve in practice. Staff need to discuss their attitudes together, being sensitive to situations where patients are not fully valued as human beings. These attitudes can be developed to some extent, for instance, by exercises involving staff in picturing themselves as recipients of the services they provide, and considering in what ways individuality, dignity and respect are threatened – often inadvertently – by the way the service is delivered and by the actions of the staff. However, it must be acknowledged that some people are temperamentally unsuited for this work, and more attention must be given to weeding out such individuals (Davies, 1982), some of whom perhaps unknowingly relish the power 'to determine where, when, how and with whom residents eat, sleep, sit, bath and go to the toilet' (Lipman *et al.,* 1979).

The application of the principles of normalization to work with elderly patients with dementia is particularly welcome, providing as it does a framework for the scrutiny of the services provided, and challenging principles that build on those outlined above, in the light of which staff are encouraged to question current practices and procedures, and a clear vision for future development. These principles are very helpfully spelt out in this context by the King's Fund (1986) publication *Living Well into Old Age*, which sets out the key principles and their implications both for the service received by the individual client and for the overall pattern of service provision. A commitment by staff to such an agreed set of values and principles forms the best basis for the practice of high-quality RO or any other approach.

An implication of such a commitment is that efforts must be made to enrich the environment as much as possible. It can never be acceptable to say 'they aren't aware of their surroundings – it doesn't matter how bad they are'. The physical and social environments are to be of high quality, because of the value placed upon the person with dementia, as a person of worth, of full human value, with the whole range of human needs. The ward, home or centre must be one to which it is worth being orientated, offering many opportunities for valued experiences, personalized help with special needs, a place where choices can be made and are respected, where it does matter whether it's Tuesday or Thursday, because each day is different and offers a variety of interesting, worthwhile activities an events, a place centred around the individual needs of the clients, adapting to them, rather than expecting the clients to adapt to the service offered. A good social environment which is client-centred, warm and supportive can go some way towards compensating for poorer quality physical facilities. No approach or technique can compensate for a poor social environment. If there is not the willingness to work for a richer, fuller, more rewarding environment for patients with dementia, then the attitudinal problems are fundamental, and must be dealt with before any real change will be possible.

THE LEARNING POTENTIAL OF PEOPLE WITH DEMENTIA

Although perhaps originally lacking a sound theoretical foundation, several writers have viewed RO from a behavioural or relearning perspective (e.g. Woods and Britton, 1977; Hussian, 1981; Holden and Woods, 1988; Hanley, 1984). Yet it is of course a learning difficulty that is at the heart of the cognitive changes associated with dementia! Is Reisberg (1981) correct in saying that re-education is of little value with people with dementia? Clearly, relearning will always have its limitations with patients with severe memory impairments. However, there is substantial evidence that some learning ability may be retained in dementia (see Holden and Woods, 1988, for a review). Morris (1989) suggests that if material can be learned, then the rate of forgetting may be relatively normal.

The RO literature provides further evidence for specific relearning in verbal orientation in single cases reported by Greene *et al.* (1979), Patterson (1982), Woods (1983) and Hanley (1986). Similarly, in relation to spatial orientation, Hanley (1981), Gilleard *et al.*, (1981) and Lam and Woods (1986) have shown that a number of patients with dementia show clear learning during a simple training programme in finding various locations around the ward or home.

Hanley (1984) argues that in verbal learning, cued recall is a useful technique; some experimental studies have suggested that patients with dementia function at near-normal levels in word learning when cued with the first few letters of the word at the time of recall. Downes (1987) has doubts about cued recall, based on the extensive research on cued recall in amnesia. He suggests that the higher levels of correct performance on tests of verbal orientation with cued recall do not indicate the person actually *knows* the day, date or whatever. The experience for the patient is one of 'guessing', rather than the normal reconstructive process involved in temporal orientation (Brotchie *et al.*, 1985). In a sense, the person with dementia reaches the correct answer through external cues, whereas the unimpaired individual is more likely to use internally generated cues. Both may achieve the same answer, but by a different process. Achieving a goal by a different route is a perfectly acceptable goal of neuropsychological rehabilitation. However, the goal has to be more than answering correctly a test of verbal orientation, if it is to have any practical significance for the person's life – a point that will be developed further in the next section.

In similar vein, doubts have been expressed as to whether the observed gains in verbal orientation relate to rote learning, from repeated presentation of the items to be tested. Again, there is the suspicion that the relearning lacks real substance. Similar considerations apply as with cued recall. In addition, it should be noted that whilst some items (the place, the Prime Minister, the year) lend themselves to rote learning, others most certainly do not (the time, day, date). Having rehearsed any number of times 'Today is Tuesday' will be of no service the following day! In the single case reported by Woods (1983) these changing items were being learned alongside those where rote learning would have been possible.

One of the themes to emerge from studies on both verbal and spatial orientation is the specificity of the learning achieved. Generally, only what is taught is learned, with little generalization to other items or locations, unless very close in content to a taught item. Maintenance of improvements is also problematic. Both these features add to the ease with which specific training effects may be demonstrated (with specific gains and rapid reversals of treatment effects), but are less desirable in the practical context.

With regard to generalization, two approaches should be considered. One is to consider carefully the most important goals for the particular patient, those that will have most impact on his or her quality of life, and concentrate the training effort on this. The second approach is to teach a more general skill, such as the use of a particular memory aid (e.g. a diary), rather than using the person's limited learning capacity to retain information that could readily be obtained from this external source. Maintaining improvements may also be facilitated by incorporating memory cues and aids in the learning process (e.g. Hanley, 1981; Woods, 1983) or by regular booster sessions. In the face of a condition with a natural history of dementia, it is unrealistic to expect training to be for a brief once-and-for-all period. An environment is needed which supports and reinforces the improvement in functioning which has been shown to be possible in structured settings.

It is important to recognize that some learning ability is useful from a behavioural perspective, but that the potential for behavioural change is not limited by this factor. At its most basic level, behaviour is seen as a product of the interaction between a person and his or her environment. Some change can occur by the person adapting to and learning about their environment. Much more can be achieved by structuring the environment so it elicits more appropriate behaviour from the person. In this way many familiar, well-learned sequences of behaviour can be drawn out from the repertoire the person has accumulated over the years, without any new learning being necessary. Thus on an outing, a trip to the pub, say, patients often show quite different behaviour from that seen on the ward. Patients who sit and say nothing all day in the large institutional 'waiting room' type of lounge, begin to chat with each other when placed in a smaller, more homely setting. Memory aids, cues and prompts can help fill in some of the gaps in the person's function, and elicit a higher level of function. Holden and Woods (1988: 26–38) provide a review of studies illustrating the sensitivity of the behaviour of the person with dementia to the many facets of the environment. Together, the person's potential ability to learn and responsiveness to the people and cues in their surroundings, provide some scope for approaches seeking to increase the person's level of functioning. Training programmes need to be carefully targeted and structured to maximize the potential for learning, and cues and prompts need to be used in a consistent manner continually to maintain any changes.

THE CLINICAL SIGNIFICANCE OF THE RESULTS OF RO

A number of controlled studies have shown statistically significant changes in verbal orientation associated with RO. Many studies have also attempted to show changes in level of functioning; here positive results are the exception rather than the rule. Although concerns have been expressed that real changes might be missed because of the relative inadequacy of the measures of function used, clearly in these group studies such changes are rarely evident. Hence critics of RO have questioned, for example, the point of knowing what day of the week it is if you're still incontinent just as often. Downes (1987) similarly asks whether even the gains that are identified, in verbal and spatial orientation, actually occur in 'real life' rather than being confined to the test situation. These are valid criticisms; statistical significance is a good start in an area such as this where therapeutic nihilism has been the order of the day, but once this is established then the clinical validity of the approach must also be demonstrated.

The important work in this area has been carried out by Hanley (1986; 1988) in a series of creative single-case studies applying RO to particular problems patients were experiencing. One example was of an 84-year-old patient who was taught to use a diary and watch to keep track of day and time. Not only did her scores improve on a verbal orientation test, but she also kept many more 'appointments' (e.g. having her hair done, collecting the newspaper, etc.) than she had previously. In a further case, the patient was taught to use a notebook to keep track of personal information of great significance to her, particularly regarding her husband's death. Again, improvements were noted on both the test of verbal orientation and the 'real-life' problem, in that she became much more consistently aware of the facts of her husband's death. In this case, it should be noted that the patient herself had asked for help in remembering this. Similarly, in relation to spatial orientation, the 80-year-old patient reported by Lam and Woods (1986) became very upset and tearful about her inability to find her way about the ward. The test of spatial orientation used involved her finding locations on the ward in random sequence, rather than learning a particular route around the ward. Although not assessed formally, the training appeared to reduce the patient's distress, and a brief retraining period was similarly successful when the patient moved from the hospital to an old people's home.

These cases, and the others reported by Hanley (1988) are clearly insufficient to satisfy the critics as to the clinical validity of RO. They do demonstrate a useful way forward, however, where targets for intervention are carefully selected to be of importance for the individual concerned and where a small, realistically attainable step could make a real impact on the person's quality of life. For one patient, it might be learning to find the toilet; for another, living in the community, learning to keep track of the days so as to be ready for the day-centre transport at the appropriate times might be important. Whatever approaches are used, the experience from RO research is that individualization is necessary if clinically valid results are to be achieved and that goals need to be precisely and specifically relevant and appropriate for the individual patient. Group studies need to be carefully designed to allow this individualization of goals, and more refined measures of real-life behaviour used, if they are to establish the clinical validity of approaches to working with people with dementia.

EFFECTS ON STAFF AND CARERS

From RO's earliest days, it has been suggested that it has a beneficial effect on those employing it, perhaps increasing staff morale, job satisfaction and improving attitudes. Schwenk (1981) claims 'it is not clear whether RO is therapeutic for the staff or the elderly'. When studies have mentioned such changes in staff, they are unfortunately seldom backed up by the type of empirical data reported for the patients (e.g. Baines *et al.*, 1987). Attitudes especially have proven difficult to measure, and Bailey *et al.* (1986) attribute to measurement problems their failure to identify a change in attitudes to elderly people amongst staff using RO over a 5-month period.

Apart from work on showing that staff do (or sometimes do not) practise RO techniques more efficiently after training (see Holden and Woods, 1988: 70–3), the main finding to date indicating a definite effect on staff arises from the comparative study on RO and reminiscence reported by Baines *et al.* (1987). They showed that staff knowledge of individual residents increased dramatically after 4 weeks of being involved with the residents in small-group sessions. The effect was not specific to either type of group, but was specific to knowledge about group members. Staff showed no increase in the information they knew about other residents with whom they worked. This finding is of some importance, in that getting to know residents better is a prerequisite of individualized care.

Even less attention has been paid to the possible effects on family carers of using such techniques. Of related interest is the intriguing study reported by Greene *et al.* (1983). RO sessions were carried out at a day hospital for patients living at home with relatives, who were unaware of what treatment the patients were receiving. Improvements in the relatives' self-rating of mood were noted coinciding with the point in the study where the patients were included in RO sessions. A corresponding deterioration in relatives' mood accompanied the cessation of the RO sessions. Although no attempts to replicate this effect have been reported, it does open up the possibility that changes in the patients' cognitive and behavioural functioning related to RO could have an effect on the wellbeing of their family carers.

In that the quality of life of most people suffering from dementia is heavily dependent on those supporting them on an informal or formal basis, much more emphasis should be paid to evaluating the effects of interventions on staff and carers. Changes here may well have important indirect benefits for the patients who, too often, have been seen as the sole focus of attempts at evaluation. Looking for changes in patients without considering the context in which they live and are cared for is to take too narrow a perspective.

REALISTIC EXPECTATIONS

The difficulties posed by dementia are so challenging that everyone would be delighted if some simple solution could be found. Some have looked to RO for the magic answer, perhaps because at times its effects have been oversold. With a condition where nothing works, something that works a little, for some sufferers may, relatively speaking, appear to have 'dramatic' effects. But with false hopes, inevitably there is a reaction. 'Approaches other than RO should be explored in view of the lack of strong evidence that RO is universally beneficial to the elderly' (Schwenk, 1981). If we begin to entertain the belief that any approach can have universal applicability and benefit then naturally there will be disappointment. The research to date on RO suggests that interventions do not fundamentally change the nature of the condition, but that under the right conditions the person may be helped to function at a higher level, and to be less disabled by the impairment he or she has. In the author's view it is better to work for relatively small, attainable goals and to be pleasantly surprised if progress allows higher-level goals to be set, rather than to become despondent, striving to reach unattainable goals. It is sometimes argued that if real improvements in the person's overall condition are impossible, then perhaps the decline could be slowed down (e.g. Holden and Woods, 1988: 272–3). However, the evidence for this more limited goal is as yet lacking. Dementia, like life itself, is at times an irresistible force, with the same inevitable end point as life. As in life, much that is good and worthwhile and valuable can be achieved along the way, which even the shadow of the ending does not render meaningless.

THE WAY FORWARD

If there are no approaches of universal benefit, perhaps the best way forward is to focus on the individual and use a range of ideas and approaches according to the individual person's particular strengths and needs. As discussed previously, the best conditions for learning and the clinically important targets for intervention are most appropriately identified on an individual basis. This approach, described as individual care planning (Holden and Woods, 1988) or goal planning (Barrowclough and Fleming, 1986), involves a thorough understanding of the whole person – abilities, interests and resources as well as needs and deficits. A plan is drawn up, which aims to meet some of the person's needs, using the person's strengths as far as possible. Aims are broken down into small clear, precise steps, and progress is monitored regularly. Often one member of staff takes on the responsibility of being key worker for that person, to further increase the personalization of care. Such an approach is only feasible where the attitudinal issues discussed above have been considered, and in an environment that is supportive and flexible. The individual care plan draws attention to those areas where a small change can make most difference to the person's life, where their limited learning ability can be best used, and the means by which the person's optimal level of function can be elicited and maintained.

Where do more general approaches like RO or reminiscence fit into this scheme? Essentially they offer a wide range of techniques and methods that can be selectively applied to an individual's needs. Some needs occur in many patients, so it is helpful to have a well-established repertoire of ideas to draw on in the care-planning process. The application to needs involving verbal and spatial orientation is obvious. Other areas can benefit from RO's methods also. For example, a need for increased communication is often identified. RO can contribute strategies such as the use of small groups, the use of a specific focus, the use of prompts and – even when impairment is severe – sensory stimulation, through music and touch, for example. Reminiscence, in addition would offer the use of memorabilia, prompts concerning previous events, lifestyle, personal memories and so on. Validation therapy, as implemented by Morton and Bleathman (1988), could bring the use of structured ritual, group singing and emphasis on the patient's comfort as ways of nurturing small group interaction. The respectful appeal to the person's accumulated wisdom and experience in the choice of discussion topics (e.g. what advice would you give to a couple thinking of getting married?) is a further useful strategy from their work.

A question of great concern to many front-line staff, which often has to be addressed in developing a care-plan, is how best to respond when the person with dementia says something that is obviously inaccurate and confused. Staff are often uncertain whether to argue, correct the person or 'go along with it'. The frequency with which this question arises indicates that RO, for all its limitations, does have relevance to some of the critical areas of work with dementia sufferers. Holden and Woods (1988) are clear about the advice RO offers: never agree; correction is sometimes useful, but must be tactful and gentle; distraction may often be used; but, best of all, respond to the feelings that you hear underlying the words, which may represent a coherent message being communicated, obscured by the inaccurate words being used. Staff are encouraged to select the appropriate strategy according to the person and the situation.

Often staff are initially surprised that RO 'allows' anything other than correction, assuming the person must at all times be reorientated to reality. The totality of the approach is not confined within its name! It is often thought that validation therapy stands in contrast to the RO approach, by moving away from repeated correction (Morton and Bleathman, 1988). In fact, there is common ground. In Feil's (1982) book she states:

The Validation worker is always honest. The worker always tries to recognise and be aware of feelings. Acknowledge with words and physical movements that the person's feelings are true. Share out loud the need to return to universal longings in times of stress. Validate the feelings. Forget facts.

(Feil, 1982)

Holden and Woods (1988) in their guidelines on dealing with rambling and confused talk, encourage staff to: 'Acknowledge the feelings expressed – ignore the content.'

The important point from the care-planning perspective is to select the response best suited to the particular individual's needs, based on an understanding of the whole person – not a response to a diagnostic category, or to a level of impairment. For instance, some sufferers may not be able to accept any correction, as it may stretch to the limit a fragile preservation of a self-image as a competent, capable person. Others may welcome correction in order to find a way through the miasma of puzzling experiences in which they feel lost and perplexed. Others may welcome correction from staff, but not from a close relative, where it is seen as arising from the previous relationship pattern and not as an accurate reflection of reality.

If this way of drawing potential strategies from the insights of various approaches to the needs of the individual can be adopted, research can move on from comparing the lack of effectiveness of rival approaches towards a finer level of analysis of the usefulness of certain components of them in tackling common needs of groups of individual patients, drawing out reasons for individual variation in response to particular strategies.

Whilst combining the best of various approaches is clearly attractive, some might argue the result runs the risk of being hopelessly eclectic. However, if subsumed within a framework of a service with a commitment to positive attitudes and values and an individualized care-planning system, the dangers of a lack of purpose, drive and direction can be avoided, whilst bringing the full range of methods and techniques to bear in tackling a condition so pervasive and devastating in its effects.

REFERENCES

Bailey, E.A., Brown, S., Goble, R.E.A. and Holden, U.P. (1986) '24 hour reality orientation: changes for staff and patients', *Journal of Advanced Nursing* 11: 141–51.
Baines, S., Saxby, P. and Ehlert, K. (1987) 'Reality orientation and reminiscence therapy: a controlled cross-over study of confused elderly people', *British Journal of Psychiatry* 151: 222–31.
Barnes, J.A. (1974) 'Effects on reality orientation classroom on memory loss, confusion and disorientation in geriatric patients', *Gerontologist* 14: 138–42.
Barrowclough, C. and Fleming, I. (1986) *Goal Planning with Elderly People*, Manchester: Manchester University Press.

Bower, H.M. (1967) 'Sensory stimulation and the treatment of senile dementia', *Medical Journal of Australia* 1: 1113–19.

Brook, P., Degun, G. and Mather, M. (1975) 'Reality orientation, a therapy for psychogeriatric patients: a controlled study', *British Journal of Psychiatry* 127: 42–5.

Brotchie, J., Brennan, J. and Wyke, M. (1985) 'Temporal orientation in the presenium and old age', *British Journal of Psychiatry* 147: 692–5.

Buckholdt, D.R. and Gubrium, J.F. (1983) 'Therapeutic pretence in reality orientation', *International Journal of Aging and Human Development* 16: 167–81.

Burton, M. (1982) 'Reality orientation for the elderly: a critique', *Journal of Advanced Nursing* 7: 427–33.

Cosin, L.Z., Mort, M., Post, F., Westropp, C. and Williams, M. (1958) 'Experimental treatment of persistent senile confusion', *International Journal of Social Psychiatry* 4: 24–42.

Davies, A.D.M. (1982) 'Research with elderly people in long-term care: some social and organisational factors affecting psychological interventions', *Ageing and Society* 2: 285–98.

Downes, J.J. (1987) 'Classroom RO and the enhancement of orientation: a critical note', *British Journal of Clinical Psychology* 26: 147–8.

Drummond, L., Kirchoff, L. and Scarbrough, D.R. (1978) 'A practical guide to reality orientation: a treatment approach for confusion and disorientation', *Gerontologist* 18: 568–73.

Feil, N. (1982) *V/F Validation: the Feil Method,* Cleveland: Edward Feil Productions.

Folsom, J.C. (1967) 'Intensive hospital therapy of geriatric patients', *Current Psychiatric Therapies* 7: 209–15.

—— (1968) 'Reality orientation therapy for the elderly mental patient', *Journal of Geriatric Psychiatry* 1: 291–307.

Gilleard, C.J., Mitchell, R.G. and Riordan, J. (1981) 'Ward orientation training with psychogeriatric patients', *Journal of Advanced Nursing* 6: 95–8.

Greene, J.G., Nicol, R. and Jamieson, H. (1979) 'Reality orientation with psychogeriatric patients', *Behaviour Research and Therapy* 17: 615–17.

——, Timbury, G.C., Smith, R. and Gardiner, M. (1983) 'Reality orientation with elderly patients in the community: an empirical evaluation', *Age and Ageing* 12: 38–43.

Gubrium, J.F. and Ksander, M. (1975) 'On multiple realities and reality orientation', *Gerontologist* 15: 142–5.

Hanley, I.G. (1981) 'The use of signposts and active training to modify ward disorientation in elderly patients', *Journal of Behaviour Therapy and Experimental Psychiatry* 12: 241–7.

—— (1982) *A Manual for the Modification of Confused Behaviour,* Edinburgh: Lothian Regional Council Department of Social Work.

—— (1984) 'Theoretical and practical considerations in reality orientation with the elderly', in I.G. Hanley and J. Hodge (eds) *Psychological Approaches to the Care of the Elderly,* London: Croom Helm.

—— (1986) 'Reality orientation in the care of the elderly person with dementia – three case studies', in I.G. Hanley and M. Gilhooly (eds) *Psychological Therapies for the Elderly,* London: Croom Helm.

—— (1988) *Individualised Reality Orientation: Creative Therapy with Confused Elderly People,* Bicester: Winslow Press.

Holden, U.P. and Woods, R.T. (1988) *Reality Orientation: Psychological*

Approaches to the 'Confused' Elderly, 2nd edn, Edinburgh: Churchill Living-stone.

Hussian, R.A. (1981) *Geriatric Psychology: A Behavioral Perspective*, New York: Van Nostrand Reinhold.

King's Fund (1986) *Living Well into Old Age: Applying Principles of Good Practice to Services for Elderly People with Severe Mental Disabilities*, London: King's Fund.

Lam, D.H. and Woods, R.T. (1986) 'Ward orientation training in dementia: a single-case study', *International Journal of Geriatric Psychiatry* 1: 145–7.

Letcher, P.B., Peterson L.P. and Scarbrough, D. (1974) 'Reality orientation: a historical study of patient progress', *Hospital and Community Psychiatry* 25: 11–13.

Lipman, A., Slater, R. and Harris, H. (1979) 'The quality of verbal interaction in homes for old people', *Gerontology* 25: 275–84.

MacDonald, M.L. and Settin, J.M. (1978) 'Reality orientation vs. sheltered workshops as treatment for the institutionalized aging', *Journal of Gerontology* 33: 416–21.

Morris, R.G. (1989) 'The neuropsychological aspects of dementia', *Current Opinion in Psychiatry* 2: 66–71.

Morton, I. and Bleathman, C. (1988) 'RO: does it matter whether it's Tuesday or Friday?' *Nursing Times* 84 (6): 25–7.

Patterson, R.L. (1982) *Overcoming Deficits of Aging: A Behavioural Approach*, New York: Plenum.

Powell Proctor, L. and Miller, E. (1982) 'Reality orientation: a critical appraisal', *British Journal of Psychiatry* 140: 457–63.

Reisberg, B. (1981) *Brain Failure: An Introduction to Current Concepts of Senility*, New York: Free Press/MacMillan.

Rimmer, L. (1982) *Reality Orientation: Principles and Practice*, Bicester: Winslow Press.

Schwenk, M.A. (1981) 'Reality orientation for the institutionalized aged: does it help?' *Gerontologist* 19: 373–7.

Stephens, L.P. (ed.) (1969) *Reality Orientation: A Technique to Rehabilitate Elderly and Brain-damaged Patients with a Moderate to Severe Degree of Disorientation*, Washington DC: American Psychiatric Association.

Taulbee, L.R. and Folsom, J.C. (1966) 'Reality orientation for geriatric patients', *Hospital and Community Psychiatry* 17: 133–5.

Woods, R.T. (1983) 'Specificity of learning in reality orientation sessions: a single-case study', *Behaviour Research and Therapy* 21: 173–5.

—— (1989a) 'People with dementia – making life worth living', *Care Weekly* p. 9, 17 February.

—— (1989b) 'People with dementia – tuning-in to the world', *Care Weekly* p. 12, 3 March.

—— (1989c) 'People with dementia – a framework for reality', *Care Weekly* p. 16, 10 March.

—— and Britton, P.G. (1977) 'Psychological approaches to the treatment of the elderly', *Age and Ageing* 6: 104–12.

Chapter 9

Reminiscence and life review with persons with dementia: which way forward?

Bob Woods, Sara Portnoy, Donna Head and Gemma Jones

SUMMARY

Reminiscence-based activities have become extremely popular in residential homes, hospitals and day centres which provide services for elderly persons suffering from dementia. This popularity seems to arise not so much from convincing empirical evidence of the effects of reminiscence, but rather from it now being implicitly recognized as a valued and enjoyable experience for both elderly persons and staff.

This was not always so. Until recently, reminiscence was seen as a negative attribute of older people: dwelling in the past and repeating stories about the old days was seen as a sign of regression (Coleman, 1986). Butler's (1963) paper on the concept of 'life review', a task to be accomplished in the final phase of life, was important in helping reminiscing and life review to be seen in a positive light. Thereafter, the positive functions of reminiscing began to be described both in terms of personal adaptation, and interpersonal or social benefits (Anderson, 1983). It is now recognized that reminiscing is not confined to the elderly, or cognitively impaired elderly, and that it is helpful at any age, particularly during times of transition and change.

The problems involved in evaluating reminiscing-type activities are discussed, and thereafter two studies are described. The first compares the effect of two reminiscence groups, held in different centres, with control-group activities. The second study describes how to collect and conduct life reviews with elderly persons with dementia and discusses the usefulness of three tools developed for this study.

INTRODUCTION

In this chapter, reminiscing and life review will be discussed as related concepts that can be specifically applied to many settings pertaining to the care of persons with dementia. After defining the concepts, a brief literature review will be given, showing the origins and development of these concepts, up to their present diverse applications. Although the usefulness of reminiscing and life review seem intuitively obvious, it is difficult to measure their benefits objectively with quantitative research methods. These difficulties will be discussed and thereafter two studies will be reported, one on reminiscing and the second on life review.

DEFINITIONS

Reminiscing and making sense of one's life are ongoing processes. They are normal and occur in each of our lives. Reminiscing seems to occur increasingly frequently as persons become older, and, whenever events occur that need to be understood and incorporated into the fabric of one's life. The term reminiscing usually refers to the vocal or silent recall of events in a person's life, either alone, or with another person or group of people. 'Intense reminiscing' often involves the use of eidetic imagery, or seeing with the mind's eye (Taylor *et al.*, 1983). The term life review is usually used to refer to the process of reviewing, organizing and evaluating the overall picture of one's life, in order that a person can come to see their life as a unique story, the thread of the story being the person's own hope and expectations of themselves.

Triggers must also be mentioned because of their implicit and explicit use in reminiscing. Taylor *et al.* (1983), define triggers as 'any form of stimuli (concrete or abstract) that help to prompt memory recall. Music, photos, food, poems, faces, colours, objects and smells are all triggers.' These may be used deliberately by staff to facilitate or access particular memories in persons with dementia, or, they may be used spontaneously during conversation. Random environmental events often serve as triggers and questions alone are often sufficient to prompt and focus recall as well.

RELATIONSHIP BETWEEN REMINISCING AND LIFE REVIEW

The life review is a particular subset of general reminiscing activity. Whereas reminiscing tends to occur generally as short, semi-random, spontaneous, frequent bursts of recall, the life review is a form of structured reminiscing that helps a person to formulate their life story according to the hope and goals they have set for themselves. As such, the life review requires more insight, guidance and energy to accomplish than general reminiscing, particularly with persons whose memory and attention is beginning to wane.

Health care professionals are in a unique position to facilitate either of these processes, with normal healthy elderly persons, as well as those who are experiencing varying degrees of disorientation. However, expectations for persons who are disoriented are naturally different, and less stringent than for unimpaired individuals.

The social, or interpersonal functions of reminiscing include: the development of relationships, entertainment, a mode of relaying history and acquired wisdom for educating and entertaining the younger generation and, as a traditional method for leaving a legacy to extended family members. The personal or intrapersonal functions of reminiscing include status enhancement, identity formation, the resolution, reorganization and reintegration of one's life, the creation of a sense of personal continuity, self-entertainment, and self-expression (Anderson, 1983). McMahon and Rhudick (1964) identified additional uses of reminiscing including, the glorification of the past, maintenance of self-esteem, reinforcement of identity, allayment of anxiety associated with signs of decline and the reminder of approaching death and preparation for death. They concluded that reminiscing is a successful adaptation to old age and that modern society should attach more significance to this behaviour and provide more opportunity for its legitimate expression.

LITERATURE REVIEW

Traditionally, only persons who were esteemed because of their public functions or special contributions, had their life stories recorded biographically or autobiographically. This process of 'committing it all on paper' implicitly necessitates an ordering and reviewing of one's life. Whatever benefits result from such a process were limited to only a few exceptional persons, usually upper-class, educated ones. Later, collective biographical studies were recorded by Frenkl (1936), Progoff (1975), Annis (1967); and Birren (1980) has developed a method of teaching autobiographical recording techniques. This was the beginning of recording the life experiences of the ordinary man. The concept of the life review as a therapeutic process is relatively new, and although it has evolved through the work of many persons, the development of a more holistic concept of medicine is generally attributed to Robert Butler. In 1958 he began a programme of intensive psychotherapy for inpatients with psychiatric disorders, in an attempt to expand 'medical surgical–custodial care programs'. In 1960 Butler stated that the significance of the family situation required greater participation of family in the therapeutic process. This led to a new emphasis on obtaining a full history from various family members in addition to the traditional medical history obtained from patients. By 1963, Butler postulated the universal existence of an inner experience or mental process in older people, namely that of reviewing one's life. His work helped to remove the mythology that reminiscing in the elderly is a pathological sign associated with 'senility'. He advocated that physicians take the time to listen attentively to their patients' reflections, above and beyond the standard methods used to evaluate the mental and physical status of old people, in order that the often marvellous characteristics of

'the survivors' could be included in the growing understanding of and interventions for the aging process (Butler, 1980–1).

By 1974, Butler had formalized the life review concept and associated it
with health in old age. Health has mental, social and physical components
of wellbeing in his theory. He differentiated between the intrinsic characteristics of the aging process and the reaction of the elderly to their
lives. For some, life review is a constructive re-evaluation of the past
leading toward personality reorganization which can lead to peace and
serenity. For others, working through unresolved conflicts creates and
reinforces depressions, regret and despair. Butler (1963) suggested that the
role of the professional in aiding the aged with life review, is to set 'self-
acceptance' as a goal for the older person. Lewis and Butler (1974) found
that life review, by its very nature, evokes a sense of regret and sadness at
the brevity of life. Most persons however, 'seemed to have the capacity to
reconcile their lives, to confront real guilt, and to find meaning, especially
in the presence of acceptance and support from others'. Lewis and Butler
(1974) state that the success of the life review depends upon the outcome
of the struggle to resolve issues of resentment, guilt, bitterness, mistrust,
dependence and nihilism. Thus, the success of life review is difficult to
measure since many of these processes can occur within a person without
overt signs of change or success which a health care worker, only temporarily present, could measure. Although Butler did not carefully describe an
exact method or tools for conducting the life review, his work was an
encouraging starting point for other researchers.

Nurses and social workers have been quick to respond to the use of life
review in their work settings. Publications in these fields include: Pincus
(1970); Ebersole (1976); Kiërnat (1979); Dietsche (1981); Ellison (1981);
Ryden (1981); Gerfo (1981); van Amelsvoort Jones and Zeiss (1984) and
Coleman (1986). Many of these studies report individual case examples as
opposed to large-group studies. The importance of individual case studies
cannot be overemphasized in light of our need to know what the range of
individual differences are, before global generalizations are made. Such
descriptive work formed a foundation for more complex empirical studies
of group work with reminiscing, which are currently being conducted.

Projects to develop materials to aid general group reminiscence started
in the late 1970s. Although originally designed for the whole range of
older persons, these projects had a special relevance for persons with
dementia, who particularly benefit from the stimulation to reminisce which
such materials provide.

In the UK, the Department of Health and Social Security (DHSS)
funded a project team, led by Mick Kemp, which attracted a great deal of
media attention. This team's work led to the *Recall* pack of six tape–slide
sequences published by Help the Aged (1981). This pack covers the years
1900–80 in a way intended to be relevant to the perspective of current

generations of older people. Music, archive sound recordings and accounts of everyday experiences from the past recounted by the elderly themselves, are blended with appropriate slides. These slide–tape sequences can be used as entertainment in their own right, but small excerpts are ideal for starting discussion with small groups of people with dementia.

Other packages of pictures, music, reproductions of newspaper front pages and so on, soon became available both in the UK and America (Holden, 1984). Although health care workers are advised to develop materials relevant to their particular clients, it is these attractively produced and readily available packages that are most often used in practice, and which have done much to encourage the use of reminiscence with dementing persons, in a wide variety of settings.

The growing popularity of reality orientation (RO) also played an important part in encouraging small-group work with dementia sufferers. Activities that were simple and yet did not seem childish were hard to find. Holden (1979) and Catmull and Ling (1981) pioneered the use of memorabilia, pictures and music to stimulate reality-based discussion in such groups, whilst others began to describe reminiscence group therapy as a prime focus for small-group work (Norris *et al.* (1982); Lesser *et al.* (1981)).

Given the oft remarked upon inability of people with dementia to remember what they had for lunch, whilst being able to talk freely about events in their childhood, it is surprising that it took so long for reminiscence to be 'discovered' as a method for working with persons with dementia. It is now known that persons with dementia do have a decreased ability to remember events from the past, when compared to normal elderly persons. However, this remote memory is often more intact than recent memory. Morris and Kopelman (1986), conclude that persons with dementia show impairments in virtually every type of memory process measured. Their ability to talk about events that happened long ago better than recent ones, probably arises from: (1) the richness of association of certain personal memories with strong affective components, (2) from repetition of certain key memories over the years (songs, names, places) and (3) possibly from certain memories being stored in different areas than those that are damaged in the most common dementing illnesses (many persons can still sing even though their speech is virtually limited to occasional phrases).

Thornton and Brotchie (1987) identified two published evaluative studies of group reminiscing with persons with dementia. The Kiërnat (1979) study included twenty-three nursing-home residents, all described as 'confused', in twice-weekly reminiscence groups conducted for 10 weeks. The findings showed that residents attending the groups most often showed the greatest improvement in behaviour, as measured by a behaviour rating scale. With moderately cognitively impaired residents in an old people's home, Baines *et al.* (1987) compared reminiscing groups with RO groups, and a 'no-treatment' control group. A cross-over design was used, so that one group had reminiscing sessions following by RO whilst the second group had RO followed by reminiscing. A number of assessment measures were used, but generally, the second group showed the most improvements over the untreated control group in both cognitive and behavioural functioning. Although the authors attributed these results to RO having a facilitative effect on reminiscing subsequently, it is also possible that one group was simply more generally responsive than the other, despite the random allocation of the residents to the groups. Baines *et al.* also assessed staff knowledge of residents, and found it dramatically increased following both RO and reminiscing. Attendance at the reminiscing sessions was very high and residents were rated by staff as having derived a great deal of enjoyment from the groups. There was a trend for residents' morale to increase following the reminiscence group, but to drop following the RO group, perhaps reflecting the painful aspects of awareness of a lonely reality for some residents.

Clearly research on reminiscence and life review with dementing people is in its infancy. In the next section the difficulties in evaluating group interventions are discussed generally. Thereafter, one study on group reminiscing, and a second study on conducting life reviews are presented.

EVALUATING GROUP REMINISCENCE AND LIFE-REVIEW ACTIVITIES

How should the effectiveness of group interventions be evaluated for persons with dementia? The answer depends upon the specific aims of such activities and to what extent the identified aims of the approach can be measured. What should be clearly avoided is simply looking at change with whatever measures come to hand. Research into RO has been bedevilled by the use of inappropriate evaluation techniques.

First, one must have an idea about what behaviours normally occur, how often, and what would constitute a desired change. For example, if a resident normally sits in a communal lounge all day, and does not speak to his or her fellow residents more than two brief sentences a day, it does not make sense to sample his or her conversation or social interaction in the lounge every minute for 4 hours after a reminiscence group. First of all it would be most logical to see whether his or her behaviour in the group setting changes over time. Does the total amount of communication increase? Does the content of his or her verbal contributions change? Does communication between residents, as opposed to conversation directed at the group worker, increase?

After examining changes occurring within the group, it is reasonable to start examining changes in behaviour immediately following the group. It might be sensible to start by encouraging only those persons participating in the reminiscing group to sit together at a table with cups of tea, and see whether or not they continue to socialize and reminisce with one another in the absence of a group worker. Only when such changes have been measured does it make sense to look beyond the time period immediately after the group session, for more global, diffuse changes. Otherwise, a researcher is looking for a needle in a haystack.

What goals are realistic then? Can one really expect a reminiscing group session held once a week to change the course of the person's disorder? Could it ever improve activities of daily living (ADL) such as the person's ability to wash, dress or go to the toilet unaided? And yet some evaluation studies based on comparing the effects of a reminiscing group with a control group, measured before and after on a behaviour rating scale, set precisely such expectations.

Haycox described reminiscence as:

> another way to bring back errant self-awareness ... as the older person recounts stories from the past, he tends to become again what he once was. For a demented patient reminiscence light up the mind and illuminates the darkened threads and connections.
>
> (Haycox, 1983)

This description gives the impression that the persons might show improvements in personal memory, awareness and self-esteem. However, there is no reason why one of the standard memory and orientation tests, which ask who the Prime Minister is, what day of the week it is and so on, should be at all sensitive to such changes. Indeed, even if a test were available that could tap into the subtle 'threads and connections' would this be measurable during the group session, or would such changes persist thereafter? Would we require such changes to persist before judging reminiscing activities to be worthwhile?

Norris suggests that it is important not to make unrealistic expectations as to what can be achieved:

> to hold the attention of a confused old person who spends most of their day wandering around the ward mumbling incoherently, for 10 seconds, can be seen as a remarkable achievement when compared with what would otherwise be the norm for that person.
>
> (Norris, 1986)

This suggests, again, that initially it is best to evaluate what is actually achieved in the group session, rather than looking for changes outside the group.

Norris also emphasizes tailoring goals specifically for each individual resident. Similarly, Holden and Woods (1988) see reminiscing and RO groups, as means to achieve specific goals set out in the care plan for a resident. For example, in a case study by J. Reed in 1988 (reported in a personal communication to the author), one 83-year-old lady with dementia, Mrs N, was specifically included in a reminiscence group because she was isolated and withdrawn in the day centre she attended. The aim was to help her become more socially involved in the group. As the sessions went by, this was achieved, and there was a marked increase in the number of relevant contributions Mrs N made to staff and other group members (see Figure 9.1). Ideally, then, there should be measurable goals for the group as a whole, and for individuals in the group.

It is unrealistic to expect patients with dementia to show general global improvements arising from participation in reminiscing groups. If only subtle benefits such as improved affect during the group, the chance to socialize with other residents, and the opportunity to have others listen to excerpts from their life occur, is it worth pursuing reminiscing-type activities? Our opinion is that any activity which can be easily taught to staff, and enjoyed by both residents and staff, and which stimulates interest,

Figure 9.1 Total relevant contributions by an 83-year-old dementia sufferer to staff and other clients in a 10-minute period during each reminiscence session (group leaders were not aware of when the observations were being made)

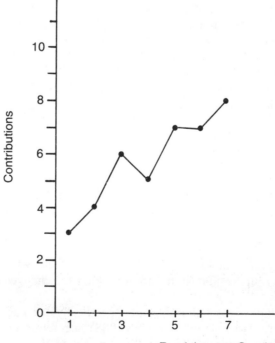

attention and interaction, at least during the time in which it is being carried out, is surely worth doing alongside other activities. There are precious few means of eliciting some of the dementing persons's retained skills and abilities which do not seem childish. In addition, there are the effects on the staff involved; any approach which helps staff to be more knowledgeable about individual residents, that encourages staff–patient interaction based on respect for a person, and a real interest in their contribution, must be welcomed. Unlike changes in patients, there is real hope that staff retain what is learned about the residents within the reminiscing sessions, and continue to utilize it thereafter during other daily tasks and care-giving activities.

Staff knowledge of particular patients may be assessed by questionnaire (Baines *et al.*, 1987), but other aspects of assessments are best explored initially by detailed observation and recording of what occurred during the group session. It is important to determine how this compares with staff- and patient-behaviour interactions in situations outside the group. The application of this method of assessment is illustrated next in a small descriptive study of reminiscing sessions in two day centres.

STUDY ONE: REMINISCING VERSUS OTHER GROUP ACTIVITIES IN TWO DAY CENTRES

Introduction and methods

Six, 1-hour, once-weekly, reminiscence sessions held in two day centres were the focus of the study. Six patients from centre A and four from centre B were observed in detail during reminiscing groups and during control-group activities. One member of staff was chosen at random at each centre and was also observed in detail during the reminiscing group and control-group activities. To ensure the best comparison, control activities which occurred on the same day, but at a different time from the reminiscing group were selected for observation.

In centre A the control activities were participation in a target game, charades and a drawing game. In centre B the activities were basket weaving, knitting and puzzle books. The reminiscing groups at both centres focused on the individual's personal life experiences: school days, work and interests, rather than on historical events, except where such events impinged directly on the group members' lives. The age of the subjects ranged from 60 to 98 (mean 78.5; s.d. 10.0). Patients in both groups showed clear cognitive impairment on tests of memory and orientation and would fall within stage 2, the moderate stage of dementia on the rating scale of Hughes *et al.* (1982). Group A consisted of four females and two males; group B had three females and one male.

Group A was located in a day centre catering for elderly people with dementia living in the community. It was run by a local authority social services department, and despite having thirty participants daily, it had a homely atmosphere, and was decorated as a home, with carpets and comfortable chairs, rather than as an institution. Group B was held at a centre for elderly people living in hospital. Not all persons at this centre had dementia, although all of those participating in the study did. The environment here was more clinical with vinyl floor covering and without easy chairs.

Reminiscence, and a variety of other activities were very familiar to staff in centre A, but not at centre B. In centre B, staff generally had a supervisory role, rather than facilitating participation in activities. Activities at centre B were more likely to be of a repetitive nature with little or no emphasis on small-group work.

The two reminiscing groups, whilst having a similar focus, did differ somewhat operationally. Essentially the sessions with group A involved only six persons, were more structured, and involved more planning and preparation than those of group B. Group A sessions were led by two of the authors (SP and DH). Group B sessions were led by workers from a reminiscence theatre group called Age Exchange, who were conducting sessions in several hospitals and homes. They conducted their reminiscing group with twelve persons, from which four were selected for specific observation. Table 9.1 shows comparable summaries of the two groups.

Table 9.1 A description of reminiscing groups in two different settings

	Group A	Group B
Type of facility	community day centre	geriatric hospital, day centre
Group leaders	2 psychologists	3 actors from Age Exchange
Aims	explicitly defined	implicit
Size	6 elderly persons 3 staff	12 elderly persons up to 12 staff
Seating	planned	not planned
Group members	all cognitively impaired	mixed, all persons in wheelchairs
Preparation for group	Specific agenda, regular liaison with staff	no fixed agenda, reliance on spontaneity and intermittent help from staff
Role playing	used regularly	used regularly
Subgroups	2 elderly persons	6 elderly persons

Measurements were made during four of the six reminiscing sessions in groups A and B. In group A by making video recordings during the group sessions. For group B, time-sampled direct observations were made consisting of four, 2-minute blocks of measurements per session. The measurements obtained for both groups were: (1) the number of contributions made per minute by each individual and (2) to whom the contributions were addressed. The experimenters scored the videos, and a 90 per cent agreement between observers was obtained with the direct observation method used.

Results

There were marked differences between the two groups. In group A, elderly persons made as many verbal contributions during reminiscing sessions as they did in the control activities, whereas in group B, persons interacted much more during the reminiscing group sessions than during control activities, where communication was rare (see Figure 9.2) (see Head *et al.*, 1990).

In both groups, the majority of interactions during reminiscing sessions were directed towards members of staff. In group A, interactions during control activities were more evenly split between communication directed towards other elderly persons and staff. In group B, virtually no interactions between elderly persons were recorded during the reminiscence sessions or during control activities.

Staff communication with elderly persons showed interesting changes with time. In group A, the staff member tended to address most of her comments to the elderly persons as opposed to the group workers, although this was variable. Initially, in group B, the staff member spoke more to other staff and the group workers, but this declined as the sessions progressed. The amount of communication directed towards patients steadily increased (see Figure 9.3). Interestingly, this increased communication carried over to the control activities also (see Figure 9.4).

Discussion

These results raise a number of issues regarding evaluation. First, reminiscing groups were better at facilitating communication than control activities were in group A, but not in group B. The nature of the control activities provided at each centre must be of some significance to the outcome, as well as the overall atmosphere and ethos of the centres.

The importance of assessing baseline levels of functioning cannot be overstressed. The staff member, as well as the elderly group of participants at centre B simply had much more scope for positive change. In essence, the usefulness of reminiscing faced a much stiffer test at centre A, because

Figure 9.2 Mean number of contributions per minute made by elderly group members during reminiscence sessions and during the alternative group activities

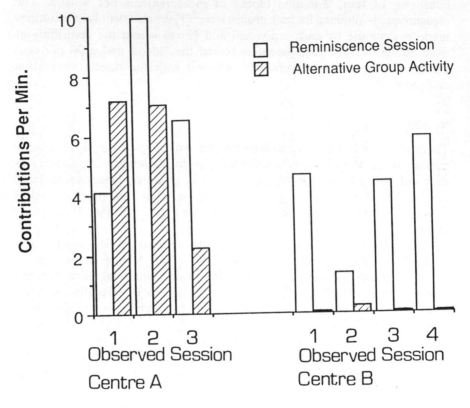

small-group activities were already occurring there. The total amount that elderly persons spoke to each other was not increased in either of the reminiscing groups, despite efforts, particularly in group A, to encourage interaction among the elderly people, by breaking up at times into smaller groups. It may be that the course of only six sessions was too short for such social interaction to develop where none existed before, and that inter-actions between people with dementia take longer to establish than between healthy elderly persons.

Interactions did occur in group A during control activities, but these tended to be one-word utterances, or brief phrases, whereas contributions during reminiscing sessions were more elaborate. This finding indicates the need for qualitative measures for recording the content of interactions, in addition to measuring the total number of utterances. Qualitative measures could also be used to examine non-verbal features such as touching and

Figure 9.3 Contributions per minute made by a staff member in centre A and a staff member in centre B during reminiscence sessions: to other staff and to elderly group members

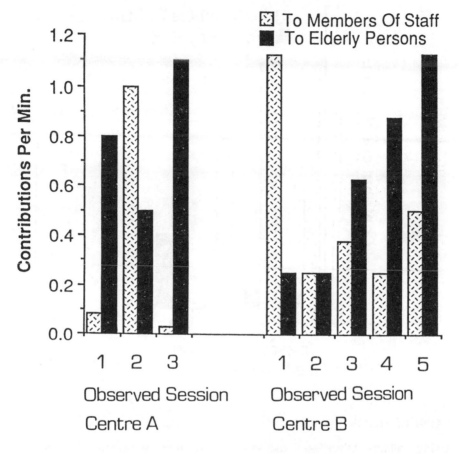

smiling. Content analysis for humour, spontaneity, listening and reciprocity, would provide a fuller understanding of communication patterns in such reminiscing groups. Cartensen and Erickson (1986) warn against focusing only on quantitative measure of interaction. They showed that most, of an apparent dramatic increase in social interaction following a simple group intervention, arose from increased ineffective vocalizations, including nonsensical and unreciprocated speech. Future studies need to direct more attention towards analysing both qualitative and quantitative aspects of group communication.

Figure 9.4 Contributions per minute made by a staff member in centre B:
to elderly group members, and other staff during the alternative activities

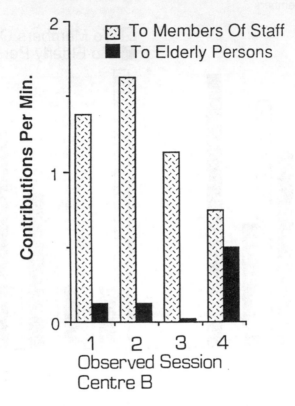

Observed Session
Centre B

CONCLUSIONS

Using reminiscence-based activities with persons with dementia is
becoming increasingly popular, and although there are many qualitative
case studies, and short reports, there is little yet in the way of published
evaluative research. The opportunity should be taken to evaluate reminiscing and other small-group activities realistically, rather than setting up
expectations for dramatic reversals of the dementing process. Instead,
questions need to be asked about: (1) how best persons with dementia
might benefit from such activities, (2) what techniques are most useful for
achieving particular care plan goals and (3) which specific methods for
particular subtypes of patients should be applied. From the experience of
running a number of reminiscing groups, we have identified particular
factors which warrant consideration for the running of future groups. The
first is to keep groups small and to pre-plan seating arrangements so that
persons with sensory and other handicaps are sitting next to group leaders

or staff members in order to minimize the effects of their handicaps. This also allows for maximum opportunity for them to communicate. The use of triggers, or prompted recall, through music is particularly effective.

Some patients do not benefit as much as others from a group-reminiscing approach. These include persons with uncorrectable visual and auditory problems, and those who could not be distracted from a rambling train of thought. Reminiscence is only one of a number of activities that are likely to prove useful with dementing people, and there is an obvious need to develop other approaches. Reminiscing group activities have the advantage of not appearing to be inappropriate or childish, but it is important to remember Coleman's (1986) warning that some older persons definitely do not like to reminisce. Individual differences in preferences for activities need to be taken seriously.

Much remains to be learned about the best ways of responding to a demented person, given their loss of a coherent time structure for their past. How firmly should a time structure be adhered to if a demented person talks as if their children are still babies? Is it helpful to keep inter-jecting 'Your children are grown up now, aren't they?', or should the group workers allow an older person to relish the reliving of an experience, and let them continue to speak in past time? No doubt the answers will differ somewhat between persons and settings, but at long last, such issues are being considered seriously and are being examined empirically, as researchers are comparing the benefits of RO, reminiscing and validation therapy for persons in various stages of dementia (Morton and Bleathman, 1988).

Perhaps the major benefit of research on reminiscing activities will be to shed light on the best ways of communicating with persons with dementia.

STUDY TWO: CONDUCTING LIFE REVIEWS WITH INSTITUTIONALIZED ELDERLY PERSONS WITH DEMENTIA

Introduction

This study was conducted in Vancouver, Canada, by Gemma Jones, Ellen Zeiss and Suzanne Taylor. The aims of this study were threefold. The first was to determine whether it was possible to conduct life reviews with persons who were in mild to moderate stages of dementia; the second, was to test the tools developed for collecting and recording life reviews during pilot work; and the third aim was to decide whether it would be appropriate to assign first-year nursing students the task of completing a life review as part of their introduction to care for the elderly. This latter aim was in response to complaints from nursing students that it did not seem meaning-ful to collect only extensive physiological data on elderly persons, and reports that some residents had objected to being asked in detail, about such things as toilet routines when the students had not asked any questions about their life.

Methods

Twenty residents in mild to moderate stages of dementia according to the Hughes *et al.* (1982) dementia rating scale, and the rating scale of Feil (1982) were selected from two extended-care hospitals. Residents and their families gave consent for their participation in this study, and also for tape recordings, and in some instances, video recordings to be made. The study protocol was approved by the ethical committees and management in both hospitals.

Six male and fourteen female residents (mean age 83.3; range: 61–100) were interviewed between five and ten times each, over the course of 3 months. The levels of care required by these persons ranged from those who could ambulate independently, but needed supervision and help with activities of daily living (ADL), to those persons who needed total nursing care and were confined to wheelchairs.

Visits and interviews were conducted in a variety of settings and for various durations. Generally, they were held in the resident's room, in the hospital lounge and gardens. Each resident was taken to a cafe or to the canteen at least once. Occasionally, a family member of the resident was present at our request, to help confirm factual details of the life review, or to help provide information about which 'triggers' would be most helpful in eliciting a response.

Usually the interviews were conducted by one person, but occasionally a second interviewer was also present to help create the atmosphere of a social visit. Some residents were happy to have written copies of their life

Figure 9.5 Condensed guideline questionnaire

LIFE REVIEW STUDY

Childhood:
–games played, where, hobbies
–favourite: toy, teacher, food
–where grew up – what you wanted to be
–family stories, traditions
–celebrations, holidays, pets, movies
–helping Mum, Dad
–schooling, clubs, religious beliefs and
  practices

Memories of People:
–parents, brothers and sisters
–grandparents
–relatives
–friends
–teachers, actors, heroes

Figure 9.5 continued

Adolecence:
−entering high school, graduation from
−clubs, activities, music/play instrument
−favourite books
−best friend(s) − activities, hobbies
−part time jobs
−interest: clothes, cars, dating
−first car, a radio programme, T.V.

Memories of Places
−holidays, vacations
−hideaways
−your bedroom, home
−where you have lived

Courting or Early Adult Years:
−people dated
−first pay cheque, salary
−when move out of parents' home
−entertainment − movies, walks
−furnishing first 'home'
−like to do things alone
−where and how met spouse

Memories of Events and Pets:
−holidays, vacations
−celebrations
−family pets

Marriage:
−how long did you know your spouse
  before marriage
−age at marriage
−wedding, best man, maid of honour
−planning for wedding
−first home as married couple
−adjusting to marriage
−surprised to have married person
  you did

Other Memories:
−historical events
−how viewed self
−being a Canadian
−coming to Canada, Vancouver

Children:
−how many?
−special events in their lives
−help from spouse in raising children
−like being a parent
−positive and negative aspects
−child's first words
−children moving out of home

Favourite Things:
−people
−places
−events

Work and Avocations:
−belong to clubs or organizations
−belong to church/ch. programmes
−involved in politics
−type of work
−change in work

*Hardest times and things that might
have happened differently:*

Health:
−major illnesses
−generally healthy

Advice:
−getting along with others
−about: marriage, raising children
−about: work, handling tough financial
  situations
−preparing for retirement

Source: G. Jones/E. Zeiss/S. Taylor − June 1982.

history given to their families, but a few chose to relate their stories with a 'for your ears only' proviso. Refreshments were always provided during the interviews in order to add to the atmosphere of a social visit. The number of visits varied, depending on how long it took to cover the details of a person's life, and on the way the resident responded to the interviewer.

The tools

Four tools were developed from pilot work prior to the onset of this study. The first was an extensive guideline questionnaire consisting of sample questions covering fourteen aspects of a person's life. The second was a condensed guideline questionnaire (Figure 9.5), with key questions and topics to cover in the fourteen subsections of the life history. A general life-course trajectory was developed for use as a checklist for the interviewer, so that the major topics which had been discussed during each visit could be recorded, and so that any gaps in the life history were immediately evident (Figure 9.6). The fourth tool developed was a historical-setting graph (Figure 9.7) which is a chronological list of major historical events from 1890 onwards. With this tool, a person's age could be plotted next to the historical events, thus making it easier for the interviewer to have reference points for the cohort and perspective any given resident would have had during their lifetime. For example, the Great Depression would have had an entirely different impact on someone if they were a child, or if they were parents, trying to find the money to run a family themselves. This historical-setting graph also provides reference points upon which questions can be based, particularly for those persons who had a great interest in political events. Often persons with dementia cannot remember how old they were at the time of particular events; with this graph, the interviewer can help to fill in some of these embarrassing memory lapses.

Only the historical-setting graph, and the life-course trajectory sheets were taken to the visits or interviews. The interviewers were thoroughly familiar with the questionnaires and did not need to refer to written questions during the actual visits. Notes on the content of the visit were made during and immediately following the interview. These were later expanded when the tape recordings and video recordings were transcribed.

Findings

It was possible to collect life histories from a wide spectrum of residents with dementia, and the process was a satisfying one for both the researchers and the residents. None of the residents disliked having their story elucidated, but rather found it to be an enjoyable experience and wished that the interviews would continue. Several families of residents continued to collect more details of the person's life story, and to collate them with

Figure 9.6 General life-course trajectory

GENERAL LIFE-COURSE TRAJECTORY					
Date of event	Degree of significance	Topic heading	Check	Special notes	Date(s)
		birth			
		childhood			
		primary school			
		secondary school			
		peers			
		pets			
		work			
		friends			
		courting			
		family			
		neighbours			
		childrearing			
		hobbies			
		vacations			
		job changes			
		significant losses			
		'favourite things'			
		health			
		grandparenting			
		celebration days			
		retirement			
		beliefs, values, feelings			
		cumulated wisdom, advice to others			
Interviewer:					
Interviewee:					

family photograph albums. Some family members said that they were glad of the chance to continue collecting life histories because it gave them a pleasurable activity to do during their visits, rather than being at a loss as to what to say and do during visits, and coming to resent them.

Several major patterns were observed during the course of this study. There was a distinct tendency for persons to relate their stories either

Figure 9.7 Historical-setting graph

Dates	Historical Events	Age
1860	American Civil War Sir J.A. MacDonald (1867–1873)	
1876	First Provincial Taxes Alexander Mackenzie (1873–1878)	
1880	Sir J.A. MacDonald (1878–1891) C.P.R. completed	
1890	Sir John Abbott (1891–1892) Sir John Thompson (1892–1894) Sir Mackenzie Bowell (1894–1896)	
1900	Spanish American War Sir Charles Tupper (1896–) Boer War Sir Wilfred Laurier (1896–1911)	
1910	Perry reaches North Pole Sir Rob. Laird Borden (1911–1920)	
1914	World War I 424,000 Canadians served, 60,000 died	
1917	First Federal Taxes, Halifax Harbour Disaster	
1920	Roaring 20's Arthur Meighen (1920–1921) First cars & trucks, prohibition W.L. Mackenzie King (1921–1926) Depression Arthur Meighen (1926)	
1930	W.L. Mackenzie King (1926–1930)	
1932	C.B.C. founded by Richard B. Bennett (1930–1935)	
1934	Bank of Canada established	
1940	W.L. Mackenzie King (1935–1948) World War II Louis St. Laurent (1948–1957)	
1944	June 6, D-Day, (41,000 Canadians died in war)	
1950	Korean War	
1951	Old Age Security Act J.G. Diefenbaker (1957–1963) Recession, T.V.	
1959	St. Lawrence Seaway opened	
1960	Space Program begins Lester B. Pearson (1963–1968)	
1962	Canadian 'Alouette' launched/Trans-Canada Highway opened	
1963	J.F.K. Assassination Viet Nam	
1967	Expo 67 P.E. Trudeau (1968–1980) 1st Heart Transplant	
1980	Joe Clark (1980) P.E. Trudeau (1980–)	

TIME

factually, giving a concise, specific answer to a question, or, what we call, creatively. Creative answers were those that had a lot of descriptive detail, and that sparked associations to other events, such that the resident continued to speak candidly without many additional prompts for information. Female residents related the emotional content of memories more readily than male residents did. However, the men tended to recount snippets of historical information to landmark personal events in their lives whereas female residents would often relate an event that occurred with reference to the age of their children, i.e. 'That happened when the girls were only about 4 or 5 years old.'

Residents often said that reminiscing about these things 'brought them back very clearly', and that they could actually see images related to their memories in their 'mind's eye', when they thought of them. Some residents did not even seem to be aware of our presence while they were recounting stories; their eyes were bright and focused on some point that seemed far away.

It sometimes happened that if a resident had been talking and thinking about a particular period in their life, that they mistook similar stimuli in the hospital environment for events or situations that had happened in past time.

A few individuals told particular sequences of their life stories over and over again, in a pattern we called 'loops'. Two types of loops seem to occur. The first type involved telling stories about periods of great hardship and unresolved crises repeatedly, and the second type involved telling stories about events which had a great meaning for the person in terms of retaining their self-esteem. Many of these stories related to traumatic times during the wars. With persons who kept telling the same story over and over again, even when asked a new question, three strategies were used to try to break the loop. First, specific 'triggers' were used as salient distractors to break the loop. If this were not successful, we tried to talk to the person about their 'favourite things', from an inventory that was being collected during the visits. Last, we tried saying to a person, 'I notice that [this] story is very important to you. I would like to write it down in great detail. Please repeat it to me slowly, making sure you tell it to me as completely as possible.' In two instances, this careful notation of a story that was frequently repeated, served to completely reduce the repetition of the particular story.

Age regression also occurred during the interviews. Three of the ladies insisted that they actually were the age they had been, at the time of the events they were recalling. When an enquiry was made to one lady, who insisted that she was 14 years old, 'But didn't you marry SW, become a school teacher and have a family?' she replied 'I didn't marry SW did I? No, I couldn't have.' Later during the interview she did mentally advance in years and talked about her children.

It was apparent that persons in moderate stages of dementia fluctuated frequently, both in having lucid moments and in their use of tense as they were recounting stories. One lady changed tense even within the same sentence: 'My husband is the most wonderful person you could ever imagine; he is so good with the children; I don't remember when he passed away.'

It is important to recognize that when residents cannot remember the factual content of parts of their life accurately, important affective components of the memories are usually communicated instead. This example is particularly illustrative.

Nursing staff reported that 83-year-old Mr N kept referring to having three sons, when in fact he had three daughters. Mr N was thought to be psychotically ill, as well as demented. Two of his daughters lived in other provinces, and his wife and one daughter lived a great distance from the hospital and could not visit often. Staff were puzzled about how to respond to Mr N's references to his sons; should they confront him with the reality of having three daughters every time he mentioned his sons, should they pretend that he had three sons or should they distract him and change the topic? When Mr N's life story was examined in more detail, it was found that he had been a farmer in Greece. He ran the farm on his own, and had actually hoped for three sons to help him run the farm. Instead he had three daughters. He eventually gave up the farm and emigrated to Canada. Throughout his life, he had never spoken of his disappointment at not having had sons in order to be able to continue running the farm. Now that he had dementia, and was showing clear signs of behavioural disinhibition, he finally started speaking of the sons he had wanted so much. This life-history information helped to put Mr N's comments into perspective, and he was clearly not psychotic. Eventually, instructions were written in the nursing care plan, advising staff to empathize with Mr N whenever he mentioned his sons, and to say to him:

> Three sons could really have helped you do all of the hard work on the farm, it must have been hard for you to hide your disappointment all of these years. Did any of your daughters ever show an interest in the work on the farm? Tell me about the farm. What did you grow? Did you have any animals? Was it a big farm?

Abbreviated versions of the life histories were placed in the residents' charts and were used by staff in one extended-care unit to develop more detailed nursing care plans, such as the one designed for Mr N, for other residents. After the study had been completed, inservice seminars were held with the nursing staff, to explain how some of the difficult behaviours exhibited by some residents related to their life histories; events or situations that occurred in the hospital were mistaken for events or situations that had happened in the past.

CONCLUSIONS

Based on a review of the literature and on the findings of this study, the following conclusions can be drawn and recommendations made.

Life review is a useful tool that can be used as an adjunct to the assessment and the planning of nursing care interventions with persons with dementia. Although life reviews have traditionally been conducted with the sentient elderly, they can also be conducted with elderly persons with dementia. The process of conducting life reviews seemed to be enjoyable for both the residents and the interviewers. Some families also appreciated the opportunity of continuing to collect the life reviews in order to keep some of the stories available for the grandchildren, and also as a meaningful activity to do during visits.

Following these findings, the collecting of life reviews from patients in geriatric settings was added to the curriculum for first-year nursing students. They found it to be a meaningful and worthwhile activity, and it helped them with other aspects of collecting physical data from the residents.

It is our recommendation that reminiscing and life-review activities should constitute a part of the assessment and care-giving provided by nurses and other health care professionals involved in providing care for the patient with dementia. Life reviews can be conducted systematically, and can be easily taught to students.

One criticism of conducting life reviews, made by staff, was the amount of time it required, when they were already feeling overburdened by their work loads. Although life reviews were conducted during official visits in this study, there is no reason why such information cannot be collected on a daily basis while persons are being assisted with activities of daily living. All sorts of activities can be used as triggers to enquire about the life of a person. For one lady bathing, recalled memories of a favourite swimming hole; for another gentleman, eating green beans was a reminder of years of gardening; and for another lady, choosing a colourful dress to wear triggered thoughts of a mother's special care. In our clinical work subsequent to this study we found that reminiscing and collecting life review information can be readily obtained during activities of daily living, and that speaking about pleasant memories, rather than trying to speak about the weather or meaningless pleasantries, often elicited enthusiastic responses from residents with dementia.

REFERENCES

Anderson, B. (1983) 'Reminiscing', MA thesis in counselling psychology, University of British Columbia, Canada.
Annis, A.P. (1967) 'The autobiography: its use and value in professional psychology', *Theory of Counselling Psychology* 14: (1) 9–17.

Baines, S., Saxby, P. and Ehlert, K. (1987) 'Reality orientation and reminiscence therapy: a controlled cross-over study of elderly confused people', *British Journal of Psychiatry* 151: 222–31.

Birren, J. (1980) *Guided Autobiography Program*, Los Angeles, Cal: Andrus Gerontology Centre.

Butler, R.N. (1960) 'Intensive psychotherapy for the hospitalized aged', *Geriatrics* 15 (9): 645–53.

—— (1963) 'The life review: an interpretation of reminiscence in the aged', *Psychiatry* 26 (1): 65–75.

—— (1974) 'Successful aging and the role of the life review', *American Geriatrics Society* 22 (12): 549–55.

—— (1980–1) 'The life review: an unrecognized bonanza', *International Journal of Aging and Human Development* 12 (1): 35–8.

Cartensen, L.L. and Erickson, R.J. (1986) 'Enhancing the social environments of elderly nursing home residents: are high rates of interaction enough?' *Journal of Applied Behaviour Analysis* 19: 349–55.

Catmull, M. and Ling, G. (1981) 'Memories are made of this ...', *New Age* pp. 20–3, Summer.

Coleman, P.G. (1986) *Ageing and Reminiscence Processes: Social and Clinical Implications*, Chichester: J. Wiley.

Dietsche, L.M. (1981) 'Facilitating life review through group reminiscence', *American Journal of Nursing* 81 (9): 573–41.

Ebersole, P. (1976) 'Reminiscing', *American Journal of Nursing* 76 (8): 1304–5.

Ellison, K.B. (1981) 'Working with the elderly in a life review group', *Journal of Gerontological Nursing* 7 (9): 592–5.

Feil, N. (1982) *V/F The Feil Method*, Cleveland, Ohio: Edward Feil Productions.

Frenkl, E. (1936) 'Studies in biographical psychology', *Character and Personality* 5: 1–34.

Gerfo, M.L. (1981) 'Three ways of reminiscence in theory and practise. *International Journal of Aging and Human Development* 12 (1): 39–49.

Haycox, J.A. (1983) 'Social management', in B. Reisberg (ed.) *Alzheimer's Disease: the Standard Reference*, New York: Free Press.

Head, D.M., Portnoy, S. and Woods, R.T. (1990) 'Reminiscence: is it worthwhile?', *International Journal of Geriatric Psychiatry* 5: 295–302.

Help the Aged (1981) *Recall*, London: Help the Aged Education Department.

Holden, U.P. (1979) 'Return to reality', *Nursing Mirror* 149 (21): 26–30.

—— (1984) *Nostalgia Series*, London: Winslow Press.

—— and Woods, R.T. (1988) *Reality Orientation: Psychological Approaches to the 'Confused' Elderly* 2nd edn, Edinburgh: Churchill Livingstone.

Hughes, C.P., Berg, L., Danziger, W.L., Coben, L.A. and Martin, R.L. (1982) 'A new clinical scale for the staging of dementia', *British Journal of Psychiatry* 140: 566–72.

Kiërnat, J.M. (1979) 'The use of life review activity with confused nursing home residents', *American Journal of Occupational Therapy* 33: 306–10.

Lesser, J., Lazarus, L.W., Frankel, R. and Havasy, S. (1981) 'Reminiscence group therapy with psychotic geriatric inpatients', *Gerontologist* 21: 291–6.

Lewis, M. and Butler, R.N. (1974) 'Life review therapy: putting memories to work in individual and group psychotherapy', *Geriatrics* 29 (1): 165–73.

McMahon, A. and Rhudick, P. (1964) 'Reminisching: an adaptional significance in the aged', *Archives of General Psychiatry* 10 (3): 292–8.

Morris, R. and Kopelman, M. (1986) 'Memory deficits in Alzheimer-type dementia; a review', *Quarterly Journal of Experimental Psychology* 38a: 575–603.

Morton, I. and Bleathman, C. (1988) 'Reality orientation: does it matter whether it's Tuesday or Friday?' *Nursing Times* 84 (6): 25–7.

Norris, A. (1986) *Reminiscence*, London: Winslow Press.

—— and Abu el Eileh, M. (1982) 'Reminiscence groups', *Nursing Times* 78: 1368–9.

Pincus, A. (1970) 'Reminiscence in aging and its implications for social work practise', *Social Work* 15: 47–53.

Progoff, I. (1975) *Intensive Journal Workshop Manual*, New York: Dialogue House Library Publ.

Ryden, M. (1981) 'Nursing in support of reminiscence' *Journal of Gerontological Nursing*, 7 (8): 461–3.

Taylor, S., van Amelsvoort Jones, G. and Zeiss, E. (1983) 'Collecting and conducting life reviews', *Proceedings of the 1st Annual Gerontological Nurses Association, Victoria, B.C., Canada*, 2: 114–18.

Thornton, S. and Brotchie, J. (1987) 'Reminiscence: a critical review of the empirical literature', *British Journal of Clinical Psychology* 26: 93–112.

van Amelsvoort Jones, G. and Zeiss, E. (1984) 'Encouraging reminiscing in the institutional setting', *Perspectives* pp. 12–13, Winter.

Chapter 10

Music therapy in the management of dementia

Ruth Bright

INTRODUCTION

The general aims and objectives of music therapy are to meet the
emotional, social and spiritual needs of our clients, whether they are
children or adults and no matter what their particular problems may be.
These aims and objectives are the same whether we are working in rehabilitation, in maintenance for a stable condition or in support and maintenance
in a degenerative condition such as dementia.

Thus we hope, through the therapeutic applications of music, to improve
or maintain self-esteem, to enhance remaining cognitive and social skills,
provide emotional support for both sufferer and family, improve intimacy
and general relationships between staff and patient, patient and patient, and
between sufferer and family either at home, in hospital or in a nursing
home. In summary, our aim is to improve the quality of life, for sufferer and
carer alike.

In reaching this goal, there are some basic assumptions, founded upon
careful observations over some 30 years:

1   That there is some limited capacity for re-learning (see Raaijmakers,
    Chapter 3, this volume).
2   That memories of early and strongly emotional events may be retriev-
    able.
3   That musical memories appear to be better retained and more readily
    retrieved than verbal memories, although these music memories may
    lead to some verbalization.
4   That despite a dementing process some attempts at problem solving
    are evident, i.e. attempts to work out which way up a garment goes, trying
    to recall who a visitor is, trying to express feelings of affection, anger,
    bewilderment and so on.
5   That creativity, although obscured by cognitive losses, is not totally
    obliterated.
6   That a person who has been pleasantly occupied for the 45 minutes or

so of a music therapy session will behave for a while afterwards in a more-than-usually relaxed or alert manner.

DEFINITIONS

Music therapy (MT) may be defined as: 'The planned use of music to improve the functioning in their environment of individuals or groups of persons who are suffering from intellectual, physical or social disadvantage,' (often summarized as 'The planned use of music to reach non-musical goals with those who are disadvantaged.') It is clear from both these definitions that MT looks at the whole person – body, mind and spirit – as well as the milieu in which the person lives. Second, it is important to recognize that the music is used as a means to an end, not as an end in itself.

MT is based upon assessment of need, to which the client will – if possible – contribute, and the music intervention is planned in order to reach the goals associated with those perceived needs. Ongoing evaluation takes place to determine the success or failure of the interventions, changes being made in accordance with the result of evaluation and reassessment.

The need for assessment and evaluation to be done by all those involved in the client's care and/or treatment makes it seem important, in the author's opinion, that music therapists work as members of a clinical team, or – if this is impossible – maintain the closest possible communication with other members of that team, in hospital or community, as well as with the family.

It must be noted that MT differs from recreational and educational music in the aspects of aims and objectives, assessment and evaluation. Although recreational music may bring some benefits to the participant in relaxation, achievement, social relationships and so on, these are a matter of chance and not of intention. For instance, going to a public concert may promote release of anxiety, but the concert was not planned by the organizers with that in mind, and no assessment of concert-goers is made to determine what music would be 'good for them'! Similarly, it may be recommended that a patient being discharged from a psychiatric unit join a choir or amateur music group in order to meet social needs, but the organizers of that group do not arrange their programmes in order to meet the needs of that individual, nor do they formally evaluate the member's social progress as the rehearsals continue, changing the choir's repertoire or activities if necessary!

APPROPRIATE SITUATIONS

MT will be helpful in any situation in which dementing persons are being cared for – in the family home, in day centres, day hospitals, acute assessment units, long-term units such as nursing homes, state institutions where there are psychogeriatric units.

THE STAGES OF DEMENTIA

Today there are many different rating scales which are used to assess the level of dementia and the rate of deterioration of a client. Possibly in time a particular scale may emerge as the 'winner', but at present dementia teams vary widely in their choice of a tool, and even the DSM 111 criteria which support a diagnosis of dementia have come under criticism (Jorm and Henderson, 1985). Folstein's mini-mental state set of tests is widely used (Folstein *et al.*, 1975), but its administration and its interpretation vary. In some establishments the assessment of cognitive function is done by an occupational therapist, elsewhere by an expert clinical psychologist. In some hospitals the admitting medical officer carries out a short form of assessment (sometimes his own invention) to make a rapid assessment of function, and unfortunately the wrong classification which may result from this rough-and-ready assessment often 'sticks', to the detriment of the patient.

The author is not generally involved in the initial assessment of cognitive functioning and often views with scepticism the label which is placed upon a patient when it is known that the assessment was carried out by a person untrained in psychometric assessment. Doubts are especially strong when it is known that the client suffers from visual or other sensory losses or even a minor degree of depression, since this diminishes powers of concentration (Goodwin and Guze, 1979), and thus diminishes the capacity to respond adequately to lists of questions.

We also know that a depressive illness can present as dementia in the elderly (Frances and Teusink, 1984) and this knowledge further reinforces the need for caution in interpreting test results as indicating a dementing process or a particular stage in that process.

Alexopoulos' 'Cornell scale for depression in dementia' has proved useful, in that it relies upon observations by carers and not upon responses of clients to questions, making it appropriate for dementing persons; it has been shown to provide a reliable means of measuring depression in those who are non-verbal, and the author and colleagues have for that reason used it to assess depression in persons with aphasic resulting from a stroke (Alexopoulos *et al.*, 1985).

When statements are made in this chapter about the level of dementia shown by a client, the mode of evaluation is through Reisberg's descriptive scale (Reisberg *et al.*, 1982; 1985).

Reisberg emphasizes that any descriptive tool should be used only after other pathologies have been excluded, so that, for example, a person with work-related failure of memory and concentration would not be assessed as being at stage 3 of a dementing process until (a) other organic illness and (b) depression had been excluded. All factors must be taken into consideration so that, for instance, a difficulty in handling complex household tasks which – in a younger person – would suggest stage 4 of a dementing process may, in a very old frail person, suggest merely a pronounced manifestation of normal aging.

Some of the clients seen by the author in the psychogeriatric units referred to below would fit into the Reisberg stage 5 (moderate dementia of the Alzheimer type – DAT), in which help is needed not only in carrying out complex household tasks but also in selecting suitable clothing. Others fit into stage 6 (moderately severe DAT) in which there is incontinence and need for help with tasks of personal hygiene. From time to time, clients are seen who are in stage 7 (severe DAT), i.e. persons who have almost no verbal output, no ability to carry out purposeful activities, persons for whom it can be said that the brain has ceased to tell the body what to do. Although on rare occasions there will be a physical response to music such as a foot tapping, a change in posture or eye contact, these are not common – see discussion below – but this does not mean that music is therefore a waste of time and money.

LITERATURE ON MUSIC THERAPY IN THE DEMENTIAS

There is very little literature on MT in the dementias, apart from a book published by an American firm (Bright, 1988). When one hears the matter discussed, there is usually little attempt to explain what is meant by 'a demented client' so that it is impossible to tell whether the ideas suggested would be appropriate for any given individual or client group. The literature associated with remotivation therapy and validation therapy does, however, refer to the value of music.

HOW IT BEGAN

MT is useful for all ages and all types of disability, but work with children is the best known and perhaps the most common. There appears to be greater community 'guilt' over illness and disability in children, so that funds for MT for children seem to be more readily available than for work in equally devastating losses in the elderly.

With the growing public awareness of Alzheimer's disease and other dementias, we can hope for greater public finance to be available for work in MT for these conditions. New knowledge about links with Down's syndrome and Alzheimer's disease (Heston, 1982) may enhance this possibility, since the interest in music of Down's children is well known.

The interest of the present author in MT for elderly people started at the end of 1959, when work in long-stay wards in a major psychiatric hospital began, and this interest has continued ever since (Bright 1972; 1984; 1986a; 1988; 1989). Gradually there has been in the community and in the medical and paramedical world a recognition that music can be not merely recreational but therapeutic as well and that the two uses of music are different.

CHOICE OF MUSIC

We must be aware of major differences in choice of music for older people: when we are working with children we are, in a sense, working with a clean page – there are few if any established preferences or associations. But with elderly dementing subjects the associations and preferences from earlier years are crucial to our being able to make contact. We are therefore compelled to find out, if possible, what music was preferred – by asking family members or by trial and error. We need to find out whether the background of the individual is such that he or she prefers 'pub or party singalong' music, church choir items, background dinner music, ballroom dancing melodies or serious symphony orchestra repertoire.

Although many elderly people enjoy modern music, it is important when working with dementing clients that the music presented initially should be familiar. Reaching a creative spark or an awareness of current music can be attempted in later sessions if this seems appropriate.

RATIONALE

Work with dementing subjects through MT has developed gradually as a consequence of increasingly rigorous observations of how people with differing degrees of pathology respond to music, in different treatment situations. (In individual interviews, family interviews, patient group sessions, in co-operation with other therapists and so on.) These observations have been supported by extensive reading and study with the opportunity for study visits to the UK, the USA, New Zealand and several parts of Europe.

The author is, in consequence, moving towards a more clear-cut rationale and framework for MT in the assessment and management of the dementias and this rationale is closely linked to the basic assumptions already set out at the beginning of this chapter.

The author is supported in the belief that, in most dementing persons, music function is spared to a greater extent than are most cortical functions. Hopefully, further investigations of brain function and structure will reveal more about the individual differences in DAT patients which will account for this sparing. It is relevant here to note that many researchers report that affect remains relatively intact. Since the emphasis of MT in DAT is upon music with affective connotations from the past, the connection between these observations appears obvious. (See discussion below).

The cortical functions which are intact may be more readily accessible through the use of music than through direct questioning because of lessening of anxiety and depression in the musical milieu. It also seems probable that the adverse effects of partial aphasia are eliminated, since music function is centred in the hemisphere opposite from the speech hemisphere.

The emphatic use of music can bring to the sufferer an unparalleled experience of success. Music provides a person with an activity in which he or she can feel competent and 'with it', in marked contrast to the general sense of bewilderment which characterizes much of life in DAT.

For some clients, this experience of success permits supportive conversation, analogous to grief counselling, to take place. The family may well benefit from occasional or regular participation in this process, to assist in the resolution of their own guilt, anger, grief and loss.

DISCUSSION OF REASONS FOR RESPONSES TO MUSIC IN DAT

The precise reasons for the effects of music itself are not known and it is inappropriate to enter here upon discussion as to whether harmonic structure or sequence as such produce particular responses. In the context of DAT it is, in the author's belief, the associations and memories from the past which are important.

1   Studies of glucose metabolism in the brain suggest that exposure to music does promote a high metabolic rate (Mazziotta et al., 1982).
2   We are using old and well-established memory traces, dating back to childhood and early adult life. This in many cases applies to behaviour as well as to cognition so that the restless and/or aggressive person will often behave normally in a music session – sitting quietly for many minutes.
3   Music may evoke tears and sadness but it is improbable that the music 'makes' someone unhappy. What almost certainly happens is that music 'takes the lid off' what was there below the surface, and ventilating emotion in a supportive atmosphere gives a sense of relief, not despair.
4   As noted above, music brings an experience of success and this has beneficial effects in lessening overall feelings of failure and depression which are so common a feature of dementia (Feinberg and Goodman, 1984). There are also often positive changes in staff attitudes, the sequence being:
    'I saw Mrs X actually smiling and singing this morning – I did not know she had it in her – I must spend more time trying to get to know her'.

5   Dementia may involve the parietal lobes (Crystal *et al.*, 1981) with consequent loss or distortion of body image. Persons who need physiotherapy and whose body image is impaired may be helped to understand what movements are required of them through the facilitation of appropriate music. (This applies also to persons with aphasia, who are unable to understand verbal commands.)

6   Gates and Bradshaw (1977) have noted a general differentiation between music centres and speech centres in the non-dominant and dominant hemispheres, respectively. Persons with some forms of aphasia are able to sing words of songs despite their loss of propositional speech; whether this is the same mechanism as that which permits aphasic DAT subjects to sing words of songs is not certain, but it may well be that it is hemispheric differentiation which accounts for the phenomenon. The self-esteem which results is certainly the same, and, for a few patients, the singing has led to verbal expression of ideas and feelings which were otherwise incapable of ventilation:
     One lady, who had spoken only in 'word salad' for over a year, came over to the keyboard when the song was played to which she and her husband had danced during their courtship, and said clearly 'I am frightened, there is something wrong with my head – I think I am going crazy!'

7   The involvement of relatives in a happy music experience, whether in hospital/nursing home or in their own home, enables the relatives to see once again the person they felt they had lost. This may bring sadness because it is only temporary, but it is none the less worthwhile. Visiting is observed to increase and this in turn lessens family guilt (where visiting had previously diminished because of emotional responses to the loved person's dementia).

Obviously there are limits to what we can achieve. However well-conceived and executed, no MT programme can restore lost cells, but we can help people to function at their best instead of their worst, even if only for a short time.

POPULATION

The author has worked with dementing clients of all ages and with a wide variety of causes for their condition:

- Alzheimer's disease of early or late onset.
- Post-stroke dementia from a single cerebrovascular accident.
- Dementia resulting from several small strokes – multi-infarct dementia.
- Huntington's disease and other degenerative neurological conditions in which dementia may occur.
- Dementia resulting from 'old' tertiary syphilis.

- Normal-pressure hydrocephalus, pre- and post-shunt.
- Dementia resulting from traumatic brain damage (motor vehicle accidents, space-occupying lesions or following surgery for these).
- Alcohol-related brain damage in Korsakoff's syndrome.
- Dementia combined with psychiatric illness, both acute and chronic states and in drug-overdose brain damage.

N.B. The patients in the last two groups tend to be younger than the others, aged from mid-teens to middle-age.

SPECIFIC AIMS AND OBJECTIVES FOR MUSIC THERAPY IN DEMENTIA

Our objectives will be in the following areas:

- Building and rebuilding social bridges between people (patient/patient, patient/staff, patient/family).
- Providing opportunities for decision-making, problem-solving, albeit in minor matters.
- Emphasizing the client's remaining positive attributes and strengths rather than concentrating upon losses.
- Reducing (temporarily) aggression.
- Reducing (temporarily) wandering and restlessness.
- Encouraging mobility in the inert and apathetic.
- Reinforcing awareness of orientation in time, person and place, by positie affirmation and avoiding confrontation.
- Comforting and supporting sufferer and family in times of anger, despair, etc.

We are working necessarily in the context of diminishing function and MT must take this into account. Otherwise there will be unreal expectations as to what can be achieved and this will in itself breed despair for both patient and therapist. In the final stages of DAT it may be that we shall see no outward responses, but can we be certain that there is no inner awareness of familiarity and comfort?

THE THERAPEUTIC MILIEU

We have to make several decisions about music sessions – How often? How many people? Where? What time of day? How to select participants?

Size of the group depends upon degree of deterioration of clients – for some, individual work must precede groups and may continue permanently either because this is all the person can cope with, because it provides a needed opportunity for counselling-type intervention, or because it provides a wonderful change from the herd-like life found in some institutions. Other patients can cope only with three to five people but othes may cope with ten people. But this is the upper limit – it is impossible to provide the individual attention necessary for therapeutic interactions for any larger group. Once a week is acceptable for a music group; it helps to mark out one day as different from others. Other groups will probably take place on other days – but if not, then music can (given the availability of the therapist) take place more often.

The place is important – the music group should not be interrupted by nursing routines nor should it probably take place in a room associated with other activities such as eating or sleeping. But if the dining room is the only available area, then chairs should be set up to give a different atmosphere from eating meals. For bedfast patients a portable instrument such as an accordion or electric keyboard is useful.

The session should last about 30–45 minutes, not including time for gathering people together, so that to set aside a total of 1 hour works out about right. (But for individual work, 10 minutes may be all the person can tolerate at first. Ongoing evaluation of concentration, etc. is vital.)

Participants should be selected so that there is not too great a disparity in level of functioning. The 'better' patients may enjoy for a while being helpers, but in most units set aside exclusively for dementia, few potential helpers are available. It is better for all concerned to have people together who are functioning at more or less the same level, to avoid frustration for participants and therapist alike.

CHOOSING THE MUSIC

1   As was mentioned above, we must aim initially at least in finding music which is familiar, either by asking relatives or by playing a wide variety of pieces and observing responses. Being aware of ethnic, educational, religious and other cultural factors helps us to avoid blatant errors – there is not much point in playing Scottish Presbyterian hymn tunes to a Hindu Pakistani!

2   Non-musical cues can promote choice and discussion, so that e.g. passing round a rose reminds people of gardens, wedding bouquets, romantic love, other songs mentioning roses. Seashells remind people of childhood holidays, mantelpiece ornaments, tongue-twisters ('she sells seashells on the seashore...') and perhaps the song 'Pearly shells'. And so on – the imaginative therapist will devise many ideas linking objects with memories and music, all of them promoting self-esteem and the dignity of choice.

3   Music can help to promote physical activity and creativity. We sway to a waltz, tap our toes to a march almost without realizing we are doing it, and all such responses can be used to encourage purposeful activity.

Some people may be able to enjoy simple folk dances, even if these consist only of walking in a ring holding hands and changing directions when the music changes.

For some, the imagination is sufficiently intact to enable the person to move with pictorial music – 'Pretend you are a tree swaying in the breeze' – but assessment must precede such work if we are not to set up yet one more failure situation.

EVALUATING THE OUTCOME OF MUSIC THERAPY PROGRAMMES

The work described here, however, has been done without research funding, and estimates of outcome have depended upon observations of nurses who happened to be with the patients following the session. Fortunately they were co-operative in making these evaluations. One must, of course, beware the fallacy *post hoc ergo propter hoc.* People may behave differently following an MT session for reasons which are coincidental and quite unconnected with the MT. But from observations by nurses and from their consistent enthusiasm for the sessions which have taken place in the wards for many years, it seems reasonable to believe that the beneficial outcome is not mere 'happenstance' but is influenced by the events of the therapy programme.

Nevertheless the atmosphere of any one session may be influenced by such non-musical factors as:

- The advance of the dementing process.
- The personality of the subject(s).
- The arrival of a new and disturbed patient in the war alters behaviour of the others, or an old patient may be going through a difficult time.
- An event in the ward can upset people severely even though they appear to have forgotten about it. When a patient hung himself – and it was suspected that several patients had seen this – a number of people (staff and patients alike) were distressed and even disturbed for some time afterwards. This affected all sessions adversely.

In order to provide some evaluation of outcome, a simple rating scale was developed by the author for a four-person weekly group of dementing subjects, the programme taking place immediately before lunch for 4 weeks. The *target behaviour* was that of socialization at the lunch table, this being selected because nurses would be present and thus able to observe changes in behaviour over the mealtime. A 5-point scale was used to measure changes in communication, verbal and non-verbal:

+2 much better than usual
+1 somewhat better than usual
  0 unchanged
−1 somewhat worse than usual
−2 much worse than usual

The results are compatible with findings by Odell at a psychogeriatric unit in Cambridge, UK, where nurses noted a decrease in agitation and aggression in the ward following MT sessions (Odell, 1983).

If we assume that there is some capacity for relearning, comparable with that described in Korsakoff's psychosis, in which there is also a short-term memory deficit (Butters and Cermak, 1980), then it is worth using the stimulation of MT to facilitate the relearning of pleasant emotional responses, in this milieu.

A final comment on evaluation: does *everyone* enjoy music therapy? Only about 5 per cent of any given patient population in a psychogeriatric ward reject attendance at the music session once they have reached the room and are aware of what is to happen. This group of non-attenders rejects most other groups activities in the ward.

It seems advisable to allow people to say 'No!' to group music because to refuse to do something may be a rare luxury! But see also notes below on recruitment.

SPECIAL NEEDS

A few older people, dementing and otherwise, find music hard to tolerate because of hearing impairment, especially as a consequence of recruitment, the phenomenon associated with sensorineural deafness in which sounds are magnified, with the result that loud sounds, especially unexpected ones, cause physical pain. This is described by DeWeese and Saunders (1960) whose text has a photograph illustrating most graphically how a man winces in pain as a loud sound is fed through earphones.

These authors also point out that recruitment accounts for the irritability of an older person who at one moment cannot hear what is said to him but at the next moment (when the speaker increases volume only a little) says angrily 'There's no need to *shout* at me!' Reactions of staff may well be 'If she is deaf, how can sounds be too loud; she is just being difficult!'

As with the pain response described above, the person with normal cognition can explain what is happening, but the dementing person is probably unable to do so and so may reject attendance at a music group for no *obvious* reason.

Yet another hearing abnormality which may influence enjoyment of music is that of diplacusis, found in Menière's disease, in which the sufferer hears the same musical note at a different pitch in each ear, causing music to be a jangled noise rather than a source of pleasure. This is another possible reason for rejecting music but also one which a dementing person will find it difficult or impossible to explain.

ASSESSMENT AND DIFFERENTIAL DIAGNOSIS THROUGH MUSIC THERAPY

We note that most dementing subjects function better cognitively and socially in a MT environment than elsewhere, either because of relaxation, increased self-esteem and decreased depression or the re-establishment of old patterns of behaviour. It may therefore be possible to make a different assessment of level of impairment when MT techniques are used, as the following vignette illustrates.

A lady who was said to be suffering from moderate DAT was having individual music therapy assessment one sunny (Australian springtime) October morning. After an initial friendly relationship had been established, the song 'September in the Rain' was played, but no specific verbal introduction to that song was given nor was the title mentioned. At the end the patient was asked 'Well, how was that for you?' She smiled somewhat wryly and said 'Well, it seems more like *October* in the *Sun* to *me!*' (The response expected from a socially adept but disorientated DAT subject would have been 'Very nice, thank you!' or a similar socially-correct but informationless rely.) It was thus clear that she was not only recalling the name of the song but could see that the title was inappropriate for both the weather of the day and the time of year, indicating an awareness of her surroundings and of season of the year which was incompatible with the provisional diagnosis made elsewhere. It emerged in conversation during the MT interview that she had been 'encouraged' (forced?) to leave her own home because of frailty and was being moved to a nursing home in the country in order to be close to an older sister whom she did not even like. Clearly there was a degree of memory impairment but far short of justifying a diagnosis of moderate dementia.

In a very similar assessment a woman, said to be suffering from severe DAT, proved to have suffered recent multiple losses and crises. She had developed pneumonia and been placed in a nursing home where she was unhappy; a male friend with whom she had gone out each Saturday for many years died suddenly. While she was in the nursing home a long-standing woman friend had died but the patient had not been told 'for fear of upsetting her'. The upset of news of her death would have been nothing compared with the shock she received when a letter arrived from a law firm telling her she had inherited her friend's estate, when she did not even know the friend was dead. It was obvious that there was a degree of impairment in memory, and it is perhaps not surprising that a superficial assessment of her incoherence, forgetfulness and inappropriate social behaviour labelled her as 'severely demented'. Nevertheless, following the revised assessment, she was maintained, once more in her own home, and with the assistance of meals on wheels and domiciliary nursing for some 3 years until a heart attack made it impossible for her to continue to live alone. In the hostel to which she then moved, she remained the 'life and soul of the party' on many occasions, enjoying life in these protected surroundings.

It was pleasing to see these ladies 'improve' from a rating of 5 or even 6 on the Reisberg scale to a level of only 3 and 4. Such re-assessment and intervention is not achieved by MT alone but by team consultation in which MT plays a significant part, together with follow-up support services in the community.

In some cases it is appropriate for MT assessment to precede assessment by others, if only because it tends to produce a more positive attitude towards the patient.

In summary, MT assessment can help us make a differential diagnosis or assist in the estimation of the level of cognition, thereby helping to prevent misdiagnosis and misplacement.

SAMPLE PROGRAMME

(N.B. for more detailed information and ideas see Bright, 1988.)

We will assume that a lady with moderate DAT – stage 5 on the Reisberg scale – has been referred for assessment and inclusion in MT programmes. Assessment would be on an individual basis (a) to ascertain musical preferences if not known from the family and (b) to assess cognitive function. Sensory losses of hearing and sight are assessed by observation since these affect all behaviour; it is especially important to find out whether the patient normally wears glasses, and, if not already known, this is achieved by conversation rather than direct questioning – 'I'm lost without my glasses these days – how about you?'

Preferences

Not ascertained by asking questions but by playing music popular in the country of the patient's upbringing when she was in her early adult life (say aged 18–25). 'This piece was popular when you were growing up – see if you can sing it with me.' (One of the skills of the MT is to have an extensive repertoire of music known by heart, and to transpose to a suitable key to enable people to sing readily.)

Title completion is also used, (starting with an easy one such as 'It's a long way to ...' but going on to more complex tasks). After each piece is played some leading comments are made which draw the patient into conversation, thus gradually building up a life history as well as forming an estimate of capacity for verbal interaction and the degree of orientation in time and place.

'That song was being played about the time you were bringing up your children – did you have an awful struggle through the depression years?' and then, 'How are they getting on right now?' These and other directions for conversation interspersed with appropriate music helps us to see whether the person is in touch with today's world or lives only in the past.

Orientation

We can also use songs which mention colours to see how observant the person is of the surroundings, and songs with numbers mentioned in the words can be used as a starting point for assessment of arithmetic skill. The lady described above, who had suffered so many losses, was asked (after various songs including numbers had been played) 'I was asked the other day to count backwards from 100 by 7s and I found it quite difficult – how do you think you would get on?' and away she went immediately with the sequence correctly all the way to 65, when we told her she could stop!

The assessment may be continued, if appropriate, in a group so as to observe social skills which are lost or retained and so on.

Assessment and evaluation

Ongoing assessment and evaluation in the music group also reveal pathology in such remarks as 'I needn't bother to go to lunch when we finish today; my insides have all rotted away. I'm going to die soon anyway.' We also note changes in agitation, comments which reveal anger and frustration, new remarks about the family which suggest the development of paranoid ideation and so on.

Although the assessment actually continues throughout the initial session, and ongoing evaluation through all subsequent sessions, the patients perceive the activity only as an opportunity for music, for fun, for private conversation in an individual session or at the end of a group session, for expression of feelings of whatever nature.

Assuming that this assessment does not reveal any contra-indications, such as recruitment, then plans are made for sessions to continue, individually for one, two or three occasions and then group sessions if this seems advisable.

In setting up a group it is important to arrange a small number of participants in a circle, where each member can see and hear what is going on. The precise details of the programme are determined by the ethnic origin of the clients. The suggestions below are assuming an Anglo-Saxon background; changes for other ethnic groups would involve selection of appropriate music and perhaps different seating of men and women depending upon the cultural norms of that society.

Ongoing assessment group sessions would include:

Quizzes ('Can you think of a song about red?' 'Is there a tune beginning with the letter "A"?' 'Does anyone know what flower is mentioned in this song?').

Theme sessions (music from a particular country, from a particular musical 'show', etc.).

Movement to music, especially joining hands in the circle.

Musical instruments, if these are acceptable to the group members and not perceived as childish.

In all of these activities we are noting responses to the music and between clients, rhythmic responses to music and other matters.

Sample individual programme

If the patient has newly arrived – allow a few days for settling in. Choose a time of day when the patient is not already worn out, but – if it is known that he or she is in an angry mood early in the morning – avoid this too, unless one wishes to find out whether music will effect changes in this.

1 Introducing oneself is important – 'I have come to play some music to you; sometimes it helps us to feel more settled to hear something familiar. You don't have to sing; just listen at first!'
2 Play a piece which relatives suggest is a favourite and talk about it for a minute or two.
3 Play music reinforcing the season of the year or any festival such as Christmas, a famous horse race – the Derby in the UK, the Melbourne Cup in Australia and so on. Talk about this briefly.
4 Play music which stimulates movement – a waltz, and hold one of the patient's hands while you continue to play and sing.
5 Title completion, as already described above. 'That lovely waltz, "My Sweet Little Alice Blue ...".' Then if a correct response is given or when you have given the answer, 'Can you see anything blue in the room/out of the window (or whatever)?'
6 Play a piece which suggests hopefulness, peacefulness or whatever mood seems to be needed and encourage a response to this if possible by unchallenging conversation.

We must note that in the early stages of a relationship one may get no verbal responses at all; we should not despair – but rather rejoice if and when there is a response! The session may last only 5 minutes or continue for half an hour, but it is vital to stop while you are ahead!

Maintenance group-work

This is very similar, but – since it may be assumed that people will be together for a lengthy period of time, as in a long-stay unit, introductions of one patient to another can be attempted, in the hope that repetition of these each week may result in learning. Songs can be used for some names, and in any case provide an excuse for talking about names. Some elderly people do not wish to use first names, but it is the author's experience that women with dementia may have forgotten their married names and thus actually respond better to first names. Men seem in any case to prefer first names, although one should always investigate this. One such person when addressed as Mr Smith, replied 'What's all this B ... S ... of Mr Smith – I'm *Bill*!'

As already mentioned, some persons with dementia reject musical instruments, probably because they represent too clearly the idea of a second childhood. But in long-term groups, where there is a stable population, one can introduce *good-quality* instruments as a fun thing to do, and they are acceptable. Ideally we should have large adult-type instruments rather than tiny toy-type; large bongo or conga drums (if money permits their purchase) are ideal. Triangles are difficult to manage because they demand two-handed co-ordination, unless one can arrange for stands to be made on which to hang the main instrument. Simple folk dances, too, are more attainable in a stable group, even though we must avoid being over ambitious.

Probably our programme has taken about 45 minutes of varied activities, carrying out a plan of a mixture of socialization, physical activity, quizzes, conversation. But it is important that we are not so wedded to a prearranged plan that we prevent spontaneity. The opportunity to be themselves may be the most valuable thing we can give to our clients, and if this involves letting half our planned programme go, then so be it!

The farewell is important since in it we express plans to meet again and thanks for the achievements of each member.

One of the features which dementia shares with malignant diseases such as cancer is that sufferers are always on the receiving end of care, never having the opportunity to help others. Anything we can do in MT sessions to give to our patients a sense of having done something for someone else is of value in raising self-esteem and self-worth.

Who does all this?

It must be acknowledged that some smaller establishments may not be able to employ a full-time music therapist. A sessional therapist is an appropriate person to do the work here described. In some places a diversional therapist or a trained volunteer can do at least some of the work in groups, even if not skilled in assessment. But this must be regarded as a stop-gap measure only. For maximum benefit we must be able to offer a professional service. Only a qualified music therapist who has special interest in dementia and who has understanding of both the capabilities and the limitations of persons in various stages of a dementing process can use music to its utmost.

SUMMARY

The principal goal of MT for the dementing client is to improve self-esteem and the quality of life. Through music we may be able to facilitate such changes as are open to our clients, making the most of the capabilities remaining to them and diminishing the effects of reactive depression and despair.

Because of the capacity to respond to music – through old learning, old social responses or other reasons – the client has an experience of success and a consequent increase in self-esteem which appears to be effective even in those who are incapable of describing their feelings or the reasons for them.

Additional 'spin-offs' from music therapy include the following:

- Staff attitudes may change towards patients, perhaps even diminishing their own work stress (Bright, 1986b).
- Family attitudes may also change, bringing greater sense of happy involvement in the care of a sufferer and a diminution of guilt and anger.
- By taking part in music based interaction, the therapist may become a facilitator in family/staff relationships, through clinical teamwork with a clinical psychologist, psychiatrist, nurse, physician and others.
- Informal evaluation through empirical observations contributes to global assessment of clients. This evaluation may also contribute to decisions about placement e.g. a decision as to sending a patient to a particular nursing home which is known to have a proper MT programme rather than one which has not.
- Including in the discharge summary notes on the patient's musical preferences, to assist in the settling-in process in the new placement.

Finally, it is worth noting Hines' comments about the value of psychotherapy in complex phenomena (Hines, 1982), that a belief in science should not lead to rejection of highly complex subjective elements involved in psychotherapy. Nor, Hines continues, should we ignore the difficulties which arise because of the unrealistic expectations of funding authorities that all treatment can (and must?) be scientifically proved.

It seems reasonable to extrapolate these remarks to the practice of MT in dementia of the Alzheimer-type,

(a) since we are dealing with emotional responses to the advances of dementia we are truly involved in psychotherapy, and
(b) the responses and interrelationships of patients, staff and family are indeed complex phenomena!

CONCLUSION

The author believes that MT is of paramount importance in the assessment, care and management of dementing persons and as such should be regarded not as an 'optional extra' or a luxury to be funded when all else has been arranged, but as an essential part of the therapeutic armamentarium.

ACKNOWLEDGEMENT

I am grateful to Professor Tom Arie, of Nottingham University, for his expositions in Australia of non-threatening ways of estimating cognitive function and orientation. The author's own approaches owe much to the emphatic style which he demonstrated.

REFERENCES

Alexopoulos, G.S., Abrams, R.C., Young, R. and Shamoian, C.A. (1985) 'Cornell scale for depression in dementia', New Research Section, annual meeting of the American Psychiatric Association, Dallas, USA, and personal communication.

Bright, R. (1972) *Music in Geriatric Care*, Sydney Australia: Angus & Robertson, now Sherman Oaks, CA: Alfred International, pp. 10–16.

—— (1984) *Practical Planning in Music Therapy for the Aged*, Sherman Oaks CA: Alfred International, (various sections on dementia and grief).

—— (1986a) *Grieving*, St Louis: Magna Music, pp. 72 ff., p. 148.

—— (1986b) 'The use of music therapy and music activities with demented patients who are deemed difficult to manage', special issue of *The Clinical Gerontologist*, pp. 131–44.

—— (1988) *Music Therapy and the Dementias*, St Louis: Magna Music.

—— (1989) 'Why does this happen? Discussions on geriatric care', Music Therapy Enterprises, Wahroonga, NSW, Australia.

Butters, N. and Cermak, L.S. (1980) *Alcoholic Korsakoff's Syndrome*, New York: Academic Press, p. 31.

Crystal, H.A., Horoupian, D.S., Katzman, R. and Jotkowitz, S. (1981) 'Biopsy-proved Alzheimer's disease presenting as right parietal lobe syndrome', *Annals of Neurology* 12: 186–8.

DeWeese, D.D. and Saunders, W.H. (1960) *Textbook of Otolaryngology*, St. Louis, MO: C.V. Mosby, pp. 307–8.

Feinberg, T. and Goodman, B. (1984) 'Affective illness, dementia and pseudo-dementia', *Journal of Clinical Psychology*, 45: 99–103.

Folstein, M.F., Folstein, S.E. and McHugh, P.R. (1975) 'Mini-mental state. A practical method of grading the cognitive state of patients for clinicians', *Journal of Psychiatric Research* 12: 189–98.

Frances, A. and Teusink, P. (1984) 'Elderly patient's confusion confounds diagnosis and treatment of depression', *Hospital and Community Psychiatry* 35(11): 1091–3.

Gates, A. and Bradshaw, J.L. (1977) 'The role of the cerebral hemispheres in music', *Brain and Language* 4: 403–31.

Goodwin, D.W. and Guze, S.B. (1979) *Psychiatric Diagnosis*, Oxford: Oxford University Press, p. 230.

Heston, L.H. (1982) 'Alzheimer's disease and Down's syndrome: genetic evidence suggesting an association' *Annals of New York Academy of Science* 396: 29–37.

Hines, F.L. (1982) 'The effectiveness of psychotherapy: problems of research in complex phenomena', *American Journal of Psychiatry* 139: 204–8.

Jorm, A.F. and Henderson, A.S. (1985) 'Possible improvements to the diagnostic criteria for dementia in DSM 111', *British Journal of Psychiatry* 147: 394–9.

Mazziotta, J.C., Phelps, M.E., Carson, R.E. and Kohl, D.E. (1982) 'Tomographic mapping of human cerebral metabolism: auditory stimulation', *Neurology* 32 (9): 921–37.

Odell, H. (1983) Personal communication re: music therapy at Fulbourne Hospital, Cambridge UK.

Reisberg, B., Ferris, S.H. and DeLeon, M.J. (1982) 'The global deterioration scale, for assessment of primary degenerative dementia', *American Journal of Psychiatry,* 139 (9): 1136–9.

——, —— and Franssen, E. (1985) 'An ordinal functional assessment tool for Alzheimer's type dementia', *Hospital and Community Psychiatry* 36 (6): 593–5.

Chapter 11

Dynamic psychotherapy with elderly demented patients

Carol Hausman

SUMMARY

This chapter describes a type of psychotherapeutic treatment of patients with Alzheimer's disease that has been largely absent from the literature and from practice – psychodynamic psychotherapy – which addresses the internal factors that determine a patient's way of adapting and finding restitution. The benefits as well as the obstacles to dynamic psychotherapy with Alzheimer's patients are explored. Principles underlying the treatment, and modifications of traditional techniques for this special population, are described. The chapter concludes with three case studies.

INTRODUCTION

The current psychotherapeutic practices for both Alzheimer's disease patients and their care-givers are described, followed by a description of some of the affective conditions that are prevalent in these patients. Next, the goals of psychotherapy in general are presented, followed by an examination of the obstacles and strengths which determine the extent to which the goals can be met when working with patients who are demented. Obstacles in the patient, the care-givers and in the therapist are examined.

The process of dynamic psychotherapy with demented patients is then described, along with modifications of traditional techniques that are necessary for this special population.

Three case studies – one in which dynamic psychotherapy was not appropriate, and two in which it was – are used to illustrate the use of dynamic psychotherapy with demented patients.

In recent years there has been an abundance of information about the dementing illnesses that afflict the elderly and that are irreversible. The major one of these dementing illnesses – perhaps the only one whose name has become a household word – is Alzheimer's disease, or senile dementia of the Alzheimer's type. There are undoubtedly more books, journal articles, workshops and conferences on Alzheimer's disease than on any other aspect of aging. Estimates of the number of older people who are its victims vary. Miller and Cohen (1981) state that about 5–7 per cent of people at age 65 have senile dementia of the Alzheimer's type, and that the incidence increases with age. Research into the causes and course of the disease is being conducted at an unprecedented pace, with new data reported almost daily in the professional as well as in the popular press. Symptom descriptions are common knowledge. Diagnostic techniques are becoming ever more sophisticated.

TREATMENTS CURRENTLY USED

What is sparse in the gerontological literature is a focus on the treatment of the actual patient with Alzheimer's disease. As of yet, there is no known effective treatment to address the brain deterioration of this disease, the physiological processes which cause the primary symptoms. Efforts to treat the effects of the disease – the secondary symptoms – have largely been of three types: environmental, managerial and behavioural.

Environmental and managerial treatments include vital attention to the care-giver; vital not only for the care-givers' wellbeing in their own right, but also because caring for the care-giver is a way of caring for the patient. Nurture and support of care-givers makes them more available for the difficult task of caring for a demented patient. We can help care-givers express their feelings about their impaired relative, their fears that the same thing may happen to them and their anger and frustration when they feel helpless in the face of this disease. We can invite them to join groups in which they will find out that they are not alone, and in which they learn how other families managed in similar situations. (Hausman, 1979). In addition, we can counsel them on how to respond to their demented relative, how best to arrange the environment, how to find good substitute care-givers, how to chose doctors, day centres and nursing homes.

Attention in the literature that is directed to the Alzheimer's patient him or herself most often focuses on pharmacologic interventions, environmental manipulation, behaviour modification and reality orientation.

Pharmacologic treatments aimed at agitation, sleeplessness, depression, anxiety and paranoid ideation can improve the quality of life of a person suffering from Alzheimer's disease. Manipulating the environment – making it safer and more orderly, while reducing overstimulation – makes the world more comprehensible and helps a demented person feel more in control of it, particularly at the beginning and middle stages of the disease. Behaviour modification can train the patient himself to keep more order in his or her life, and can sometimes alleviate embarrassment by such factors as incontinence, wandering, forgetfulness, dangerous kitchen practices – giving the patient more of a sense of control and providing the patient the maximum amount of independence for the longest possible duration.

Reality orientation, too, is aimed at a feeling of control to enhance self-worth and reduce embarrassment and confusion.

Each of these types of treatment not only makes the demented patient feel better, but also makes him or her appear more 'normal' and thus more acceptable to others. Other people will tolerate, even welcome, their demented friends and relatives if they don't appear too demented.

The focus of these treatments – behavioural, environmental, managerial – is primarily on external stressors and behaviour. The focus of this chapter, however, is on treatment of the internal factors which determine each person's way of adapting and finding restitution. This focus has been absent from the literature on the treatment of Alzheimer's disease.

AFFECTIVE CONDITIONS IN ALZHEIMER'S PATIENTS

Every older person's experiences, ways of managing impulses, and internalized representations help determine his or her ways of coping with the changes that inevitably accompany aging. Long-unresolved internal conflicts often re-emerge with vigour in old age and make demands on ego resources and defences. Because those ego resources and defences are less and less strong and available in Alzheimer's patients as the disease progresses, an overwhelming percentage of demented patients develop emotional diseases – depression, anxiety, paranoia – secondary to their dementia.

There are additional reasons that account for the extent to which Alzheimer's patients develop emotional diseases.

The feeling of mastery over one's self and one's environment is a prerequisite for mental health. Dementia leads to a diminished sense of control and hence to feelings of helplessness, fear and dependency.

The capacity to adapt to change is one of the determinants of whether an older person will develop psychopathology. Alzheimer's patients lose that flexibility.

The ability to invest in others, so important to successful aging, is lost by people with Alzheimer's disease, as they become preoccupied instead with the loss of their essential selves.

Ability to mourn for the past as well as for current losses, freeing a person for further growth, is another factor correlating with successful aging. Alzheimer's patients often become fixated on the past, unable to mourn appropriately, and therefore unable to come to terms with the past, accept its successes and failures, and go on with the present.

The need to be able to redirect psychological energy from lost functions into other areas – or the defence of sublimation – is much harder for people whose reasoning ability, mobility and powers of organizing their environment are diminished. They become unable to shift energy into new relationships and interests, another essential ingredient of successful aging.

People who are confused by their environment and do not understand what is happening around them often become suspicious. They hear others talking but cannot sort out what is being said. Those with hearing and visual losses often fill in the missing information themselves. This process can lead to suspicion that others are plotting to institutionalize them, use their money, make important decisions for them. Alzheimer's patients use the same dynamic – filling in the missing blanks. Fear, suspiciousness and alienation of others often result.

These tragic accompaniments to the dementing process – loss of control, suspicious and accusatory behaviour, preoccupation with self, inability to sublimate or mourn, fixation on the past – lead to withdrawal and isolation, which in turn lead to exhibition of more demented behaviour.

USE OF DYNAMIC PSYCHOTHERAPY AS AN INTERVENTION FOR AFFECTIVE CONDITIONS COMPLICATING ALZHEIMER'S DISEASE

One of the primary avenues of addressing and resolving internal stress is individual psychodynamic psychotherapy. However, starting with Freud (1924), psychodynamic psychotherapy was considered inappropriate for older people. Other types of psychotherapy – supportive, cognitive, pet, art, movement, group – were used frequently. But it was assumed that the elderly did not possess the prerequisites for dynamic therapy – a high level of cognitive resources, psychological sophistication, a capacity for introspection and the ability to develop a therapeutic alliance (Cath, 1982).

In the years since Freud, therapists have found that the non-demented elderly are indeed responsive to psychodynamic psychotherapy, and this modality has been used with increasing frequency and success. But therapists, as well as family members and patients, still question its use with the demented elderly.

To determine the appropriateness of the use of dynamic psychotherapy with the demented elderly, several questions must be posed: What are the goals of psychotherapy with Alzheimer's disease patients? What are the obstacles to engaging in dynamic psychotherapy with this population? What strengths do these patients have that may substitute when the usual prerequisites for engaging in dynamic psychotherapy are missing? How might we conduct dynamic psychotherapy with demented patients? What special techniques might be used?

GOALS OF PSYCHOTHERAPY

In dynamic psychotherapy, goals are the same with the Alzheimer's disease patient as with any other patient: (1) a relationship in which the patient feels cared about; (2) emotional outlet or catharsis; (3) enhancement of self-esteem; (4) minimization of psychological and behavioural problems; (5) increase in coping skills; (6) enhancement of role functioning; (7) a sense of control; (8) the ability to grieve over losses of roles, capacities and significant others; (9) development and maintenance of the most mature and productive defences possible while shedding inappropriate defences; (10) the development of insight.

These goals can be met with greater or lesser success in all patients, demented or not, depending on the abilities and receptivity of the patient, the relationship between the patient and therapist, the support of people in the patient's environment, and the therapist's skill. With Alzheimer's patients, the possibility of reaching the goals depends on additional factors as well: (1) the degree to which the disease has progressed; (2) the point in the progression of the disease at which the patient and therapist begin working together; and (3) the patient's pre-morbid degree of psychological sophistication.

The first three goals mentioned above – establishing a relationship in which the patient feels cared about, having an emotional outlet, self-esteem enhancement – can almost always be met to some extent, no matter what the patient's condition, given adequate support and a good therapist–patient match. A patient whose treatment begins while even minimum verbal skills are available, can be helped to reach the goals of minimizing psychological and behavioural problems, increasing coping skills and role functioning, achieving a sense of control, and grieving over losses. The earlier in the progression of the disease the therapy starts, the more successful will be the attainment of these goals. Development of insight is more complicated, for it can only be reported by a patient when his or her verbal skills are reasonably intact, but it is impossible to know whether or not insight which can no longer be verbalized can actually take place. The question of defences will be discussed in more detail later in the chapter.

OBSTACLES

When engaging in dynamic psychotherapy with Alzheimer's disease patients, obstacles arise in three areas – the family, the therapist and the patient.

The family

Family members are often resistant to a suggestion of any kind of psychotherapy for their demented relative. They see the patient as unable to comprehend, communicate or remember. How can what they understand as dynamic psychotherapy possibly be useful to someone with these limitations? Given these doubts, and the burdens already undertaken by them in caring for their demented relative, how can it be worthwhile to spend

money and energy on trips to a therapist that could be used for more practical services?

At later stages in the disease, the patient may not even recognize the
therapist's name. How can the family feel that therapy can be meaningful if
the patient recognizes the voice, touch, office and affect, but not the name
of the therapist?

The care-giver may feel that the therapist only sees the patient at his or
her best, and has no understanding of the extent of stress the patient gener-
ates on a 24-hour basis. Counselling with the care-giver to try to address
these feelings becomes yet another burden and expense.

Once therapy is underway, the patient may manifest the defence of
splitting, which can cause particular resentment in the care-giver. Splitting
is a primitive defence mechanism which actually stems from infancy, when
the good and bad aspects of mother are seen, and internalized, as two
different beings. All but very psychotic people are able to integrate these
two aspects of mother and self, but at times of stress and emotional trauma,
many people temporarily revert to a form of splitting in which they see
some people as all good and others as all bad.

This defence is particularly common to Alzheimer's patients. It becomes
a problem when it causes the patient to see the therapist as the good object,
and the main caretaker as the bad object. Even the best-intentioned caretaker is likely to feel anger and resentment when this happens. The anger,
combined with the doubts and burdens already mentioned, may cause
unconscious or conscious sabotage of the treatment by the care-giver.

Sabotage may take a passive–aggressive form such as last-minute
'unavoidable' cancellations, forgetting appointments, late payment; or it
may take the active form of sudden termination. When resistance occurs in
patients, it is a routine part of the therapeutic process, but when it occurs in
the care-giver, it is a different matter.

The therapist

Countertransference phenomena exist in all therapists, no matter how well-
analysed they are. When recognized and understood, countertransference is
a very useful tool. Countertransference has come to have a broader
meaning than the classical definition – relating to the patient as if he or she
were a significant person from the therapist's past. It includes all the feelings aroused in the therapist during the clinical work.

Unexpected and often unrecognized countertransference problems
abound with geriatric patients. The therapist's own child–parent relationship is likely to be a factor. Feelings of hostility, frustration and helplessness
often come into play when working with patients who have irreversible illness
and will not get better.

With Alzheimer's patients, countertransference phenomena multiply. In the therapist's mind the question – 'Will this happen to me?' – keeps arising. Patients of background and education similar to the therapist's intensify such identification. The deeply rooted archaic feelings of helplessness that we all have become intensified when working with demented people.

Some activities called for on the therapist's part when working with an Alzheimer's patient are far from what a therapist normally does in the course of his or her work, and make the therapist feel more like a caretaker than a professional. I recall a home-visit patient early in my practice whose room was in such disarray that I was convinced it had a profound negative effect on the organization of her thinking. Before we could engage in any kind of therapy, the room had to be straightened, and I was the only one around with enough motivation to do so. Another patient had two instances of incontinence during sessions, which annoyed me and embarrassed her. We were able to co-operate in finding a solution – plastic liners on my chairs. We discussed and used the problem and its solution in the therapy as an example of her feeling that she was too great a burden. The opportunity to discuss this openly and honestly with me at the time she felt she was overburdening me, became a very helpful model in her subsequent dealings with her care-givers on the same issue.

Resentment over the need to spend many extra hours talking to doctors, nursing-home personnel and adult children; anger when and if the patient doesn't recognize you or know your name; frustration about the need to arrange transportation, make home visits and deal with third-party reimbursement restraints – all such feelings tempt the psychotherapist who works with Alzheimer's patients to yearn for a practice composed of easy neurotic young people who come on time, stay for 50 minutes, and talk clearly.

Inexperienced therapists dismiss demented patients too soon because of their own self-concept problems when they find themselves doing more of these case management tasks and less of the 'therapy' they were trained to do.

The patient

The two major obstacles within the Alzheimer's disease patient when engaging in dynamic psychotherapy are in the areas of communication and defences.

The application of psychotherapeutic techniques needs communication channels, and the normal channels are impaired in Alzheimer's patients. After all, the target of psychological techniques is the brain, and the brain of Alzheimer's patients is permanently impaired. Injury to the cerebral cortex means injury to the autonomous ego functions of thought, memory, speech and perception. Lost, to one degree or another, are: the ability to abstract; the ability to compare and thereby think in 'as if' terms (so necessary when working with transference phenomena); the existence and use of the observing ego; the ability to be accountable for one's acts; the ability to problem-solve.

Because of all these losses and changes, the demented patient often calls in inappropriate primitive *defences* which can compound the problem of engaging in dynamic psychotherapy. Rather than try to change, a demented patient clings to and tries to be even more of the way he or she was before. At this stressful time, he or she may have a need for the very defences which are being threatened. 'An aggressive ambitious person may try to defend against the threat of loss of control by becoming even more aggressive and controlling. The compulsive person may become more rigid and set in his or her usual ways.'

The primitive defence of splitting, described above, in which everything and everyone is seen in extreme terms, often comes into play during the course of this disease. Projection, with its accompanying accusatory behaviour, and withdrawal, which feels passive–aggressive, alienate those whose support is needed. Loss of secondary processes causes regression to primary process thinking and the need for immediate gratification, sometimes snowballing to aggression, psychotic symptoms (delusions and hallucinations), combativeness, and other catastrophic reactions. These lead to further alienation of care-givers (not to mention alienation of the therapist). The defence of denial, so useful to so many with this disease, is less available. The defense of sublimation, discussed above, is often diminished.

STRENGTHS

Many clinicians have observed that demented patients can be reached affectively long after they cease to be able to be reached cognitively. The affective responses in the limbic system seem to be the last to go (Verwoerdt, 1981), which may be the reason that a person's lifelong style of affect seems to remain intact except in the very late stages of this disease.

The skill of recognition, which remains long after the ability to recall, can be worked with.

A person's ability to form relationships, at least in all but the last stages of this disease, can be utilized, and is a major component of therapeutic action.

The transference often develops very rapidly in demented patients, and is another strength which can be used.

CONDUCTING PSYCHOTHERAPY

The Alzheimer patient's ability to benefit from psychotherapy will depend mainly on the relationship with the therapist. The earlier in the progression of the disease this relationship is formed, the better the chance of using it to help bring about movement toward the other goals. Many demented people develop relationships with the therapist easily and quickly because of their unmet need for someone who is accepting, empathic and trustworthy. Sometimes people who have endured multiple losses have to test the relationship, to ascertain that it *is* trustworthy. If the relationship feels safe, non-threatening, accepting, honest and respectful, the patient will be able to move toward the highest level of functioning possible for him or her at the particular stage of his or her disease. If such patients are not afraid, they will be able to hear interpretations better, try new ways of coping with a minimum amount of defensiveness, know that their efforts to communicate will not be criticized. They will learn that when they try to maintain control, or to grieve, they will have an empathic ally. A patient can accept painful information from a therapist he or she has learned to trust.

Knowing that the demented patient can still be reached affectively gives direction to the treatment. When the therapist reacts to the patient's feelings, the patient will know he or she is cared about. The therapist does not try to change the patient or to get him or her to operate in a cognitive mode that has been lost. Such acceptance of the patient as he or she is is in stark contrast to the approach of many family members, who have a poignant investment in getting the patient to be the way he or she used to be. Our investment is in improving the patient's current emotional state.

Usually, a therapist working with demented patients has to be able to relate well to primary process thinking in order to receive the patient's communications, particularly in the initial stages when establishing a sense of trust, but also in later stages when dementia is more severe. Secondary process responses at times may actually increase distress because they may remind the patient of his or her losses and thereby increase anxiety and depression. (Anyone who has watched a family member try to get a demented patient to remember a date or an event, will know exactly what I mean.) For this reason, reality orientation is often contra-indicated with this population at the moderate and severe stages.

A therapist can find ways to use the patient's skill of recognition in the treatment. When we know our patients well, we know about their experiences, their environment and their affective style. We can name their people and recite their stories for them. We can name feelings that the patient can no longer name, and we can relate these feelings to events from the patient's past with which he or she is familiar. Memories are triggered. Patients will recognize what we name, and will respond to this recognition, long after they themselves can bring the subjects forth verbally. Afterwards, when the patient enters our office, he or she may not be able to say where he or she is, but will recognize that it is a place in which he or she feels accepted and understood. The relaxation that accompanies this reaction can be seen in patients' faces.

In the use of transference, the major difference between working with demented and non-demented older people lies in the extent to which we interpret the transference. We do expect the transference itself to be one of the mutative factors, but not necessarily the interpretation of it. The amount of interpretation depends, as it always does, on the amount of cognitive capacity the patient has, as well as on his or her psychological sophistication.

Although it seems paradoxical, the most common type of transference – placing the therapist in a parental role – can take place with patients who are older than their therapist. Allowing a temporary dependency when we are placed in the parental role enhances the patient's feeling of safety. The patient will see the therapist as a strong, powerful figure who provides the protection and power he or she can no longer provide for him or herself. Because such patients trust the therapist, they can allow themselves to receive strength and power and ally themselves with it.

Goldfarb advocates 'accepting the patient's delegation of oneself as parental surrogate'. He states:

> Once done, the therapist as parental surrogate accepts the patient's belief that he will be of help to the patient as he hoped the ... actual parents ... would be ... The therapist can use his status to suggest to the patient constructive action which yields success.
>
> (Goldfarb, 1975: 135)

The use of this power is very delicate and care must be given to prevent its abuse. Suggestions given by the therapist can range from ways to proceed in interpersonal relationships to use of the bathroom on a regular basis. In the best of circumstances, the patient, having identified with the powerful parent/therapist, takes ownership of the suggestions, and takes pride in his or her successful behaviours.

At other times the patient treats the therapist as if the therapist were his child, spouse or sibling. One patient with whom I worked admonished me for the infrequency of our meetings, just as she did her own daughter. I addressed her feelings of abandonment and longing, and was able to show her that she was actually displacing feelings towards her daughter onto me. In this case I had an opportunity to work with the daughter as well, and was able to teach her to reply in an empathic rather than a defensive manner to her mother's accusations, without increasing the frequency of her visits. Empathy enabled the daughter to become an ally in understanding her mother's feelings, rather than being seen as the unfeeling enemy who abandoned her.

We cannot interpret transference in the classical way with people who have lost the ability to compare and engage in 'as if' (metaphorical) thinking. When that is the case, we can use the transference in the way we use it with children and primitive patients – by acting it rather than interpreting it. We can be the strong parent when that is needed, or we can be the loving child. As the first example above illustrates, sometimes the patient will believe that he or she has some control over us, and through that power re-establish some of his or her lost self-esteem and mastery. Regression to grandiosity will take over. When he or she was a child, after all, if his or her grandiose self was responded to positively by his or her parents, he or she would have had a growth in self-esteem. In the transference, this can be enacted or re-enacted, for a positive emotional experience.

In the transference we can at times view the patient as he or she was in the past and as he or she wants to be viewed. We become a carrier of his or her past. The initiation and repetition of his or her stories proves that we've heard them and remember them. This frequently permits letting go of the constant repetitions about which families tend to complain.

In general, in psychotherapy with demented older people, there is on the therapist's part more activity, more informality, more flexibility and more creativeness. There is also more eclecticism, for the therapist must have behavioural, cognitive and supportive skills to call upon when necessary, along with the skills for conducting dynamic treatment. For example, supportive psychotherapy skills are often useful during the initial stages of therapy when the relationship is being established. Behavioural-therapy skills are often useful when a trusting patient is willing to try a new way of doing something that will enhance his or her own independent functioning.

Ventilation of strong feelings should be encouraged during the psycho-therapy sessions. We will not always know exactly what feeling the patient is expressing. But when they cry, if we can stay with them and not deny their feelings by telling them they shouldn't feel that way, an important catharsis can occur. As with other patients, the demented older person can get past the feeling and on to other things.

The therapist must search for places within the session where the patient can make decisions, and thus move toward some sense of mastery. For example, encouraging the patient to decide where to sit, whether the shades are up or down, whether to keep the door open or closed, whether to take a walk or stay in the room for the session, are all important areas of control for someone who no longer feels confident about making decisions. When using an agenda for the session – written or verbal – the patient can be the one to decide the order in which to cover the items.

Family members report a carry-over of feelings of mastery. We can of course teach caretakers to search for similar areas of control at home to reinforce the patient's self-esteem.

Life review is a part of all therapy, but with older people, and particularly demented older people, it is important to conduct the life review in a systematic way. Organization of the life review can be facilitated by props such as outlines, pictures, maps and diaries. Among the goals of life-review therapy are seeing and valuing the patient as he or she was in the past and helping return to him or her some of the sense of mastery and self-worth that he or she had formerly. Life-review therapy also facilitates the mourning process, for it helps the patient to grieve and to be liberated from the past, thereby enhancing his or her ability to face the present (Butler and Lewis, 1974; Hausman, 1980).

In our time with the demented patient, we must try to give rather than ask for. This means as many declarative statements as possible. It means refraining from asking 'why' or 'what' to the extent we do with non-demented patients. Questioning can feel to the demented patient like having his or her deficiences underlined. Questions put the patient on the spot and increase his or her anxiety. Instead of asking, the therapist must find ways to give – to suggest to the patient how he or she feels, to remind him or her about people from the past, tell him or her about experiences between the patient and us. We must not be afraid to be wrong. After all, hitting an emotional chord once in a session is not a bad score. When that emotional chord is touched it is obvious, for tension is visibly reduced. Thoughts expressed by the patient after this special moment are often very clear communications; with further clarification by the therapist further relief and relaxation take place. This is comparable to the 'moment of insight', so gratifying for any therapist and patient, no matter what the patient's age or cognitive capabilities.

SPECIAL TECHNIQUES

Many special techniques can be used to enhance the therapeutic process with elderly patients who have dementing illnesses. Each therapist invents his or her own repertory of devices. Some that have been found useful follow.

More frequent and shorter psychotherapy sessions often bring about better results with this population of patients. Meeting with the patient two or three times per week for 15 to 30 minutes, rather than the usual once per week for 50 minutes, can enhance emotional and cognitive carry-over from one session to the next, and the ability to recognize both the therapist and the material might be greater. Regular scheduling of therapy sessions can give needed structure to the patient's week, and are often the only regular place the patient has to go. Sessions of greater frequency with shorter duration are often possible for patients who can get to the therapist's office on their own, or for patients seen in institutions.

Sessions held at the patient's best time of day are more productive. To get to know the patient's full range, it is helpful to have an occasional session at other times of day as well. This is also useful for increasing the therapist's empathy with the caretakers.

Use of short, simple sentences enhances the demented patient's comprehension. As in all therapy, minimizing the amount the therapist says at any one time is a wise practice.

Keeping the therapy session as a place where deficiencies are not pointed out and where details are not corrected enhances the patient's ability to feel safe and protected.

For patients who find it confusing and overstimulating to make choices about the way the session is conducted, doing things the same way each time can enhance the sense of security.

Periodic verbal summaries throughout the session, done by the patient if possible, or by the therapist if necessary, help keep the focus on the work at hand.

A notebook containing the agenda for the next session and written summaries for each session allows the patient to refresh his or her memory. The notebook is for the patient to take home. If there is danger of the patient's losing it or forgetting to bring it to the next meeting, it can be written in duplicate or photocopied.

Many therapists have found it helpful to make phone calls between sessions, and particularly before each session, to remind the patient of the therapist's existence, that the session is about to take place, and to remind him or her to look in his or her notebook to review what was discussed last time and what you might be talking about this time.

The use of pictures for focusing on a topic is helpful in preventing rambling and in bringing out deep feelings. It is important to find pictures with which that particular patient can identify. The pictures from the 'senior apperception test' are sometimes useful for this purpose (Bellak and Bellak, 1973). Even better, their own scrapbooks, photographs and momentos, or an album created in the therapy sessions, can be used for this purpose.

Telling stories – from the patient's own past, or analogies and fables or something from the newspaper that is relevant – stimulates memories and feelings and helps to organize thinking. In addition, as was mentioned above, sometimes the therapist's telling the patient's story convinces him or her that someone important values that story and is holding it. Knowing that the memory is held by the therapist may decrease the patient's need to be overly repetitive.

Certain behaviours on the therapist's part that would not be appropriate with non-demented patients might be therapeutic with this population – like touching, hand holding, eating together. Eating is an emotionally and socially charged experience. Those patients who are seen on home visits often have no opportunity to serve in the role of host without great performance anxiety. Serving tea to a non-judgemental, important person with whom the patient has learned he or she can relax can enhance self-esteem as well as functional ability. At other times, having coffee in the therapist's office or in a restaurant relaxes the patient enough to bring forth memories and feelings that might not otherwise emerge.

Special techniques are unique to each patient and to each therapist. The main deterrent to the use of special techniques is rigidity within the therapist about how he or she is supposed to conduct him or herself professionally. The therapist who works with Alzheimer's disease patients must feel comfortable with the kinds of flexibility that enhance the relationship and bring about change.

CASE STUDIES

Because psychotherapy-outcome research is difficult to quantify and because virtually no guidelines have yet been developed for objective measures of the efficacy of psychodynamic psychotherapy with demented patients, the following case studies will illustrate the use of this modality with Alzheimer's patients. In the first case, Mr M, dynamic psychotherapy turned out to be inappropriate. In the other two cases, Mr D and Mrs K, it was an effective treatment.

Mr M

This 80-year-old patient, who had been a prominent political scientist during most of his adult life, was referred to me by his physician and brought to my office by his wife many years after the onset of his dementia. He had always protected his wife's feelings, and much of his self-esteem still rested on the gentlemanly way in which he responded to her and others, even though he could no longer form comprehensible sentences nor remember the subject as his sentence structure became more and more convoluted.

In two visits we developed a good rapport. His wife had previously told me of some of his recent losses. When I mentioned the losses, as well as his obvious memory problems and word-finding difficulties, he became frustrated and depressed – his cover had been blown, yet he had no resources to remedy the situation.

At this point I realized that proceeding in this way could turn my office and our relationship into associations with low self-esteem and inability to cope. It was not too late to help him regroup his defences and forget the momentary disturbance. He did not appear to have the capacity to work in the way I had anticipated, and we had not had a chance to develop a relationship of trust before his dementia became severe. We switched from a psychodynamic approach to some life review work, family support and environmental manipulation.

Recognizing when an approach is not appropriate is as important as recognizing when it is.

Mr D

In this case I was not the therapist. Mr D, a 74-year-old man, had been referred to me by his physician for evaluation while he was still working as an economist. His boss had become concerned with a deterioration in his work and had called Mr D's wife. In conjunction with his geriatrician and a neurologist, and after ruling out all other known causes of his cognitive losses, he was diagnosed as having senile dementia of the Alzheimer's type, senile onset. At the time of the diagnosis, I offered to see Mr D in psychotherapy, but his wife turned down the offer for him. Several months later she came to see me herself in order to explore her feelings about his condition. After a while I was able to convince her that psychotherapy might be beneficial to him as well. She eventually agreed, and I referred Mr D to a colleague whom I supervised, while I continued working with his wife with two objectives – relief and resolution for her, and encouragement for her to allow him to continue in his own therapy.

Matters were more difficult than usual in this case because it was a late-life marriage. Taking care of an Alzheimer's patient at home requires a reservoir of history and affection, and in a later marriage there often hasn't been enough time to build that reservoir. In this case, both Mr and Mrs D had been widowed earlier in life and both had high hopes for the current marriage. His Alzheimer's disease, coming about 6 years after they married, was a cruel blow. On the other hand, this case was made easier by some factors – the money spent on the therapy was his, not theirs; they had good health insurance coverage; he was still able to negotiate the public transportation system; his own son and daughter-in-law were in favour of the treatment.

Periodically Mrs D balked. She would keep returning to the point of view that it seemed crazy for him to be engaging in dynamic psychotherapy. 'When I mention Dr E, he doesn't even know who she is.' Mrs D talked about how she could send him to a geriatric day centre for almost a whole week for what one psychotherapy session cost. She started to engage in a lot of resistant sabotage – scheduling other things for him 'by mistake' at the time of his therapy house, paying the bills late. Yet all the while she kept saying he was calmer, more at peace, and even more cognitively competent after his sessions with Dr E.

Dr E reported that transference was largely to an analyst he had had 40 years earlier – a good experience from his twenties of which he had a strong emotional memory. He often confused his current therapist with the former one, even though they were different sexes. Dr E eventually pieced together a lot of what he had accomplished in his early psychoanalysis, and would bring it up herself when it seemed relevant. She always knew when she hit a responsive chord – his agitation would noticeably diminish.

Mr D was able to meet many of the goals of dynamic psychotherapy. He had a strong feeling of being cared about and valued in the relationship with his therapist. He had an emotional outlet. He was able to grieve over the loss of his first wife and of his career. He was able to use the defence of denial periodically throughout the therapy – a defence that served him well when he chose not to face his inevitable deterioration. He retained coping skills and role functioning much longer than would have been expected if one judged from his mental status examination.

One example of maintenance of coping skills was particularly interesting. Despite severe losses in memory, judgement, computational ability and ability to abstract, and despite many deficits in his ability to perform activities of daily living, he continued to use the transportation system, do the shopping and engage in sexual relations. In his therapy sessions, a main focus was on his sense of control over his life. Since Dr E and I were collaborating with the permission of both Mr and Mrs D, I was able to discuss the matter of his sense of control with his wife. She was able to reinforce some of his mastery at home.

All of these factors helped Mr D to regain some of the self-esteem which was lost when he had to stop working, and the enhanced self-esteem in turn permitted him to experience other accomplishments.

During nearly a year of successful psychotherapy, Mr D's decline seemed to slow and he and his family had many good times together. Eventually, because of wandering and incontinence and other problems which made home management increasingly difficult, he was scheduled to go into a nursing home. Shortly before his admission, he died in the hospital of another disease.

Mrs D continued in treatment for 2 months and returned a year later for three sessions. It was clear to her, to me, and to Dr E that his having continued in therapy had been well worthwhile. I also found out that the therapist had been the only person to whom Mr D had revealed his knowledge that he had Alzheimer's disease. All through the deterioration, he was able to do two things which were of utmost importance to him – continue finding his way to Dr E's office, and continue to protect his family from knowing that he knew.

Mrs K

This patient was referred to me before there was any evidence of dementia. Her ex-son-in-law, the widower of one of her two daughters, referred her to me and volunteered to pay her bill. He lived out of town. Her local daughter resented both the referral and the continuing therapy. She felt it was easy for her ex-brother-in-law to write a cheque, but that no-one understood the extent of the burden her mother was to her. This resentment was addressed to some extent by the daughter's joining a short-term group for people with elderly parents (Hausman, 1979), where, in addition to receiving support, she learned some ways to communicate with her mother and to arrange for her a more structured and manageable environment. However, the lifelong relationship between them was too poor, and the daughter was too resistant to change, for there to be much progress in her outlook or attitude during a short-term group experience.

Positive feelings developed very quickly with this 80-year-old woman, mostly because the transference was to her idealized dead daughter. However, she also saw me in a parental role at times, and sought advice on many matters. We were able to work together for 2 years before any dementia became pronounced. I was able to learn many of her memories, and subsequently to use them to lead her to important subjects and unresolved issues long after she had the ability to initiate these topics herself. Since recognition is easier than recall, she found things I brought up familiar – events from her past, events from our past together, feelings I knew she had, insights I knew could comfort her. Knowing her so well enabled me to name feelings she was currently having. When her disease progressed to the point that it was severe, I did most of the talking. I learned many things from working with her that have been useful with other patients.

Mrs K eventually went to a nursing home where we continued to meet. When I first saw her there, she did not recognize me in the new surroundings. I was frustrated at the amount of time I had to spend during each visit explaining to her who I was. Eventually, I got the idea of having one of the staff (who often resist outside therapists as much or more than the family) to approach her a few seconds in advance and say, in as enthusiastic a voice as possible, 'Dr Hausman is here!' I would watch the wheels turning in her head, and when a smile and calmness crossed her face, I would approach her and she would know me.

As her Alzheimer's disease progressed, the positive after-effects of our therapy sessions would last for shorter and shorter periods. Eventually she was no longer able to recognize me or to get any more from being with me than from being with a sensitive staff member. By this time some of the staff had become receptive to learning ways to be with Mrs K therapeutically. When I stopped seeing Mrs K regularly, I worked from time to time with them.

With both Mr D and Mrs K, termination of psychotherapy came at the time of the patient's death. This is as it often is, and should be, with Alzheimer's disease patients. When the therapist becomes an important component of the patient's increasingly circumscribed life, we must try not to become another of his or her losses.

CONCLUSION

Psychodynamic psychotherapy is a useful modality for some elderly people who are victims of Alzheimer's disease. The earlier in the progression of the disease the relationship with the therapist begins, the more chance is there for successful attainment of the goals of psychodynamic psychotherapy. Modifications of traditional techniques are increasingly necessary as the disease progresses. Many of the techniques which are helpful to the therapist can be taught to care-givers and used to improve the emotional climate between the patient and the care-giver.

REFERENCES

Bellak, L. and Bellak, S. (1973) *Senior Apperception Technique*, Larchmont, New York: C.P.S. Inc.

Butler, R. and Lewis, M. (1974) 'Life review therapy', *Geriatrics* pp. 165–73.

Cath, S.H. (1982) 'Psychoanalysis and psychoanalytic psychotherapy of the older patient', *Journal of Geriatric Psychiatry* 15: 43–53.

Freud, S. (1924) 'On psychotherapy', *Collected Papers* vol. 1, London: Hogarth Press, pp. 220–48.

Goldfarb, A. (1975) 'Depression in the old and aged', in R. Flach and C. Draghi (eds) *Nature and Treatment of Depression*, Ann Arbor, Michigan: Books on Demand, University Microfilms International.

Hausman, C. (1979) 'Short-term counseling groups for people with elderly parents', *Gerontologist* 19: 102–7.

—— (1980) 'Life review therapy', *Journal of Gerontological Social Work* 3 (2): 31–7.

Miller, N. and Cohen, G. (eds) (1981) *Clinical Aspects of Alzheimer's Disease and Senile Dementia*, New York: Raven Press.

Verwoerdt, A. (1981) 'Individual psychotherapy in senile dementia', in N. Miller and G. Cohen (eds) *Clinical Aspects of Alzheimer's Disease and Senile Dementia*, New York: Raven Press.

Chapter 12

Validation therapy with late-onset dementia populations

Naomi Feil

SUMMARY

This chapter presents the background, theory base, assumptions and implementation of validation therapy with late-onset dementia populations. The interrelationship of physical losses with developmental coping techniques is also discussed. When recent memory, mobility and sensory acuity fail, the very old disoriented person 'restores' the past in an attempt to find safety and comfort in an increasingly estranged environment, and in order to resolve their life. The validation worker empathizes with the disoriented person, acknowledging the meaning behind the behaviours and works with the emotional content of communication when the factual content is not clear. The validation approach can be used on a one-to-one basis and/or in a group setting. The specific one-to-one methods for the working with the four stages of disorientation are presented in this chapter.

INTRODUCTION

The background to the validation approach is presented first, using specific case histories and clinical studies. The validation approach is compared with reality orientation, behaviour modification and remotivation techniques. Thereafter, the goals, principles and beliefs of validation are presented. Finally, the method for catagorizing behaviours into four discrete and progressive stages is presented along with specific verbal and non-verbal interaction techniques for each stage. The chapter concludes with an overview of research pertaining to the validation approach up to the present time.

The validation approach is now practised in over 6,000 long-term care facilities, community-based support groups, adult treatment centres, and hospitals in the United States, Canada, the Netherlands, Norway and Australia. The interest in validation is not surprising since there are no pharmacological treatments or cures for dementia yet, and given the demographic projections for the dramatic increases in the numbers of elderly persons, including those with dementia. The goals of validation are to stimulate verbal and non-verbal communication in order to help restore feelings of dignity and wellbeing, and to help persons resolve the meaning of their lives.

DEFINITION

Validation therapy is three things: (1) a way of catagorizing the behaviours that are exhibited by the disoriented elderly into four discrete and progressive stages, (2) a method for communication (verbally and non-verbally) with persons in each stage and (3) a theory of late-onset disorientation in elders who have led relatively normal lives well into their seventh and eighth decades. This latter criteria identifies such elders with those diagnosed as late-onset Alzheimer's disease patients (Jones, 1987). The validation approach means accepting and validating the feelings of the demented old person; to acknowledge their reminiscences, losses and the human needs that underlie their behaviours without trying to insert or force new insights. Validating includes: reflecting a person's feelings, helping them to express unmet human needs, restoring well-established social roles (which in turn help to motivate expression of social behaviours), facilitating feelings of wellbeing and stimulating interaction with others (Feil, 1984; 1985; 1989).

BACKGROUND

The author began to develop the validation approach in 1963, whilst working as a group therapist for the 'Special program for the senile' (Weil, 1966), at the Montefiore Home for the Aged, Cleveland, Ohio. The age range of persons in this programme was between 76 and 101 years; diagnoses comprised of 'senile psychosis' and 'organic brain damage' often complicated by circulatory insufficiency. At autopsy, the majority of these residents had Alzheimer's plaques and neurofibrillary degeneration. The author, in reviewing the case histories of these residents, found that they had led normal lives until their late seventh or eighth decades when symptoms of disorientation began to appear. These residents did not respond to reality orientation, remotivation or insight-oriented group therapy; instead they would 'withdraw, vegetate and become increasingly hostile when confronted with present reality' (Feil, 1967). These observations led the author to develop a new approach which did not insist upon participation in present reality, and which did not result in such withdrawal.

VALIDATION GROUPWORK RESULTS: 1972

After 6 months of using the newly developed validation techniques to work with the disoriented residents in the group programmes already described, it became apparent that their anxiety was reduced. Validation techniques did not demand cognitive improvement, but rather accepted their loss of: (1) social controls, (2) cognitive thinking, (3) sensory acuity, (4) reflective self-awareness, (5) speech and (6) mobility. Listening to their verbal and non-verbal behavioural messages, the author found a pattern to their behaviour. Their lifelong accumulated wisdom (or crystallized intelligence, as some modern psychologists call it) was often preserved despite severe cognitive deficits. In spite of the substantial brain damage incurred in dementia, persons still try to communicate their feelings of fear and their awareness that 'something is wrong'. Because of the progressive damage to speech that occurs in dementia, such communication is often cryptic, and very symbolic. For example, an 86-year-old Russian immigrant, former housewife, began opening drawers in search of something. When asked 'What are you looking for, Mrs K?' she replied, 'I'm looking for yesterday. I must untangle the noodles in the mirrors of my mind.' Another lady of 93 years, would stop singing whenever she reached the word 'crazy' in the song 'A Bicycle Built for Two' (Daisy, Daisy). At this point, she would laugh, mockingly. When asked why she had stopped singing, she replied, 'It's better to be crazy; then it doesn't matter what you do!'

After 6 months of weekly, 1-hour group sessions, the author found that respecting and validating the accumulated wisdom of such disoriented elderly through both one-to-one (or personal) and group approaches produced diverse, favourable results. Both approaches include the use of (1) touch, (2) close eye contact, (3) a low, caring tone of voice, (4) linking the non-verbal (symbolic) behaviour to the individual's unmet human needs, (5) mirroring non-verbal behaviours and (6) matching the rhythms and repeated movements of the more severely impaired residents with one's own body movements or music.

Results of this early research (Feil, 1972) using the group approach included: (1) heightened energy during interactions using a validation approach, (2) increased verbal communication and (3) improved social behaviour and control of behaviour. In validation group settings residents: assumed new social roles (presumably through tapping memories of previous social interactions); began to communicate with each other instead of with the group worker; and they began to show caring behaviours towards each other. Feelings of wellbeing were expressed in the form of positive comments, smiling, laughing and increases in eye and body contact (Feil, 1972).

VALIDATION COMPARED TO OTHER TECHNIQUES

Three examples of a social worker's notes, made after residents had participated in 6 months of reality orientation sessions, and then contrasted to the validation approach follow:

Example one

Mrs F constantly stared into space, shouting: 'There's Mother! She's got my laundry. I have to leave this place to help her carry it.' Trying to orient Mrs F to present reality, I told her in a quiet, calm voice: 'You are 95 years old and your mother is dead.' Mrs F nodded and said to me: 'Honey, I know that and you know that. But my mother doesn't know that, and I have to help her right now.'

By contrast, utilizing validation techniques and respecting Mrs F's need to help her mother, the social worker achieved the following. 'Mrs F, your mother worked very hard, you wanted to help her, you love your mother very much don't you?' Mrs F nodded, burst into tears, sobbing: 'She was a wonderful mother. I should have helped her. She didn't have to die so young.' Mrs F knew, at some level, that her mother was dead. After she had expressed her grief and guilt, her facial muscles relaxed, her voice became less frantic, and after 6 months she no longer stared into space trying to restore images of her mother. She began to interact with the validation worker (in this instance the social worker) increasingly. Once her feelings had been acknowledged, shared with someone she could trust, and validated, the grief lessened.

Example two

Mr T is worsening after each contact. He is uncontrolled, abusive and refuses to listen to the nursing staff. He must be restrained and medicated for his own, and others' protection. Psychiatric referral requested.

Mr T unties his restraints with magnificent dexterity ... he often slides right down in the chair ... shouting 'God damn SOB let me out of here. I hate her. Stinker John! You stink.'

When using reality orientation to reason logically with Mr T the following pattern occurs.

John, you are living in a home for the aged; you can't get out of the chair because you might fall. When you shout so loudly nobody wants to sit near you. If you stop shouting we can read the paper. Look at the headline; can you read the date?

Mr T grabbed the newspaper and threw it on the floor, spitting at the social worker: 'I don't give a damn about your f—— paper! You can take your date and shove it.'

Using behaviour modification methods, and walking away whenever Mr T started to swear or become abusive and rewarding him with attention whenever he was quiet, did not work either. Mr T's swearing increased; he began kicking other residents and spitting at them and was only quiet when medicated or sleeping. Ignoring his outbursts increased his 'acting out' or negative behaviours.

Using a validation approach resulted in interactions such as that described next. 'You hate this place don't you Mr T? You can't stand anyone here. You hate this chair, being locked up like this. You can't move. You used to travel; you were a salesman, weren't you?' Mr T replied 'Damn right!' Respecting his anger and linking his aggressive behaviour to his unmet human need (the need to be useful), gradually helped to establish trust and eventually Mr T began to strike out less and to communicate more verbally.

Example three

Mrs K tried to give me some 'play' money (like for the game Monopoly) in honour of the birth of my son. To orientate her, I told her that play money has no value. Her face fell and she began to cry. The lady sitting next to her, also moderately demented, said to me: 'What do you care if it's play money. Giving makes her feel good.' It was true, Mrs K had been a well-known philanthropist in the community. She was restoring her sense of worth by giving me the money.

These old disoriented residents were not helped by remotivation techniques either. They could not relate to the objects and props that I used to stimulate awareness of present reality. Their attention span was too short. They could examine a flower for only a few moments before dropping it. They could not read the newspaper or poems used in the group. They could not look outside to establish the season of the year, yet alone remember the day or the date.

Such residents were unable to achieve new insights into their behaviours because of the cognitive damage to logical- and associative-thinking capacity. Thus, they had also lost reflective self-awareness. Reality orientation, behaviour modification and remotivation methods did not help these moderately demented persons precisely because of the damage to their logical thinking.

THEORY BASE FOR THE VALIDATION APPROACH*

Four theories have relevance to validation techniques. They are: (1) Maslow's (1968) 'universal human needs hierarchy', (2) Erikson's (1950) developmental stage theory, (3) Jones and Zeiss (1985), Jones and Burns (Chapter 5, this volume) reminiscing disorientation theory, and (4) Miesen's (1990) work on 'parent-fixation' and his adaptation of Bowlby's attachment theory to dementia.

It is beyond the scope of this chapter to discuss in detail the relevance of these theories to the validation approach in detail. However, the following brief synopsis should provide the reader with the key associations.

Validation techniques provide a means of helping disoriented elderly persons to meet the 'higher order needs' in Maslow's scheme, in addition to the custodial care that is so often the sole extent of planning care for them.

Erikson defined the final goal of lifespan development as being that of achieving 'ego integrity or despair'. This seems too global to be useful for work specifically with the disoriented elderly, and so for the purposes of using the validation approach, a ninth stage has been added; that of 'resolution versus vegetation'. Within this stage we can focus care more specifically for persons for whom the past is the predominant focus. They can be assisted to resolve their lives by care-givers encouraging them: to 'wrap up loose ends', to justify having lived and to prepare for death.

Reminiscing disorientation theory describes a mechanism for disorientation, and helps put into a larger context the importance of reminiscing with persons whose focus increasingly becomes lodged in the past. (For a detailed discussion see Chapter 5, this volume.)

Miesen has demonstrated that the dementing process activates attachment behaviour, particularly those behaviours and memories associated with memories of parents. (For a detailed discussion see Chapter 4 in this book.)

VALIDATION GOALS

The primary goal of the validation approach is to help the older disoriented person to be as happy as possible. When their struggle to resolve life is respected and validated by a trusted, significant person in present time, withdrawal inward is halted. With their dignity restored, they feel relieved and make new efforts to respond to the maximum of their ability. Buried emotions often come to light in these persons, and when these old hurts are acknowledged and validated the disoriented elderly begin to communicate (with the person(s) they trust) to the maximum of their potential. The process of validation cannot restore damaged brain tissue, but it can help to stimulate whatever capacities are dormant and yet intact.

The validation worker does not expect disoriented elderly to behave in the same way the younger adults would. The worker does not try to provide new insights into a person's behaviour, or to insert or probe for feelings that are not openly expressed, neither do they judge, analyse or hope to change the disoriented person. Rather, the worker accepts the person wherever they are at the moment, and is committed to help the person to reach their own goal, not the goals of the worker, and not to demand of the person that they become and remain oriented. The validation worker tries to reduce anxiety and to strengthen wellbeing through acknowledging the intuitive wisdom the elderly person still possesses, and by accepting them for the way they are.

ASSUMPTIONS BEHIND VALIDATION

The condition of the brain is not the exclusive regulator of behaviour in old–old age. Validation is based upon the belief that behaviour in old age does not depend solely on the condition of the brain but on a combination of the following physical and psychosocial factors: (1) damage to recent factual memory, (2) damage to eyes, ears, mobility, (3) accumulated losses (loved ones, social roles, job, identity), (4) the 'coping mechanisms' (or coping repertoire) that a person developed throughout their lifetime in response to these losses and (5) the extent to which the person has completed the developmental tasks of Erikson.

Clearly, cognitive functioning in old age is dependent on a multiplicity of factors. Neuroscientists acknowledge that some persons with considerable brain atrophy continue to function quite well whereas normally persons appear to be incapacitated with similar amounts of damage (Wells, 1977; Roth, 1984).

PHYSICAL LOSSES EMPHASIZE EMOTIONAL NEEDS

In 1950 the neurosurgeon, Wilder Penfield wrote: 'The patient, himself, can activate the memory from within, stimulating the same pattern of cortical nerve cell connections without the use of the sense organs.' Similarly, in the disoriented elderly, it seems that dim images, seen through damaged eyes in present reality, can trigger sharp, photographic-like images from the past. 'The earlier an event or image has been imprinted on memory, the longer it is retained', wrote Schettler and Boyd in 1969. Miesen's (1990) research with persons with dementia confirms that early, strong emotional memories, particularly of home and parents, seem to remain intact longest during the progression of dementia.* Brain damage can lead to a return of early, well-established patterns and images. For example, a 90-year-old demented woman with poor eyesight 'saw' her mother through her eidetic memory. A spot on the wall triggered this image of her mother, and temporarily 'became' her mother. She had to tell her mother that she loved her in order to make peace before she died, and this need must have contributed to her visual search and retrieval of her mother's image. A validation worker would accept the need of the 90-year-old lady to 'restore' her mother and would not argue with her or insist that her mother was dead, but neither would the worker pretend that the mother was alive. Often, on a deep level of awareness, the disoriented elderly know that their parents are dead, but they still need to restore them to feel safe or to tie up loose ends. The worker explores without judging by asking such questions as: 'You see your mother? What does she look like? You need to tell her that you love her?'

Damage to the kinesthetic sensory brain areas can also contribute to the reactivation of past memories in the disoriented elderly. Piaget (Ginsburg and Opper, 1969) wrote that muscles 'perform an abbreviated imitation ... the sensorimotor forerunner of verbal behaviour ... When the object is no longer present, the movements in abbreviated form are the same movements involved in the initial perception.' Body movements can take disoriented old people to the past. A slight flick of the wrist can remind a disoriented man of his work, Mrs G's shiny black purse 'became' her filing cabinet as she tried to restore her identity as a file clerk to survive feelings of uselessness in the nursing home.

Movements trigger memories as well as other stimuli such as food, music and pets. Sometimes, self-stimulation is used to trigger such memories. Mrs K could not see her hand clearly, in addition to dementia her eyesight was very impaired. She held her hand in front of her, caressing it, crooning and rocking it as though it was a baby. This is the way she restored her identity as a mother. The validation worker understood her need to restore her identity as a mother and used touch, close eye contact and mirroring of Mrs K's movements to work with her. The worker said 'You love your baby very much.' Mrs K responded and looked up at the validation worker, and began to talk and sing with her. Mrs K no longer needed to use her hand as a symbol of a baby in order to feel worthwhile, the validation worker had become a significant other for her.

When speech is damaged, body movements are all that is left to communicate with. In the disoriented elderly, body movements express three basic human needs: (1) the need for love and safety, (2) the need to be useful, to restore one's identity and work and (3) the need to communicate strong, basic emotions and to be understood. Strong (raw) emotions often spill out for the first time when a person suffers brain damage. Loss of brain functioning in certain areas leads inevitably to loss of control and disinhibition occurs stimultaneously with extreme expression of emotion. The severely disoriented old person is no longer able to conform to social rules and becomes utterly honest about the expression of their feelings (repressed or current).

It appears that current losses in present time often evoke memories of losses in the past. The losses are different, but the feeling of pain, grief, shame, fear and rage can be the same. Losses fuse into each other when memory becomes impaired. In listening to the expression of feelings of loss, the validation workers does not 'feed the fantasy' or 'buy into the delusion', they only acknowledge that the feelings are real even though the events happened long ago. For example, when Mr S, rocking and pounding away in the arm of his chair, is hammering an imaginary nail to restore his feeling of usefulness as a carpenter and the validation worker says 'You were a fine carpenter', Mr S nods and begins to talk about his work. He no longer feels isolated.

CATEGORIZING BEHAVIOURS INTO FOUR STAGES AND APPLYING STAGE-SPECIFIC COMMUNICATION TECHNIQUES

There are four, generally discrete stages in the behaviour of persons with late-onset dementia. In beginning to work with a resident the validation worker observes their behaviours, collects a 'mini-life review' (Feil, 1982), and identifies which stage a person belongs in by collecting information from family interview and the medical history.

Stage one: malorientation (characterized by confabulation and self-defensive behaviour)

Mrs R, aged 89, with pursed lips points an accusing finger at the house-keeper who has come to clean out her cluttered room. Oranges lie in the toilet bowl; Kleenex tissues are stuffed under the mattress springs; buttons, bits of dried-up food, debris, old bundles of newspapers tied up with 40-year-old hair ribbons, letters and safety pins litter the room. Mrs R is a hoarder and shrieks at the housekeeper, 'You keep out of my drawer! Thief! You stole my oranges. I had six cooling in the toilet.' If the house-keeper was trained in the validation approach she would not argue with Mrs R, but rather acknowledge that there is meaning behind her hoardings and accusative behaviours.

The housekeeper would realize that Mrs R had led a normal life until recently when she began blaming others for any little thing that 'went wrong' or that threatened her. A host of losses have overwhelmed Mrs R simultaneously, for the first time in her life. Her eyesight is worse, her left ear doesn't hear and her recent memory is fading. Her daughter moved 300 miles away last week. The more Mrs R loses, the more she blames others. She blamed others throughout her life when things went wrong, but this was within the realm of normal behaviour. Blaming was her way of coping when life became difficult, and when she could not assume respon-sibility herself for the things that went wrong. At 89, Mrs R cannot face the multitude of losses that accompany aging and a fading memory. Her blaming is much worse than it ever was. Mrs R is usually oriented to present time although she is becoming forgetful. She is an example of someone in the early, first stage of dementia, someone who is *maloriented*, not yet fully disoriented. Aware that something is 'wrong', forgetful, afraid of losing control over her life and burdened by unacknowledged feelings from the past, she hoards to keep control and blames others for self-defence.

The physical characteristics of malorientation

The following are typical physical characteristics of the first stage: eyeslits narrowed, eyes very focused and directed; general body tension; facial muscles tight; shallow breathing; direct, purposeful movements; clear speech but because recent memory is beginning to fade there are occasional lapses or repetitions in conversation; no continence, arms folded, fingers often pointing, usually clutching a purse, raincoat, cane, wallet or bags.

Emotional characteristics of malorientation

Typical emotional characteristics of stage one include: rigid (social controls) adherence to social proprieties, avoidance of physical contact or touch, intimacy and exposure of feelings; desperate efforts to hold onto old, familiar social roles; confabulation to hide her increasing confusion from others; threatened by the presence of persons who are more severely affected by dementia themselves and resistant to change because of limited coping mechanisms, and thereby overly dependent on familiar routines and defences.

Maloriented persons often express feelings of fear and insecurity by blaming others. Some persons in this stage blame others for 'poisoning' their food or for stealing jewellery or other items of strong personal value. Memory is waning, and persons in stage one often forget where they put things with the consequence that family are accused of stealing from them.

The validation worker accepts that maloriented persons cannot face so many losses and that their blaming, in this final stage of life is functional. (If Mrs R, for example, were younger, her blaming would be pathological not functional, and the worker would try to help her achieve insight and to help her develop new coping mechanisms.) In very old demented persons the validation worker uses techniques that lessen anxiety, make a person feel safer and reduce their blaming behaviours. These techniques are directed at building trust and facilitating non-threatening communication with maloriented persons.

Helping techniques for stage one

1   Listen with empathy.
2   Explore content of communication using non-threatening questions such as: *Who? What? Where? When? How?* Avoid asking *Why?* because this question implies 'cause and effect' and is cognitively the most complex question of all to answer. Since the maloriented are trying to deny the damage to their memory and logical-thinking ability, this question is very threatening for them. Maloriented persons do not want to be analysed or patronized. Avoid touch other than a handshake with these persons.
3   Use 'repetition' when in doubt, if you cannot think of a reply quickly enough, or, if you have not caught the gist of what the person was

saying. Repeat or paraphrase the key words from the person's most recent conversation.

4   People generally speak using words that relate to their preferred sense: visual, auditory or kinesthetic. It is helpful to be aware of any strong preference and to build trust by choosing words that the person would use themselves. If a person uses 'seeing' or visual words you can use words such as 'look like,' 'appear', 'imagine'. If a person prefers their auditory sense it is helpful to use 'hearing' words such as 'sounds like', 'loud', 'noisy'; persons with a strong kinesthetic sense use mainly 'feeling' words like 'hurts', 'how does it strike you', 'drive you crazy', 'hits you hard'.

5   Using 'polarity' refers to asking questions in the extreme, for example, 'When was it worst?' 'How often did it happen?' 'Was there ever a time when it didn't happen?' Maloriented persons can express anger, sadness and fear without being threatened by exposing their feelings overtly when questions are asked using polarity.

6   Reminiscence is a useful method to use with the maloriented because they do not yet confuse past and present time, although they do experience occasional confusion. Using reminiscence can help to uncover information about how a person coped in the past, for example: 'What happened when you lost your husband? Did you live alone then? What did you do to overcome the loneliness then?'

7   Using 'opposite' imagery can help persons focus on more positive thoughts. Help a person imagine the opposite to the situation they are currently threatened by.

How often do you validate someone?

In a one-to-one approach the validation worker meets the maloriented person for 5 to 10 minutes at least three times a week in long-term care settings, once a week in the community or day-care centres, and twice daily in acute-care hospital settings. In charting the behavioural changes, the worker will find that the anger gradually lessens, accusing behaviours diminish and the person become less anxious as judged by their tone of voice, muscle tone and their communications. A maloriented person will not withdraw inward if they are validated consistently. Instead they will continue to interact with family and peers without accusing others. They will save their accusations and challenges for the validation worker. They are aware that friends and family will reject them if they continue to blame them continually whereas the validation worker will not reject them, but will accept their angry feelings without confronting them.

Stage two: time confusion (characterized by a lack of awareness of the time of day, month or season and increased impairments in recent memory)

Mr L unties his restraints with dexterity. Tall, but stooped at age 94, he wanders frequently. He cannot distinguish clearly between past and present time, and, thinking of his wife he goes into Mrs T's bedroom, takes off his clothes and tries to get into bed with her, as he did for over 70 years with his wife. The nurse arrives in response to Mrs T's shrieking. In her training in the validation approach, she has recognized from the following physical and emotional characteristics that Mr L is in the second stage, and knows how to communicate with him using the six techniques described on pp. 211–12.

Physical characteristics of time confusion

Stage two is characterized by the following physical attributes: unfocused, but bright eyes; fluid movements and relaxed muscle tone; loose facial muscles; loss of sensory acuity; and often bladder incontinence. Speech is unclear, and very few specific nouns are used; a person may switch from past to present tense within the same sentence and even invent new words when they cannot find the correct 'dictionary' word. With the loss of metaphorical speech (the ability to use 'as if' constructions) already begun in the first stage, speech becomes increasingly literal and abbreviated.

Emotional characteristics of the time confused

Disinhibition increases in the second stage and persons experiencing time confusion no longer conform to social rules, and are not motivated or able to conform. With the additional damage to memory, past and present time cannot be consistently differentiated. Instead of keeping track of chronological, or clock time they make associations through the emotional tone of memories. They can jump 60 years in seconds. With eidetic vision, they restore images of people and objects from the past in order to survive the loneliness and boredom of the nursing home or hospital. This restoration of the past is functional to their survival in these environments in light of their cognitive limitations.

In the example of Mr L the nurse might encourage him to talk about his wife, about missing her and about some of his favourite memories of her. She would validate his feelings of loss. If Mr L were younger and had any chance of functioning in the community independently again, it would make sense to try to orient him to present time and place and explain that his wife was dead, but not now that he is 94 and has sustained substantial damage to recent memory.

Helping techniques for the time confused

1   Use touch liberally. Persons in stage two are not threatened by touch, but rather find it comforting. Zuckerman (1950) stated the 'previous stimulation of a group of nerve cells which has led to a state of satisfaction, increased its sensitivity to further stimulation of a like kind'. The amount of touch and the location depend upon the needs of the individual. Touching different areas triggers memories of different relationships. For example: gentle pressure on the cheek with the palm of the hand triggers feelings of a mother relationship (Buhler, 1971), whereas touches on the back of the head with a cupped hand are more likely to trigger feelings of a father relationship. Each person will respond differently depending upon their own early memories and relationships with their loved ones. Through working with touch, the validation worker can often 'become' or replace a significant, trusted person that the person in stage two is reminiscing about.

2   The use of genuine, close eye contact is very important in working with persons in time confusion because of their impaired eyesight. The worker must bend down and be very close to them for optimal interactions. Eye contact in combination with touch and a clear voice can help to stimulate verbal and non-verbal communication.

3   Use simple words to identify and talk about the emotions that persons in the second stage are demonstrating. Unlike persons in stage one, they are not threatened by this because they are not as aware of their cognitive impairments as the damage progresses.

4   In order for a worker to empathize with the resident, it is helpful if they try to match the emotion that the resident is feeling with memories of a time in their life when they experienced the same emotion.

5   Link a resident's non-verbal behaviour to their unmet human need where that is obvious. For example, if Mrs J is kissing her hand and crooning, a validation worker might gently touch her on the back of the neck, bend down and say in a soft, nurturing voice: 'You miss your baby, don't you. You love that baby a lot.' They might continue to sing a lullaby together. Such interactions can occur within a few seconds. The resident does not know who the validation worker is, but she will know that this person makes her feel safe and that her need to restore her mother has been validated. With increased feelings of self-worth she may try harder to talk, and no longer need to use her hand to symbolize a baby.

6   Because it is not always possible to determine what a resident in stage two is doing or meaning, the validation worker can use 'ambiguity' in the form of vague questions (relating to universal human needs), and non-specific pronouns (he, she, it), when trying to establish and maintain contact. The worker must try to identify the feelings that the

resident is exhibiting, even when they cannot be clearly verbally expressed. For example, Mr G points his finger into space, counting from 1 to 30 over and over. His brow is knit in deep concentration and he appears to be working hard. The validation worker moves close to make direct eye contact with Mr G and uses the ambiguous pronouns 'that' and 'it'. 'That is hard work Mr G. Does it take a long time to finish?' Mr G worked in a canning factory, counting the cans as he worked; he looks up at the worker and beams. 'Yup! Thirty cans in 30 minutes!'

Persons in stage two will never be able to participate in present reality for any length of time, in spite of intensive work with validation, because of the nature of the brain damage. However, if validated, they will interact more, talk more, express feelings of happiness and withdraw less. They will also utilize more social controls, act out less and need less restraining and tranquillizing medication. Persons in stage two also benefit from validation groups. Group work is discussed in Feil (1982) in detail and will not be covered in this chapter.

Stage three: repetitive motion (characterized by patterned self-stimulating movements and vocalizations and increasingly contractured posture)

Mr S pounds his fist against the chair. He is 92 and has lost comprehensive speech. For 63 years he was an expert cabinet maker. He sees the hammer, wood and special nails with his eidetic vision, and he uses his kinesthetic memory to move his hand to past rhythms of hammering. He is 'working' to survive the uselessness and loneliness he feels in the nursing home. The validation worker understands that he moves in order to survive and that this behaviour is purposeful for him. Mr S was oriented to present time until he was 86. His eyes failed increasingly, his knees gave out, his wife died and his recent memory became increasingly impaired. Eventually he needed to restore memories of his past work to feel safe and worthwhile.

Characteristics of the repetitive-motion stage

In this stage more damage has occurred to the eyes, ears, brain and to mobility, which is often relatively spared in earlier stages. The person in stage three continually experiences reduced levels of social contact, and, with little stimulation from the outside, withdraws inward even further. In stage three, residents cannot initiate any form of purposeful verbal or nonverbal communication with others. These persons appear to be egocentric and totally unaware of others. They stimulate themselves in the little world they have withdrawn into. Eye contact is much reduced in stage three and persons have an increasingly stooped posture, further forcing their eyes to be directed downward. Repetitive motions, rhythms, humming, pacing, clucking, moaning and singing replace verbal behaviour. Persons are no longer aware that they are incontinent and incontinence of urine and faeces often occurs in this stage. These persons re-enact former movements related to their work, for example, women in stage three can often be observed using motions resembling cleaning, dusting and waxing the furniture.

Helping behaviours for the repetitive-motion stage

1   Genuinely mirroring the repetitive movements of persons in stage three will help to establish a true and meaningful relationship. The worker knows the social history of the person with whom they are working and so can relate the characteristic movements to events and work from an individual's past. Although persons are very impaired in stage three, and may be almost blind and deaf, they still have a sense of when they are being patronized or ridiculed, and will not form a relationship if they are being treated thus.
2   Persons in the third stage express three universal needs through their movements, rather than using speech; the need for love (by folding, rocking and clucking, etc.), the need to be useful, to work (by making familiar movements to those used for work) and the need to be heard and to express their true emotions to a significant person (by shouting and swearing, etc.). The worker links the behaviour to the human need.
3   Use music and movements that are culturally meaningful. Persons in stage three may not remember the song title, but often can still sing all the words of a song, even though their speech is entirely impaired. (This is because the location of speech and music centres in the brain are located in different places, and the latter is not generally damaged as quickly as the speech centre.) The song must be familiar, with strong emotional memories, i.e. it is not helpful to sing a Jewish song in a Baptist home. Music and movements will often trigger verbal behaviours and temporary awareness of 'clock time', heighten energy and stimulate interaction, thus reducing isolation.

Stage four: the vegetative stage

In this stage, movements are minimal. The repetitive movements have stopped and there is barely enough movement to keep a person alive. The eyes are almost constantly closed in this stage. When persons in stages two and three are left alone for long intervals in care facilities, to sit in geriatric chairs without other stimulation, they progress quickly to the fourth stage. Music and touch may spontaneously trigger some verbal or non-verbal response, but it is often too late to expect proper speech or purposeful behavioural responses.

RESEARCH AND EMPIRICAL SUPPORT FOR VALIDATION THERAPY

Throughout the 28 years in which validation therapy has been used with disoriented old–old, some formal research studies have been conducted to assess its utility (Alprin, 1980; Peoples, 1982; Fritz, 1986). Two measured research studies are being conducted by The Institute for Life-Span Development and Gerontology in Akrom, Ohio and Dr Colin Sharp at South Port Community Nursing Home in Australia. Two films have been produced documenting results of validation (Edward Feil Productions, 1979 and 1986). These studies included only late-onset dementias of the Alzheimer type or related disorders. Practitioners working with both early- and late-onset dementias report 'younger people (age 40 to 80), behave differently than old–old people in spite of similar damage to brain tissue' (Edward Feil Productions, 1986). Many researchers conclude that 'the earlier the onset ... the more severe the course of the disease' (Roth, 1984).

Conducted with widely differing methodologies, together these studies provide the foundation of a body of empirical evidence supportive of the efficacy of validation therapy.

1   Feil (1972) trained observers (registered nurses and nursing assistants) at the Montefiore Home for the Aged, Cleveland, Ohio. The research team studied twelve severely disoriented nursing home residents, diagnosed organic brain syndrome with senile psychosis. They divided the twelve patients into two groups. Both groups met four times per week for approximately 25 minutes for a period of 6 months.
     Therapeutic goals were to increase positive affect and decrease negative affect in order to promote self-worth. Additional goals were to lessen demands on staff time as self-worth of patients increased.
     Results: All except one group member in the experimental group showed an increase in positive affect. Eight group members showed a decrease in negative affect. Eleven patients rated from plus 1 to 3 in interaction results indicated heightened awareness of self and an increase in feelings of self-worth in all but one group member. The charge nurse on the ward wrote: 'I found the residents less anxious on the ward as compared with those that were not included in the experimental group – and less demanding of nursing time.'
2   Alprin took a very different approach to the assessment of validation therapy. He examined its utility in the organizational level of analysis. He examined the impact of validation therapy on the therapist's attitude and behaviour as well as the disoriented very old nursing-home resident.

Alprin (1980) obtained quantifiable data with regard to behavioural changes of residents and staffs in nursing home settings. He surveyed forty-eight directors, activity personnel and social workers in sixteen homes throughout the United States who were using validation therapy with disoriented, very old residents.

Alprin reports at the conclusion of his survey: 'The evidence obtained thus far would suggest very strongly many positive changes in behavior of resident groups following validation therapy. Almost without exception, shifts in staff behaviour were in a positive direction.'

3   Peoples (1982) compared the effects of validation therapy with reality orientation in a 225-bed nursing Home. She used Hogstel's tool for assessing the degree of confusion.

> Behaviors showed qualitative improvements in behavior for seven of the ten subjects in the Validation group compared with three ofr the eight subjects in the Reality Orientation group. Attendance at the Validation group was better. Validation therapy produced significant improvement in behavior ... whereas Reality Orientation produced no significant difference.
>
> (Peoples, 1982)

4   Most recently, Fritz (1986) performed an analysis of the effectiveness of validation therapy on speech patterns of cognitively impaired very old nursing-home residents before and after Validation groups. Fritz writes:

> I found that Validation Therapy made a significant improvement on the elders' speech patterns. A computer program which measures the number of verbs, nouns, propositions, etc. that a person uses in recorded conversation, and I found that the categories of Malorientation and Time Confusion showed a significant increase in fluency levels and in lucidness, after having participated in Validation groups.
>
> (Fritz, 1986)

CONCLUSIONS

The validation worker can help prevent 'maloriented' persons (in stage one) from voluntarily withdrawing quickly or further into 'time confusion' (stage two) or 'repetitive motion' (stage three). One-to-one techniques can stave off the 'vegetative' fourth stage in those who have withdrawn inward as far as stage three.

There is no formula for working with human beings. The validation worker respects the uniqueness of each disoriented person and realizes that they are trying to survive loneliness and despair by utilizing their crystalized, intuitive wisdom and past behaviour patterns to cope. The validation worker understands their struggle in this final stage of their life and chooses to walk beside them, wherever they happen to be.

EDITOR'S POSTSCRIPT

It is important to emphasize that when the four stages of dementia were developed to form the validation approach in the late 1960s, purely on behavioural observations, there were no comprehensive stage-specific medical models of dementia to help clinical research and practice. It is reassuring to see, that practical clinical behavioural observations are converging with, and being confirmed by neurobiological advances in understanding dementia.

NOTE

*This section on pp. 203–4, and the sentence on p. 205, has been inserted by the editor. The author prefers the term disorientation instead of dementia, as used in the title and in several places in the article.

REFERENCES

Alprin, S.I. (1980) Unpublished study of staff attitudes after validation, Cleveland State University, Cleveland, Ohio, College of Education, September.
Buhler, C. (1971) 'Humanistic psychology as a personal experience', *Journal of Humanistic Psychology* 19:8.
Edward Feil Productions (1979) *Looking for Yesterday*, Cleveland, Ohio (film).
—— (1986) *The More We Get Together*, Cleveland, Ohio (film).
Erikson, E.H. (1950) *Childhood and Society*, Cleveland, Ohio, New York: W.W. Norton.
Feil, N. (1967) 'Group therapy in a home for the aged', *Gerontologist* 7(3): 192–5.
—— (1972) 'A new approach to group therapy,' research findings, unpublished paper presented to the Gerontological Society, annual meeting, Puerto Rico.
—— (1982) *V/T Validation: The Feil Method*, Cleveland: Edward Feil Productions.
—— (1984) 'Communicating with the confused elderly patient', *Geriatrics* 39: 131–2.
—— (1985) 'Resolution: the final life task', *Journal of Humanistic Psychology* 25(2): 91–106.
—— (1989) 'Validation: an empathic approach to the care of dementia', *Clinical Gerontologist* 8(3): 89–94.
Fritz, A. (1986) 'The language of resolution among the old–old. The effect of validation therapy on two levels of cognitive confusion', paper given at Chicago, November.
Ginsburg, H. and Opper, S. (1969) *Piaget's Theory of Intellectual Development*, New Jersey: Prentice Hall.
Jones, G.M.M. (1985) 'Validation therapy: a companion to reality orientation', *The Canadian Nurse* pp. 20–3, March.
—— (1987) 'Caregiving in dementia', Talk given at the Alzheimer's and Related

Diseases Symposium, Institute of Psychiatry, June 1987.

—— and Zeiss, E. (1985) 'Reminiscing disorientation theory developed from life review with the elderly', paper presented at the 13th International Congress on Gerontology, New York, 12–17 July.

Maslow, A.H. (1968) *Toward a Psychology of Being* New York: Van Nostrand Reinhold.

Miesen, B. (1990) 'Gehechtheid en dementie', *Onders in de beleving van dementerende ouderen (Attachment and Dementia. How Demented Elderly Persons Experience their Parents)*, Almere: Versluys.

Penfield, W. (1950) 'The cerebral cortex and the mind of man', in P. Laslett (ed.) *The Physical Basis of Mind*, New York: Macmillan.

Peoples, M. (1982) 'Validation therapy versus reality orientation as treatment for disoriented institutionalized elderly', unpublished master's thesis, College of Nursing, University of Akron, Ohio.

Roth, M. (1984) 'Evidence of the possible heterogeneity of Alzheimer's disease and its bearing on future inquiries into aetiology and treatment', in R. Butler and A. Bearn (eds) *The Aging Process: Therapeutic Implications*, New York: Raven Press, pp. 251–75.

Schettler, N. and Boyd, G.S. (1969) *Atherosclerosis*, Biomedical Press: the Netherlands.

Sharp, C. (1988) 'Psychological testing and monitoring and evaluation of the validation therapy programme', inception report, Hawthorn, Victoria, Australia.

Weil, J. (1966) 'Special program for the senile in a home for the aged', *Geriatrics* 21: 197–202, January.

Wells, C. (1977) *Dementia*, Philadelphia: F.A. Davis, Co.

Zuckerman, M.D. (1950) 'Neurosurgery sheds light on brain and behaviour linkages', in P. Laslett (ed.) *The Physical Basis of Mind*, New York: MacMillan.

FURTHER READING

Amaducci, A.N., Davison, B. and Antuono, S. (eds) (1980) *Aging of the Brain and Dementia*, New York: Raven Press.

Butler, R. and Bearn, A. (1984) *The Aging Process*, New York: Raven Press.

Copley, J. (1987) 'Validation therapy aids patients with Alzheimer's', *Advanced Journal of Occupational Therapy*, pp. 3–5, 11 May.

Deichman, E.S. and Kirchhofer, P. (eds) (1986) *Working with the Elderly*, Buffalo: Potentials Development.

Goroff, N. (ed.) (1981) 'Reaping from the field: from practice to principle', *Proceedings of Social Group Work* 1 and 2.

Gubrium, J.F. (1986) *Oldtimers and Alzheimer's: The Descriptive Organization of Senility*, Connecticut: Jai Press, Inc.

Hanna, T. (1987) 'What is somatics? Part three', *Somatics* VI: 57–61.

Houts, M. (1967) *Where Death Delights*, New York: Curtis Brown.

Kral, V.A. (1962) 'Stress and mental disorders in the senium', *Medical Services Journal, Canada* 18: 363–70.

Morton, I. and Bleathman, C. (1988) 'Does it matter whether it's a Tuesday or Friday?' *Nursing Times* 84(62): 25–7.

Piaget, J. (1952) *The Origins of Intelligence in Children*, New York: W.W. Norton.

Roth, M., Tomlinson, B.E. and Blessed, G. (1966) 'Correlation between scores for dementia and counts of senile plaques in cerebral grey matter of elderly subjects', *Nature* 209: 109–10.

Saha, P.K. (1986) appears in *The More We Get Together*, Edward Feil Productions, Cleveland, Ohio (video tape).

Sterns, H. (1988) Project Director, Research Study, 'Effect of validation', Rockynol Retirement Center, Akron, Ohio.

Terry, R.D. (1980) 'Structural changes in senile dementia of the Alzheimer type', in A.N. Amaducci and S. Antuono (eds) *Aging of the Brain and Dementia*, vol. 13, New York: Raven Press, pp. 23–32.

Tomlinson, B.E., Blessed, G. and Roth, M. (1970) 'Observations of the brains of demented old people', *Journal of Neurological Science* II: 205–42.

Verwoedt, A. (1976) *Clinical Geropsychiatry*, Baltimore: Williams & Williams.

Von Franz-Hillman, S. (1971) *Jung's Typology*, Zurich: Spring Publications.

Walsh, A.C. (1985) *Mental Capacity, Medical and Legal Aspects of the Aging*, Colorado Springs: Shepard's McGraw Hill.

Weil, J. (1957) 'Pertinent factors in the development of a special service department of the senile in a home for the aged', Address at the fourth Congress of the International Association of Gerontology, Merano, Italy, July 1957.

Chapter 13

An evaluation of an occupational therapy service for persons with dementia

Cathy Conroy

SUMMARY

Four pilot research projects were undertaken to evaluate the effectiveness of the occupational therapy service to demented people in our care facility. The interventions used in the research included activity sessions, dressing retraining, reality-orientation classroom sessions versus staff-attention sessions and home visiting. Although it was not possible to effectively separate the contribution of the occupational therapy service from the care and support simultaneously offered by other professionals and relatives, the majority of the demented people maintained or improved, though not significantly, their level of functioning with occupational therapy intervention in the first three studies. The home-visiting pilot study indicated that relatives had different priorities than previously assumed. These results were the impetus for restructuring aspects of the occupational therapy services provided for persons with dementia and their families.

INTRODUCTION

This chapter describes four pilot studies and the historical and professional reasons for the selection of particular interventions. Practical recommendations for occupational therapy (OT) workers with the demented elderly, emanating from the studies, are discussed at the end of the chapter.

THE SETTING

Moorgreen Hospital is situated on the outskirts of Southampton, in southern England and houses three separate units on site. One of these, the Thornhill Unit, caters for elderly people (over 65 years) with psychiatric problems. Seventy beds are available for acute and relief admissions, and forty beds for continuing care patients in the nursing home sector of the unit. The most usual diagnoses are depression and dementia. There are 900 admissions a year to the Thornhill Unit and dementia and depression are equally represented in the patients using the short-stay facilities. The Thornhill Unit is served by three full-time psychogeriatricians and ten community psychiatric nurses. Over 1,100 domiciliary visits are made each year by the medical staff. Community psychiatric nurses, psychologists, social workers and OT staff visit people in their homes before and after discharge to hospital. A 'sitting' scheme exists to enable carers to entrust their demented dependant to someone else's care for up to 8 hours per week.

THE PATIENTS

All patients in the studies described herein had a diagnosis of dementia and were familiar to the Thornhill Unit. They had been assessed at home by the medical staff and many had been visited regularly by community nurses. Patients could attend a day hospital, have a 'sitter' come in, and have relief-admission periods at Moorgreen Hospital. Patients referred from other hospitals, who had typically been wandering, taking other patient's possessions or behaving aggressively were admitted to an acute-admissions ward and were not always familiar to staff at the Thornhill Unit. The residents in the nursing home sector were known to the unit as they had already been on the acute-admissions wards or had been relief-admission patients.

The subjects in the studies ranged in age from 60 to 95 years.

OCCUPATIONAL THERAPY

During 1984–7, the OT staff consisted of 6.05 (whole-time equivalent): helpers, one enrolled nurse and one occupational therapist (the author). Three occupational therapists worked, consecutively, on a temporary basis, for 14 months, and two occupational therapists from the day hospitals helped with some of the visits and interviews described in study four (see pp. 231–3).

In 1976, when the author started to work at Moorgreen, the OT staff held regular activity sessions for the long-stay patients and carried out dressing assessments and retraining on the acute admissions ward. Reality orientation had been attempted but was awaiting further development; some home visiting by OT staff with patients prior to discharge had occurred, but such visits were more usual with the functionally ill, depressed patients. OT involvement appeared to be a collection of services that had been useful at some time in the past but not specifically for demented people.

THE RESEARCH STUDIES

The research studies undertaken sought to evaluate the types of interventions that the OT staff offered to the demented people in the Thornhill Unit, Moorgreen Hospital. The work was undertaken in the clinical setting and the usual methods of referral, screening and treatment were retained. The studies were conducted with the assistance and advice of many colleagues and virtually all of the OT staff were involved.

Study one, the engagement-level study with the long-stay patients, was undertaken because the OT staff wondered whether it made any difference if they held activity sessions or not. Likewise, study two, the dressing survey, arose from the expressed doubt that any of the patients improved. Study three, the reality-orientation versus staff-attention study was conducted because the patients were exposed to classroom RO sessions during their very short periodic stays in hospital and we wondered at the usefulness of the classroom sessions. The efficacy or benefits of RO philosophy and techniques were not under question in this study. Finally, study four, the home visiting study, examined the usefulness of a different type of visit for our OT service; one that took the initiative in sorting out problems associated with routine activities of daily living (ADL) but also enquired about individual and shared activities of the carer and the demented person.

STUDY ONE: THE ENGAGEMENT-LEVEL STUDY

Introduction

Chronologically, this was the first study. Over the years, as the Thornhill Unit increasingly focused on community support work, more OT resources were diverted away from those patients destined to live out their lives in the hospital. It was not surprising, then, that the OT staff members working with the long-stay hospitalized patients wondered if OT services were valued, and if so, how the patients benefited from them.

Many studies have commented on the lack of activity amongst the elderly in institutions (Godlove *et al.*, 1982; McCormack and Whitehead, 1981; Gilbert, 1984; McFadyen *et al.*, 1982; Jenkins *et al.*, 1977; McClannahan and Risley, 1974). Demented people appear to be less 'engaged' or active than those who are not mentally impaired. (Gilbert, 1984; McFardyen *et al.*, 1982). Activity programmes have been an intrinsic part of attempts to measure improvements in institutionalized elderly people (Bower, 1967; Mueller and Atlas, 1972; Filer and O'Connell, 1964; Loew and Silverstone, 1971; Chadwick, 1984; Wallis *et al.*, 1983; Pappas *et al.*, 1958; Cosin *et al.*, 1958). Miller, in his review of management of dementia, says: 'Contrary to common prejudice there is strong evidence that improvements in functioning can be achieved by social and behavioural manipulations although maintaining such gains may be more difficult' (Miller, 1977: 77).

The purpose of this study was to find out if patients in the long-stay sector were more 'engaged' in activities during activity sessions in the OT department than at other times. We hoped to demonstrate that patients' participation in the activity sessions was reflected by behavioural improvements.

Methods

The activity sessions took place in an activity centre, apart from the ward. Each session lasted about an hour and a half and there were two or three staff members (an enrolled nurse and two OT helpers) and between six and twelve patients. Usually the patients and staff sat around a large table. There was a recitation of day, date, place and weather and a preview of the lunch menu with each patient in turn. The staff members moved from one patient to another, attempting to interest them in pictures, puzzles, books, the newspaper, conversation or simple game or craft activities. Quizzes, singing or keeping time to music, and rolling a ball on the table surface often occurred in the sessions. Coffee, tea and biscuits were served by the hostess during the sessions.

For this study, engagement was defined as follows: 'A patient is said to be engaged when she/he is either directly engaged in purposeful activity and/or social interaction or is attending to another person/s engaged in purposeful activity or interaction.'

A time-sampling method utilizing a stopwatch (every 30 seconds for 50 minutes) was used to determine whether the patient was 'engaged' or 'disengaged'. Inter-rater reliability trials enabled the three observers to reach agreement 85 per cent of the time.

The Clifton assessment procedure for the elderly (CAPE) (Pattie and Gilleard, 1979) was used to measure any cognitive or behavioural changes in the individuals in the three phases of the study. Pattie and Gilleard define levels of dependency and eight out of ten of the patients were in high-maximum-dependency level on the behaviour rating scale and all the patients were within those limits on the cognitive rating scale.

Seventeen patients were observed consecutively as they were admitted to the long-stay sector. Measurements were completed on ten patients and this is the substance of this study. Phase A refers to the period immediately after admission, usually about a fortnight during which the patients remained on the ward. A minimum of three observations of their engagement levels were made and the CAPE (full version) was administered. Within the first fifteen activity sessions held in the OT department (phase B), seven samples of engagement levels were recorded, and again, the full

CAPE was repeated for phase B. Last, the final fortnight that the patients remained on the ward was referred to as phase A2 and engagement levels and CAPE measures were taken at this point also.

Results

In phase B, every patient had higher engagement levels (EL) during activity sessions than on the ward. The average EL in phase A (ward) was 22.42 per cent, in phase B 50.93 per cent and in phase A2 (ward) 26.92 per cent. Seven patients had higher scores on the cognitive assessment scale and seven on the behaviour rating scale during phase B. Seven patients continued to improve on the cognitive assessment scale and four on the behavioural rating scales during phase A2 when the patients were back on the wards.

In addition, as we observed the patients, we attempted to write down what they were doing. Even though this group were elderly, confined to hospital and were rated as highly dependent, the activities favoured by individuals and the amount of participation varied considerably (see Figure 13.1). (For a more complete discussion, see Conroy *et al.*, 1988.)

Discussion

The higher engagement levels during the activity sessions may be attributable to the combination of factors including: adequate space, a variety of materials and facilitation by the OT staff during the activity sessions. During the activity sessions, the staff's mandate was clear: to engage patients in activities, whereas, on the wards, patients needing physical assistance or intensive psychiatric management might be competing for the staff's attention. Engaging the patients in activities would be viewed as desirable but not a priority.

Whether the activity sessions contributed to improved cognitive or behavioural functioning is unclear but most of the patients did show slight (although not statistically significant) improvements. This could be attributed to any combination of nursing and medical interventions, and simply becoming accustomed and adjusted to their new surroundings, but planned OT intervention was the only common, simultaneous variable adjusted in this study.

STUDY TWO: THE DRESSING SURVEY

Introduction

The dressing survey was initiated because members of the OT staff wondered if their continued efforts in retraining made any difference to the

Figure 13.1 Engagement during the activity sessions (phase b)

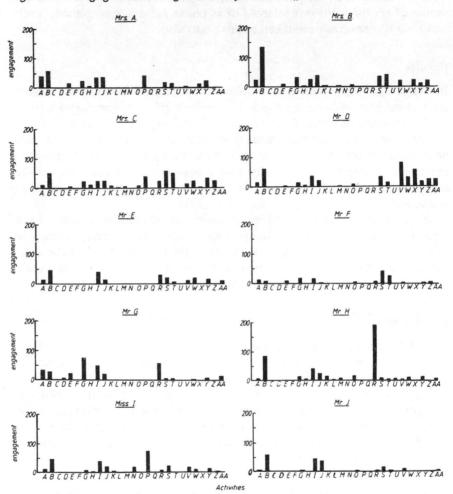

Note: The vertical axis represents the number of times (at 30-second intervals) the patient was observed engaged in an activity. The activities, represented by letters A–AA on the horizontal axis, are: A Watching or listening to staff; B Speaking to staff; D Smiling at staff; E Looking directly at observer; F Speaking to observer; G Watching other patients' activities; H Speaking to other patients; I Taking drinks; J Eating biscuits; K Walking; L Sitting down, drawing up chair; M Standing up or moving to the edge of chair; N Moving purposively; O Adjusting clothing, glasses, putting on slippers or wiping hands, blowing nose, using or folding own serviette; P Knitting; R Writing, drawing, colouring, holding a pen; S Ball games, quoits, throwing large dice, balloons, bean bag game; T Shaking percussion instrument/responding to music, exercises, clapping; U Whistling; V Looking at newspaper, magazines, pictures, scrapbook, book; W Dominoes, lotto, noughts and crosses; X Looking at, cutting, moving the greeting cards; Y Reality orientation; Z Quiz, listening to poetry, story; AA Raffia, threading chamois leathers, sanding wood, basketwork.

patients' dressing abilities. A decade ago, when the transition from long-stay to short-stay wards was being made, for people who needed only partial supervision, the sole alternative to staying in hospital was going into a local authority residential home. Usually the homes had waiting lists, and minimum standards of continence and self-care for their residents. There-fore, it was quite important that assessment of self-care skills, including dressing, be considered as part of the team's recommendation for place-ment. Furthermore, if the patient's skills were optimized, they could have a more advantageous placement.

Subsequently, the growth of many private rest homes provided a real alternative to placement in local authority residential homes. They were competing for clientele and usually asked only for assurance of continence, good nights and no problems with wandering.

The relief admission programme was developed and offered an addi-tional placement option. Demented patients were scheduled for short stays in hospital to give their carers a break. Concern for the carer shifted the emphasis from whether the demented person could dress themselves or not, to whether they could get out of a chair unaided or not. It was assumed that a carer could dress the demented person without undue stress but if the demented person was unwilling or unable to move without the aid of another person, then an elderly carer would be likely to be unable to con-tinue caring for that person at home. (Of course, other factors such as rest-lessness, co-operativeness, continence and how well they slept at night, were also significant in determining whether or not a carer was able to maintain that role for the demented person.)

The purpose of this study was to find out whether the patients' dressing skills improved when they underwent dressing assessment and retraining by the OT staff.

Methods

A record of the age, sex, CAPE information/orientation score (Pattie and Gilleard, 1981), number of admissions, type of dementia, Hachinski scores (Hachinski et al., 1975), other medical diagnoses, the number of dressing sessions, the method used for retraining, how much assistance patients required at the beginning and end of the retraining sessions and the outcome of dressing retraining were completed on eighty-three patients. Their ages ranged from 60 to 95 years with the average age being 79.84 years (s.d. 6.59). Twenty-nine of the participants were men (35 per cent) and fifty-four (65 per cent) were women. The number of admissions each patient had had to the unit at the time of the survey varied from fifty-five cases being first admissions to one individual having had twenty-one previous admissions.

Eighty of the 83 subjects were asked the twelve information/orientation questions of the CAPE (survey version). The number of correct responses varied from 0 (nine individuals) to 10 (one person). The mean number of correct answers was 3.41 (s.d. 2.51), indicating that persons were relatively cognitively impaired.

The doctors in the unit used the Hachinski scale in addition to the patient's history, to classify the diagnosis of dementia into three discrete categories. The number of persons in each category was as follows: senile dementia of the Alzheimer's type, (n=33), multi-infarct dementia (n=31), mixed dementia (n=18). One case had been admitted following a road-traffic accident and did not have a detailed history so that case was classified as other (n=1).

Results

The average number of sessions spent with a patient was six (range: 2–21).

By far, the most usual dressing technique was that of behavioural retraining; it was used in eighty of the eighty-three cases. Behavioural retraining means that a system of prompts progressing from verbal, to demonstration, to physical prompts, are employed with pauses and encouragement at each stage for the patient to carry out the task. Other behavioural techniques such as backward chaining might also be used. A specifically functional approach was used in three cases. The functional approach implies that the patient is taught a different method of dressing because, for instance, he has lost the use of an arm. Attempts were made to teach patients to use an assistive device in six cases.

The average level of dressing competence was assessed as level 5. Ratings were adapted from the functional classification system of the Medical Center Rehabilitation Hospital, Grand Forks, North Dakota, USA. The levels describe how much the patient is able to do while dressing and how much help is required. The levels are numbered 1–9. Level 1 is 'unable to assess', level 2 is 'totally dependent – the patent does not perform any of the activity' and level 9 is 'independent – the patient is able to and does perform the dressing activity independently without assistive device'. Level 5 is moderate assistance: the patient required assistance with certain items of clothing (e.g. shoes, tights, braces, zips). This was the average level of competence when people entered the study and at the final assessment. The mean score for the initial dressing session was 5.15 (s.d. 1.44) whereas the mean for the final dressing session was 5.33 (s.d. 1.63). Although this shows an improvement in the right direction, it is very slight.

Eighteen people did improve by at least one level in their dressing level score although fourteen people deteriorated and fifty-one people were maintained at baseline levels. Of the eighteen who did improve, a disproportionate number had senile dementia of the Alzheimer's type rather than multi-infarct dementia; had other medical diagnoses secondary to the dementia; scored only 2 and 3 on the CAPE I/O, and started at a lower dressing level than others who had a similar CAPE score. All except one of the people who improved in their dressing performance did so within nine treatment sessions. Only 51 per cent of those who improved had done so by six sessions, which was the average number of sessions in this survey.

In this sample of demented people there was a wide range of dressing levels for all of the CAPE I/O quadrisections (see Table 13.1) but overall, the means of the dressing assessments tended to rise with the higher score on the CAPE I/O. This supports observations by other researchers that higher scores on verbal tests tend to correlate with higher dressing perform-ance. (Weintraub et al., 1982; Wilson et al., 1973).

Discussion

The intention of this survey was to collect information about an intervention in current practice and no experimental interventions were introduced; however, two impressions were confirmed. First, we had evolved a behavi-oural technique of dressing retraining over years of work with these patients and it was heartening to read, in the course of this study, that other researchers (Rinke et al., 1978; Patterson, 1982; Schuman et al., 1981) favoured the behavioural method and allied techniques. Second, in our clinical work there was a large degree of individual variation and our clinical impression corresponded to Martin et al.'s (1986) findings, in their longitudinal investigation of forty Alzheimer patients, that although the 'total group pattern ... [showed] relatively equal deficits on measures of word-finding ability and constructional skill ... embedded in [the] group data were clusters of patients who exhibited markedly contrasting profiles of impaired and preserved cognitive abilities' (Martin et al., 1986: 605).

The results of this study show that although some people did improve in their dressing ability, the great proportion were only maintained at baseline

Table 13.1 Initial and final dressing levels of CAPE score groups: numbers in each group, range of dressing levels, mean and standard deviation

CAPE I/O score group	No.	Range		Mean		S.D.	
		I	F	I	F	I	F
Score 0 and 1	21	2–7	1–7	4.85	4.95	1.52	1.49
Score 2 and 3	23	2–9	3–9	5.13	5.69	1.60	1.86
Score 4 and 5	17	3–9	3–6	5.12	5.05	1.41	1.09
Score 6+	19	4–9	2–9	5.63	5.63	1.16	1.86

Note: I = initial dressing level; F = final dressing level.

levels. Considering the usual nihilism associated with treating demented people, this must be acknowledged as encouraging. Whether OT intervention specifically made a difference cannot be ascertained from this study, but the observations that people with medical diagnoses secondary to dementia improved more than those with just dementia, and that people with low verbal scores and initial low dressing-performance levels were represented highly amongst the improvers, suggests that their dressing performance might have improved as they felt better.

STUDY THREE: THE REALITY-ORIENTATION/STAFF-ATTENTION TRIAL

Introduction

Reality orientation classroom sessions had been part of the programme offered by the OT staff for more than 10 years (Conroy and Clarke, 1977). Sessions had been held on one or both of the short-stay admission wards for demented people every weekday morning. With increasingly higher proportions of patients comprising relief admission who were only in hospital for 13 days, we wanted to know if RO was still an appropriate intervention.

Method

The method for the present study was adapted from Woods (1979) 'Reality orientation and staff attention: A controlled study'. Seventeen individuals (twelve women, five men; mean age 78.82 years, s.d. 5.95) took part in thirty trials. Two women participated four times and seven people participated twice.

The patients were all living at home with their spouses and/or children. Their relief admissions were, by definition, scheduled in advance.

As patients arrived on the wards for their scheduled relief admissions, they were allocated randomly to either a reality orientation group or a staff attention group. Although as many as nine relief admission patients were admitted on one day, the establishment of criteria for participation in the groups, meant that no more than three entrants joined the groups in any one week. The criteria were that the patients must be able to co-operate with the testing procedures and that they must score a minimum of six points on the combined CAPE information/orientation subtest (possible score 12 points) and the concentration test (Holden and Woods, 1982: 256–7) possible score 19 points).

If a patient scored enough points to be in one of the groups for the trial, the nursing staff completed the MACC behavioural adjustment scale

(Ellsworth, 1971), and the Holden communication scale (Holden and Woods, 1982: 258–9) based on their observations within 48 hours of their arrival on the ward. Nursing staff repeated a second set of tests 36 hours before the patients were discharged. The CAPE I/O test and the concentration test were also repeated at discharge.

Both groups were held simultaneously in the activity centre, away from the wards. The groups were conducted by four OT helpers who rotated the tasks between them. The helpers were all experienced staff who had conducted reality orientation groups prior to the commencement of this study. The staff attention group was based on the description by Woods in his 1979 study: 'a discussion group with staff encouraging each resident to participate. Rambling, inappropriate or unrealistic contributions were permitted and accepted. RO materials were not used' (Woods, 1979: 503). In the RO group, subjects attended an average of 7.3 sessions whereas in the staff attention group subjects attended an average of 7.7 sessions during their 13-day admission.

Results

T-tests did not reveal any significant differences between the ages, number of sessions or scores at admission or discharge between the reality orientation group and the staff attention group.

Results showed that there was a slight but not significant decrease in the concentration test scores for both groups. There was a slight, but not significant, improvement on all other test measures from the time of admission to discharge. The greatest improvement was on the MACC behavioural adjustment scale for the group who took part in the reality orientation sessions (see Table 13.2)

There was no significant change in the CAPE information/orientation score between admission and discharge, neither were there differences in CAPE I/O scores between the RO and SA group. Most of the previous published studies (Brook et al., 1975; Powell-Proctor and Miller, 1982; Woods, 1979; Hanley et al., 1981; Johnson et al., 1981; Burton 1982; Powell-Proctor, 1981; Greene, 1984; Wallis et al., 1983) reported increases in verbal orientation with groups receiving classroom reality orientation.

The discharge CAPE I/O and concentration assessments were usually carried out in the afternoon during this trial whereas the admission CAPE I/O and concentration assessment generally took place in the mornings. This might account for the lack of increase in the verbal orientation ratings and the lower concentration scores. Analysis of covariance showed that there was a trend nearing significance ($F=4.12$, dfl, 27 p. 0.053) in the concentration scores, indicating that the discharge assessment of concentration was much the same as the admission scores.

Table 13.2 Patients' mean score on admission and discharge

	Assessments							
	CAPE I/O		Concentration		MACC		Communication	
Type of treatment	A	D	A	D	A	D	A	D
Reality orientation (n15)								
Mean	3.60	3.80	9.27	8.40	54.53	58.47	16.47	15.13
Standard deviation	1.80	2.34	3.22	4.44	6.39	7.39	6.27	7.49
Staff attention (n15)								
Mean	3.80	4	10.20	9.33	55.67	57.33	16.67	14.33
Standard deviation	1.82	2.33	4.46	4.56	7.49	8.12	8.17	7.36

Note: CAPE I/O is the Clifton assessment procedure for the elderly, survey version (Pattie and Gilleard, 1981). In this study only the information/orientation items were used. Possible score is 12. Concentration is concentration test by Woods (Holden and Woods, 1982:256–7) and the Clifton assessment procedure for the elderly reading and writing tests (Pattie and Gilleard, 1979). Possible score is 19. MACC stands for the MACC behavioural adjustment scale (Ellsworth, 1971). Possible score range is 16–80. Communication is the Holden communication scale (Holden and Woods, 1982: 258–9). The scale ranges from 0–48 with a lower number indicating better communication. A = score at admission; D = score at discharge.

However, the nurses' ratings, which were made blind, did demonstrate a difference between the admission and discharge scores and between the RO and SA groups. The RO participants showed an improvement (though not a significant one), on their mean score on the MACC behavioural adjustment scale at discharge (see Table 13.2). Folsom's original declaration of intent, in developing RO, stated that the 'emotional needs of individual patients required concentrated attention' (1968: 292). Barnes (1974) described improvements in the population he worked with that might have been attributable to changes in mood. Greene and colleagues also reported an 'improvement in the patient's mood at home as rated by relatives' (Greene *et al.*, 1983: 42). On the Holden communication scale, the mean differences between the admission scores and the discharge scores were better, though not significantly, for the staff attention group (see Table 13.2).

Discussion

In his 1979 study of realty-orientation and staff-attention groups, Woods had found that on tests of concentration, the staff attention group were significantly worse than the RO group and the control group, suggesting that 'the wrong form of attention is worse than no special treatment at all' (Woods, 1979: 506). This study did not replicate Wood's findings.

Recent reviews of reality orientation (Powell-Proctor and Miller, 1982; Burton, 1982; Greene, 1984; Hanley 1984) emphasize the limited benefits of the classroom sessions but suggest that specific behavioural or cognitive training may be more helpful.

Although the results, in terms of supporting classroom reality orientation were disappointing, it was reassuring to see that the participating patients did not deteriorate during their stay in hospital. It was disquieting to realize that nearly half the patients on the relief admissions programme were unable to participate because of the severity of their impairments and there was little in the OT programme to offer them.

STUDY FOUR: THE HOME-VISITING PILOT STUDY

Introduction

Nineteen home visits were completed to demented elderly and their carers. The demented persons were aged 65–93 years (mean age 78.05); seventeen were women and two were men. These demented people had had at least one scheduled relief admission to Moorgreen Hospital and were regularly visited by a community psychiatric nurse.

The survey version of the CAPE questionnaire was administered to obtain dependency ratings for this group. The CAPE dependency score revealed that 18 of the 19 people scored D and E (high-dependency ratings) meaning that this population of people living in the community and coming in for relief admissions, were equivalent to the patient population in the long-stay hospital wards.

The purpose of the home visit was twofold: first, to link our experiences and impressions of the patient in hospital with our impressions of their carers and home environment, and, second, to check up on how well our system of supplying activities of daily living (ADL) equipment and advice was working. It was estimated that 33 per cent of the visits would highlight further work that should be carried out by the OT department. We wanted to see if this estimate was realistic.

Methods

A semi-structured interview with four parts was designed for this study. It was filled in at all nineteen visits. The four sections of the interview are the following:

1   Factual data – i.e. type of home, people living in the house, people/ professionals/agencies who gave help, relationship of patient to carer, etc.
2   Activity profile – structure of their day, interests (previous and present)

of the carer and the demented person, activities they shared (past and present), things that were difficult and possible to do.

3   ADL inquiries assessments – toilet, dressing, feeding, access etc.
4   Action to be taken by OT.

The interview lasted approximately 1 hour and the carer and person with dementia were present. The person with dementia was encouraged to participate in the discussion. The visits were usually timed and the person with dementia was in hospital so that dressing, and if necessary, feeding and transfer assessments and the CAPE could be completed as well as determining whether home visits were possible.

Nineteen visits and interviews were completed in 10 weeks. Fifteen of the visits required some professional 'action' by the OT. Many of the homes visited already had commodes, rails or high-chairs, yet supplying or advising where and how to obtain specially adapted items and equipment was the largest single category of 'action' requested of the OTs. The next largest category was alerting other professionals, followed by giving advice during the interview. Three out of five reports arising from the interviews were concerned with activities of daily living. Asking others for further assessment and trying to obtain keys for the toilets for the disabled persons are other examples of requests for action. Of the twenty-three questions asked of the carer and their demented relative, ten items were concerned with activities of daily living, so presumably this aspect of their life together was covered in most depth, and that is likely why most requests for help were in this area.

Discussions about the patients' leisure activities, the carers' leisure activities and shared activities were often quite emotive. Carers often stated the wish that there were more activities for the demented person to do; a few carers sounded somewhat resentful or resigned to the lack of initiative demonstrated by the demented person in remaining active. Some explained the attempts they had made, often in an apologetic way, to engage their demented relative in some activity. Husbands and wives often went for walks, shopping, or out in the car together; some couples mentioned that they watched television or listened to music together. One woman listed gardening as a shared activity though 'we both used to be keen gardeners but now I bring him outdoors with me while I garden and I talk to him about what I'm doing.' One severely demented lady carried a small bag around with an orange, some yarn, a pair of tights and some nice smelling soap in it and would sometimes empty and refill the bag. Another carer would ensure that her mother-in-law had the newspaper to read each day: 'There are so few things she will concentrate on and it's very difficult to do anything if you can't concentrate.' A daughter observed that her mother often counted things and wondered if buying a counting frame for her for Christmas would be appropriate.

In one instance, a carer made a complimentary remark about a picture that his wife had coloured while in hospital.

Several times I was asked 'What do you do with them?' (i.e. demented people collectively) and occasionally I was asked what their demented relative was able to do in the OT sessions. I was relieved that some of the carers did not ask this question knowing their relative had not been included in our OT sessions, because they were 'too restless' or 'too demented' and yet there we were in their homes, asking them what activities they did!

Visits to the patients' homes helped to still any unease that our service was not doing its job optimally. A particular worry was that the necessary aids and adaptations or specific advice to enable the families to cope with the tasks of daily living had not been provided. The structure of the questionnaire reflects that preoccupation. The number of requests and the nature of the advice given suggests that there was indeed room for improvement on that front. The responses of the relatives to the questions about leisure and shared activities also indicated that this was an area in which more constructive and supportive help could be given than we had hitherto envisaged. We found ourselves acknowledging the difficulties that the carers experienced in finding something for the demented person to do and we felt that our service should be better at providing suggestions for carers.

There are some suggestions in the literature for activities for persons with dementia. Allen's work on cognitive disability, and task analysis (Allen, 1982; 1985) provides a starting point, and Earhart's (1985) description of occupational therapy groups gives very pertinent illustrations of how such concepts might be applied. Sensory integration as advocated by Ross and Burdick (1981) suggests modalities that may be particularly useful for the more impaired sector of the demented population. Levy's article (1986) on appropriate activities for various levels of cognitive disability is aimed at carers of Alzheimer's disease victims. Hasselkus and Brown describe programme planning for respite admissions in a hospital for community-based elderly persons which emphasizes 'facilitation of normal, meaningful activity and functional skills during hospitalization' (Hasselkus and Brown, 1983: 83).

OVERALL DISCUSSION

In study one, the results of the activity sessions for the long-stay patients, indicated that the provision of encouragement and materials increased their level of engagement. Cognitive and behavioural functioning scores, as assessed by the CAPE, increased and continued to increase even after patients ceased to attend the activity sessions. This implies that the improvements could not be attributed solely to increased engagement in the activity sessions.

Other factors must likewise be acknowledged to have influenced the outcome of the dressing survey in study two. The majority of the patients maintained their initial level of performance but, of those who did improve by at least one level, a disproportionate number had a secondary medical diagnosis in addition to dementia, low scores on the verbal orientation measure and had also started at a lower level on the dressing-level scale than patients with similar verbal-orientation scores. This suggests that dressing ability improved as persons felt better. All, except one of the persons who improved in their dressing performance, did so within the nine treatment sessions.

The results of the reality orientation versus staff attention study demonstrated that RO sessions were as good as SA sessions for demented people. There was no statistically significant improvement but all measures except concentration showed small increases in scores.

The goal of the home visiting pilot study was to discover whether persons within our service were getting the necessary aids, equipment and advice they needed to enable the elderly with dementia to carry on with activities of daily living at home. Fifteen out of nineteen homes visited identified further needs in this area. Carers often reported that they valued help and advice on maintaining shared leisure activities, responsiveness and awareness, more than maintaining the demented person's participation in dressing and feeding.

The contribution of the occupational therapist to the care of demented persons centres on utilizing those skills which remain intact. Observations and assessments are made to ascertain their strengths and to note areas of difficulty. Activities are analysed with a view to matching the demented persons' abilities to routine tasks of living, leisure and pursuits and social interactions. If necessary, adaptations to the environment may be made to enable the person to carry on with their usual activities. A large-faced clock or watch with bold numbers for people who have difficulty seeing, and a higher chair if it becomes a struggle to get out of the lounge chair, are common adaptations for older people. Adaptations may also be made to the way in which a task is carried out; the behavioural approach to dressing in this evaluation was an example.

Kielhofner and Burke, 1980; Kielhofner, 1985; Smith *et al.*, 1986, have made us more aware of the importance of bolstering valued activities rather than merely checking that functional skills are sustained. The findings are of our fourth study confirm that often the carers' concern about providing a newspaper or going for a walk, seemed to take precedence over striving to maintain dressing skills. Variations in carers' priorities must be recognized and incorporated in hospital-based efforts to work with families.

The carers at home indicated that they were able to sustain some shared leisure activities at home, but they were usually eager for advice on ways of increasing responsiveness and awareness. If skills such as dressing or feeding, are dealt with as efficiently as possible, carers and demented persons could have more time and energy to pursue joint activities. It is important that these priorities be acknowledged and incorporated into the hospital milieu, and during community follow-up visits.

PRACTICAL IMPLICATIONS

Various changes are being made to the OT service as a result of the evaluative research described in this chapter.

The reality orientation classes and the dressing assessments and retraining are examples of practices surviving beyond their maximum usefulness. Changes in the provision of care offered by the unit mean some old practices are no longer as useful and must be updated, if high standards of care and support are to be maintained.

Planned activity sessions do afford opportunities for engagement in activities for persons with dementia, who, apparently cannot initiate or sustain meaningful activities on their own. It may be more beneficial to offer such activity opportunities, regularly, to persons in hospital for relief admission and in the nursing home (the most impaired groups), rather than to the persons who are admitted to hospital for an episode of physical illness or for assessment for placement.

Relief admission patients and nursing-home residents were found to be nearly equivalent in the severity of their impairments. This level of disability requires a different type of approach and the utilization of different activities than OT services had been offering. We are presently experimenting with sensory stimulation methods, as suggested by Ross and Burdick (1981) in their manual.

Reality orientation classes take place only occasionally now. The presence of four patients of sufficient cognitive ability on the short-stay admission wards is considered to warrant setting up RO sessions.

The dressing assessments and retraining are being used only with people who have been referred for particular physical disabilities e.g. fractures, CVAs, etc, on the first admission of relief patients, and at six-monthly intervals for reassessing regular relief admission patients.

If the carer of a relief admission patient encourages the patient to participate in dressing at home, then we also ensure that the necessary time and support for dressing are provided during their stay in hospital. With the exception of the reassessments, we work with the patients for more than six sessions as a result of the findings of study two: the dressing survey.

As a further consequence of this research, home visits with relief admission patients and their carers have been planned. The aim of such visits is to maintain the most-valued activities when the demented person comes into hospital for relief admission.

We try to ensure, in turn, that relatives and other professionals are aware of what we have learned about the demented person's abilities, interests,

activities and responses. Only then can personalized yet realistic OT interventions with severely impaired demented people be facilitated within the
multi-disciplinary team concept.

ACKNOWLEDGEMENTS

I am particularly indebted to Dr Peter Coleman, Dr David Wilkinson, Dr
Chris Sinner, Ms Jill MacKean, Mrs Elizabeth Earwood, Professor Roger
Briggs and my husband, Ed Conroy, for their help and encouragement
during this project. I am thankful to occupational therapy and nursing staff
for their co-operation and support throughout the studies. Teaching Media,
based at Southampton General Hospital, produced Figure 13.1.

REFERENCES

Allen, C.A. (1982) 'Independence through activity: the practice of occupational
    therapy (Psychiatry)', *The American Journal of Occupational Therapy* 36 (11):
    731–9.
—— (1985) *Occupational Therapy for Psychiatric Diseases: Measurement and
    Management of Cognitive Disabilities*, Boston/Toronto: Little, Brown and
    Company.
Barnes, J.A. (1974) 'Effects of reality orientation classroom on memory loss, confu-
    sion, and disorientation in geriatric patients', *Gerontologist* pp. 138–42, April.
Bower, H.M. (1967) 'Sensory stimulation and the treatment of senile dementia', *The
    Medical Journal of Australia* 1 (22): 1113–19.
Brook, P., Degun, G. and Mather, M. (1975) 'Reality orientation, a therapy for
    psychogeriatric patients: a controlled study', *British Journal of Psychiatry* 127:
    42–5.
Burton, M. (1982) 'Reality orientation for the elderly: a critique', *Journal of
    Advanced Nursing* 7: 427–33.
Chadwick, P. (1984) 'Social stimulation and the elderly', *Nursing Times* 8: 41–2,
    March 7.
Conroy, C. and Clarke, R.J. (1977) 'Reality orientation: a basic rehabilitation tech-
    nique for patients suffering from memory loss and confusion', *British Journal of
    Occupational Therapy* 40 (10): 250–1.
Conroy, M.C., Fincham, F. and Agard-Evans, C. (1988) 'Can they do anything? Ten
    single-subject studies of the engagement level of hospitalized demented patients',
    The British Journal of Occupational Therapy 51 (4): 129–32.
Cosin, L.Z., Mort, M., Post, F., Westropp, C. and Williams, M. (1958) 'Experi-
    mental treatment of persistent senile confusion', *International Journal of Social
    Psychiatry* 4: 24–42.
Earhart, C.A. (1985) 'Occupational therapy groups', in C.A. Allen (ed.) *Occupa-
    tional Therapy for Psychiatric Diseases: Measurement and Management of
    Cognitive Disabilities*, Boston/Toronto: Little, Brown and Company, 235–66.
Ellsworth, R.B. (1971) *The MACC Behavioral Adjustment Scale: Revised 1971
    Manual*, Los Angeles, California: Western Psychological Services.
Filer, R.N. and O'Connell, D.D. (1964) 'Motivation of aging persons', *Journal of
    Gerontology* 19: 15–22.
Folsom, J.C. (1968) 'Reality orientation for the elderly mental patient', *Journal of
    Geriatric Psychiatry* 1 (2): 291–307.

Gilbert, M. (1984) 'Challenging stereotypes', *Nursing Mirror* 158 (16): 42–3.

Godlove, C., Richard, L. and Rodwell, G. (1982) 'Time for Action', Social Services Monograph: *Research in Practice*, Joint Unit for Social Services Research: Sheffield University, quoted in MacDonald, A.J.D., Craig, T.K.J. and Walker, L.A.R. (1985) 'The development of a short observation method for the study of the activity and contacts of old people in residential settings', *Psychological Medicine* 15: 167–72.

Greene, J.G. (1984) 'The evaluation of reality orientation', in I. Hanley, and J. Hodges (eds) *Psychological Approaches to the Care of the Elderly*, London: Croom Helm, pp. 192–212.

——, Timbury, G.C., Smith, R. and Gardiner, M. (1983) 'Reality orientation with elderly patients in the community: an empirical evaluation', *Age and Ageing* 12: 38–43.

Hachinski, V.C., Illiff, L.D., Zilhk, E., Du Boulay, G.H., McAllister, V.L., Marshall, J., Russell, R.W.R. and Seymour, L. (1975) 'Cerebral blood flow in dementia', *Archives of Neurology* 32: 632–7.

Hanley, I. (1984) 'Theoretical and practical considerations in reality orientation therapy with the elderly', in I. Hanley and J. Hodge (eds) *Psychological Approaches to the Care of the Elderly*, London: Croom Helm, pp. 164–91.

——, McGuire, R.J. and Boyd, W.D. (1981) 'Reality orientation and dementia: a controlled trial of two approaches', *British Journal of Psychiatry* 138: 10–14.

Hasselkus, B.J. and Brown, M. (1983) 'Respite care for community elderly', *The American Journal of Occupational Therapy* 37 (2): 83–8.

Holden, U.P. and Woods, R.J. (1982) *Reality Orientation: Psychological Approaches to the 'Confused' Elderly*, Edinburgh: Churchill Livingstone.

Jenkins, J., Felce, D., Lunt, B. and Powell, L. (1977) 'Increasing engagement in activity of residents in old people's home by providing recreational materials', *Behavioural Research and Therapy* 15: 429–34 as quoted in D. Felce and J. Jenkins (eds) (1977) 'Engagement in activities by old people in residential care', Research Report no. 150 Health Care Evaluation Research Team, Dawn House, Sleepers Hill, Winchester, Hants, England.

Johnson, C., McLaren, S.M. and McPherson, F.M. (1981) 'The comparative effectiveness of three versions of "classroom" reality orientation', *Age and Ageing* 10: 33–5.

Kielhofner, G. (1985) 'Occupational function and dysfunction', in G. Kielhofner (ed.) *A Model of Human Occupation: Theory and Application*, Baltimore: Williams & Wilkins, pp. 63–74.

—— and Burke, J.P. (1980) 'A model of human occupation, part 1. Conceptual framework and content', *American Journal of Occupational Therapy* 34 (9): 572–81.

Levy, L.L. (1986) 'A practical guide to the care of the Alzheimer's disease victim: the cognitive disability perspective', *Topics in Geriatric Rehabilitation* 1 (2): 16–26.

Loew, C. and Silverstone, B. (1971) 'A program of intensified stimulation and response facilitation for the senile aged', *Gerontologist* 1: 341–7, Winter.

McClannahan, L.E., and Risley, T.R. (1974) 'Activities and materials for severely disabled geriatric patients', *Nursing Homes* 10–13, December–January.

McCormack, D. and Whitehead, A. (1981) 'The effect of providing recreational activities on the engagement level of long-stay geriatric patients', *Age and Ageing* 10 (4): 287–91.

McFadyen, M., Prior, T. and Kindness, K. (1982) 'Engagement: an important variable in the institutional care of the elderly', in R. Taylor and A. Gilmore (eds) *Current Trends in British Gerontology, Proceedings of the 1980 Conference of the*

British Society of Gerontology, Aldershot: Gower Publishing Company Ltd, pp. 148–58.

Martin, A., Brouwers, P., Lalonde, F., Cox, C., Teleska, P., Fedio, P., Foster, N.L. and Chase, T.N. (1986) 'Towards a behavioral typology of Alzheimer's patients', *Journal of Clinical and Experimental Neuropsychology* 8 (5): 595–610.

Miller, E. (1977) 'Management of dementia: review of some possibilities', *British Journal of Social and Clinical Psychology* 16: 77–83.

Mueller, D.J. and Atlas, L. (1972) 'Resocialization of regressed elderly residents: a behavioral management approach', *Journal of Gerontology* 27 (3): 390–2.

Pappas, W., Curtis, W.P. and Baker, J. (1958) 'A controlled study of an intensive treatment programme for hospitalised geriatric patients', *Journal of American Geriatrics Society* 6: 17–25.

Patterson, R.L. (1982) *Overcoming Deficits of Aging: A Behavioral Approach*, New York: Plenum Press, pp. 70–5.

Pattie, A.H. and Gilleard, C.J. (1979) *Clifton Assessment Procedures for the Elderly (CAPE)*, Sevenoaks, Kent: Hodder & Stoughton.

—— and —— (1981) *Clifton Assessment Procedures for the Elderly (CAPE). Survey Version*, Sevenoaks, Kent: Hodder & Stoughton.

Powell-Proctor, L. (1981) 'Reality orientation: a treatment of choice?' *Geriatric Medicine* 11: 88–92.

—— and Miller, E. (1982) 'Reality orientation: a critical appraisal', *British Journal of Psychiatry* 140: 457–63.

Rinke, C.I., Williams, J.T., Lloyd, K.E. and Smith-Scott, W. (1978) 'The effects of prompting and reinforcement on self-bathing by elderly residents of a nursing home', *Behavior Therapy* 9: 873–81.

Ross, M. and Burdick, D. (1981) *Sensory Integration: A Training Manual for Therapists and Teachers for Regressed, Psychiatric and Geriatric Patient Groups*, Thorofare, New Jersey: SLACK Incorporated.

Schuman, J.E., Beattie, E.J., Steed, D.A., Merry, G.M. and Kraus, A.S. (1981) 'Geriatric patients with and without intellectual dysfunction: effectiveness of a standard rehabilitation program', *Archives of Physical and Medical Rehabilitation* 62: 612–8.

Smith, N., Kielhofner, G. and Watts, J. (1986) 'The relationship between volition, activity pattern and life satisfaction in the elderly', *The American Journal of Occupational Therapy* 40 (4): 278–83.

Wallis, G.G., Baldwin, M. and Higginbotham, P. (1983) 'Reality orientation therapy – a controlled trial', *British Journal of Medical Psychology* 56: 271–7.

Weintraub, S., Baratz, R. and Mesulam, M. (1982) 'Daily living activities in the assessment of dementia', in S.I. Corkin, K. Davis, J. Growdon, E. Usdin and R. Wurtman (eds) *Alzheimer's Disease: A Report of Progress in Research*, New York: Raven Press, pp. 189–92.

Wilson, L.A., Grant, K., Witney, P.M. and Kerridge, D.F. (1973) 'Mental status of elderly hospital patients related to occupational therapist's assessment of activities of daily living', *Clinics in Gerontology* 15: 197–202.

Woods, R.T. (1979) 'Reality orientation and staff attention: a controlled study', *British Journal of Psychiatry* 134: 502–7.

Part III

Interventions for persons with dementia in the community

EDITORS' NOTE

Many persons in the community with experience of someone who has a dementing illness, particularly a family member, are afraid that they will befall the same fate even though family histories of dementia are not common. A recent study of persons seen at the Maudsley Hospital Memory Clinic in London, UK, showed that many persons with no measureable impairment, were extremely concerned about their memory whenever it did not perform 'perfectly'.

Changes in memory functioning with aging, fatigue and emotional overexertion have not been well publicized and it is increasingly evident that prolonged 'fear of becoming demented' can have deleterious consequences for a person's physical and mental wellbeing.

The following chapters on memory training have been included because: they address the 'sociology of memory', they have the potential to help allay the fears of those worrying about having a memory impairment, and they contribute to our knowledge about what methods and interventions will help persons with early and real memory loss. Memory training is part of the ongoing psychological study of what types of memory are affected, and spared in dementia, and it has an important role to play in determining how long persons can be maintained at a given level of functioning with structured, systematic intervention.

Chapter 14

The anticipation of memory loss and dementia in old age

Eena Job

SUMMARY

From the standpoint of what might be called a sociology of memory, the author explains the synthesis she has adopted in an attempt to understand memory in old age and to deal with the practical problems experienced by many old people who have no discernible pathology.

It is argued that the aging process too often occurs in a social situation detrimental to intellectual functioning, and that the decrements interpreted as precursors of dementia may be due less to the aging process itself than to deleterious elements of that social situation.

Memory training for the aged has a role within this context if it deals specifically with problems the old people themselves regard as relevant, and if the model used for explanation makes sense to them; but dealing with low self-esteem and overcoming isolation are at least equally important.

INTRODUCTION

For 2 years the author conducted a series of workshops for the Continuing Education Unit at the University of Queensland, workshops called 'Fending off forgetfulness'. The age range of participants was from 22 to 87, and though most adult ages were represented, elderly people tended to predominate. The sample was self-selected and there was no clinical testing. It is likely that a few had some pathological condition, but the great majority were clearly 'normal' – though many had come to the workshops because of their doubts on that point. They were misinterpreting quite normal forgetfulness as the first insidious signs of dementia; and this was especially the case among those whose family history included a dementing relative, or among those whose work brought them into frequent contact with nursing-home patients or other casualties of old age.

The workshops attracted a very positive response from those with a strong sense of identity and a conviction that they were to a large degree in control of their own destiny. The author believes the programme could be adapted for those in need of greater guidance.

The workshops arose out of research into people aged 80 and over (see Job, 1983; 1984), in which the majority of respondents, despite their extreme age, demonstrated memory competence over the whole range of short- and long-term memory. Those who recalled the past vividly were also very much in touch with the present, while those few who had retreated to the past tended to confuse husbands with fathers and were hazy about how many children they had had. The author became convinced that the widely held assumption that age brings biological changes mysteriously affecting short-term memory, while leaving long-term memory not just intact, but better than ever, was little more than a myth. And a very damaging myth at that.

TOWARDS A SOCIOLOGY OF MEMORY

There are social myths about memory as there are about other crucial elements in life. Mythically, memory is a box in which information is laid down as acquired; those born with a large box are thereby gifted with a good memory. But inevitably in those living to be old there comes a time when there is no space left for recent information, and in attempting to pack more in, old memories spill over to the surface and people are reduced to 'living in the past'.

Like other social myths this simplistic model has a dangerous potential for self-fulfilling prophecy, reinforcing stereotypes about the elderly as out of touch with reality and incapable of learning something new. As we grow older we become especially vulnerable to the assumption that we are like machines that are wearing out, our creative days long past. Everything that serves to reinforce that assumption – anxiety, low self-esteem, withdrawal – contributes to the lapses we call forgetfulness, and the anxiety associated with lack of self-esteem and consequent withdrawal from society is exacerbated by crises common in old age. Old people – and indeed, young people, too – can become temporarily disoriented and confused as a result of the shock of a bereavement, a sudden change in location, the side-effects of medication, anaesthetics, external or internal head injuries, illness or depression. If such symptoms are interpreted as the first signs of an irreversible decline, we increase the likelihood of that decline.

According to the *Oxford English Dictionary* the process or condition of aging, growing old, living a long time, is 'senescence'; 'senility' refers to the disease processes that are peculiar to that period. It shall be argued that whatever disease processes may or may not be present, the social situation of most old people encourages deterioration. The term 'social construction' was coined by sociologists Peter Berger and Thomas Luckmann (1966) in the 1960s to describe a continuous interchange between society on the one hand, and individuals on the other. Society, with rules of behaviour built into it, is 'out there' when we are born, like the air we breathe; and again like the air we breathe, we take it in, internalize it, initially without question. We have to acquire a fair degree of sophistication before we begin to wonder about things like air pollution – or about whether some of the social rules and expectations we have accepted as unquestionable are conducive to our mental health.

Society as 'breathed in', as it were, has defined old age as a period of inevitable decline. Old age is stigmatized, a devalued status, as Irving Rosow (1974) puts it; and the old themselves accept the devaluation and the stigma. There are few things more conducive to poor performance, in any sphere, than a self-image of oneself as a poor performer. Added to these damaging expectations – the subjective dimension of old age – there is the objective situation of the old as characterized by loss – loss of loved ones; loss of income; loss of sensory acuity; perhaps loss of mobility; certainly loss of many opportunities for problem solving. As one distinguished geriatrician says: 'man is a problem-solving animal and without facility to have problems to solve, goes into a decline. Our society encourages and forces the elderly into becoming non-problem-solving beings' (Whitehead, 1978).

What we don't use, we lose. To retain our faculties we must use them, and to use them, we must have a stimulus to use them. Imagine a healthy and intelligent 10-year-old, deprived of physical exercise, intellectual stimulation, variety of social contacts and close emotional ties – how long would such a child remain healthy and intelligent? Yet for old people, close emotional ties are commonly – even inevitably – severed by bereavement; social contacts of any kind are reduced, often both in quantity and quality; intellectual stimulation may be entirely absent; opportunities for physical exercise limited by expectations that 'resting' is the most suitable behaviour. It is remarkable that in spite of the way old age is socially constructed, so few old people actually conform to the agist stereotype of senility. It needs to be said over and over again that those who deal with the casualties of old age are in constant danger of defining those casualties as typical of the majority. But they are not. Research has established beyond doubt that, as Hobman says, most old people most of the time 'accomplish the process of ageing with little or no recourse to their medical advisers and none to the social services. Old age is not a disease, nor is it a social problem' (Hobman, 1978).

Just as old age is not a disease, neither is forgetfulness, which is by no means restricted to the old. There is a demonstrable need for a sociological approach to the study of memory. Such an approach would present memory as more of an acquired skill than as an inborn gift, and examine the influence of environment not only on the establishment of memory habits, but as factors in any later deterioration. Memory skills are culture bound; as members of urbanized societies with formal schooling we concentrate heavily on verbal rehearsal as a means of consolidating material (often in the form of abstract propositions) in long-term memory. In doing so we may lose some of the richness of mental imagery and kinesthetic responses which are important aids to memory in other cultures (e.g. see Wagner, 1978). If at the same time we lose respect for the aged as repositories of experience, we denigrate reminiscence and deny the value of the past as a perspective for the present and the future. Contemporary moves to record oral histories is a step towards reversing this process and may lead to a re-evaluation of the memory capacities of the aged.

Replacing social myths with more accurate perceptions is necessarily a long-term project. To meet the needs of elderly people whose interpretation of their own memory problems is coloured by existing myths, it is necessary to begin with an explanation of what memory is and how it works.

A MODEL OF MEMORY

As a sociologist the author needed to achieve some sort of synthesis between conflicting theories, in a volatile field where a great deal of heat is generated by differences in interpretation and in terminology. For the workshops, her mentors in the psychology of memory were selected eclectically from authors such as Anderson (1983), Baddeley (1983), Cermak (1972), Cermak and Craik (1979), Loftus (1976; 1980), Neisser (1982), Norman (1976), Schank (1982), Schank and Abelson (1977), Seamon (1980), and Wingfield and Byrnes (1981); and to obtain some understanding of the neurological processes involved she relied heavily on the works of Sir John Eccles (1973; 1979), as well as those of Karczmar and Eccles (1972), Bergland (1985), Mark (1974) and others. The synthesis arrived at was in terms of the processing of information at several different levels, considered as a series of happenings related to the registering, storing and finding of information, rather than as box-like structures 'containing' information. In this model the terms 'short-term memory' and 'long-term memory' refer to time-related mental activities, not to containers or structures of any kind.

In short-term memory, for instance, it is not space, but time, that is short. Short-term memory deals with the present, and the present keeps slipping into the past, so it can be thought of as just another term for our immediate consciousness. The time limitations are very strict and apply to the whole human race: for the brightest among us, holding nine separate items such as digits in our heads for as long as 15 seconds will strain short-term memory to its limit.

Long-term memory has no such limitations, but it is equally busy. It is responsible for making permanent records that are available to consciousness at a moment's notice; for making sense of these records in the light of what is already stored there; and for their constant updating in the light of new information. In addition, it helps short-term memory with the third remembering task – retrieval of the information when required. So long-term memory is far from being a passive storehouse. Rather, it is more like a factory, constantly re-assembling old and new information so that it makes sense in the immediate circumstances, and linking them up together into networks of associations.

Apparently when we remember something, a cue from short-term memory activates ideas in long-term memory connected into networks by associated meanings. Activation of any one item automatically makes ready others that are closely associated with it, with lessening degrees of activation spreading from one network to another, until a pattern is found that matches the cue to our satisfaction. Some of the linkages between the networks form quite well-worn pathways, a generalized framework that saves us the bother of considering every incoming item as something entirely new. These frameworks are heavily influenced by cultural factors as well as by individual experiences. And almost all networks contain potential blockages, in the form of painful or embarrassing associations that we would rather forget.

A good memory for long-ago events is characteristic of those who are alert and observant of present-day events, and have well-established habits of thinking about their experiences – recent as well as past – long enough to consolidate them for storage. Attention is necessary for input; consolidation is necessary for storage; retrieval is necessary for output; these three steps are the crux of the matter, around which the 'Fending off forgetfulness' workshops were built.

This, the psychological aspect of memory, has its physiological counterpart in the form of networks of neurones connected up together by electrical impulses that spurt chemical neurotransmitters across the minuscule gaps separating one neurone from another. And though the brain has two separate hemispheres, and there are different, identifiable regions devoted to speech, hearing, motor activity, etc., yet the brain operates as a unit through these immensely complicated, instantaneous connectivities. Hearing something, for instance, activates not only the auditory cortex but may conjure up images in the visual cortex and perhaps initiates incipient speech movements in the throat through the motor cortex, all charged with some emotional impact generated in the limbic lobe and hypothalamus. The emotions probably emanate from memories, for the storage of which the hippocampus is a vital area. But the hippocampus is not itself the site of storage; memories appear to be stored over the brain as a whole. And once they are stored, according to some authorities they are there forever: 'There seems to be nothing that can be done to the physical brain, compatible with its continued life, that can permanently destroy memory once the initial susceptible period is over' (Mark, 1974: 76–7). That susceptible period is usually about 6 hours.

The model of memory outlined above was presented to workshop participants in simplified form as a preliminary lecture, usually beginning with the challenge 'Does anyone remember being born?' to emphasize the fact that we are born only with the equipment for memory, not with memory as such. Physiological aspects were dramatized by the use of a dissectible plaster cast of the brain. Questions were encouraged, but all that was aimed for was some understanding of general principles; the course was experiential rather than didactic and the emphasis throughout was on practice and personal participation.

FLUCTUATIONS IN MEMORY

The information-processing model in its many varieties is based on the computer as the fashionable analogy for human memory. To some extent this is legitimate, but like all analogies it is an approximation only, and the differences are crucial. The operation of a computer is logical and predictable in the extreme, while the operation of human memory is emotional rather than logical, and for that very reason, creative rather than predictable. To help people remember, we must keep in mind that people, unlike computers, are not cold electronic machines. The billions of brain cells we use when we use memory are thoroughly involved in the whole emotional business of what it means to be a living, breathing, feeling, remembering, variable, vulnerable human being. The levels at which processing of information takes place vary according to the purposes, motivation levels and vitality of the person doing the processing, resulting in fluctuations in normal performance that vary within a considerable range.

Biological rhythms

One very common cause of forgetfulness is the normal fluctuations that occur from hour to hour and day to day in our physiological levels of arousal, as indicated by pulse rate, body temperature, galvanic skin response, etc. These rhythmic variations are partly individual, partly species-wide; partly inbuilt, but at the same time highly subject to environmental influences. Such biological rhythms have been shown to affect memory (Folkard and Monk, 1978) as they affect everything else about us – which is not surprising, because the brain as part of the body is subject to normal variations in its electrochemical circuitry. These variations are highly individual, and often insufficient allowance is made for them. Expectations regarding memory tend to be very high, and often performance is judged adversely on the evidence of an occasional, perfectly normal lapse – especially as people grow older. Absentmindedness in a schoolboy may be excused on the grounds that 'he's a bit of a dreamer'; but no such tolerance is extended to forgetfulness in old age.

Figure 14.1 General causes of forgetfulness

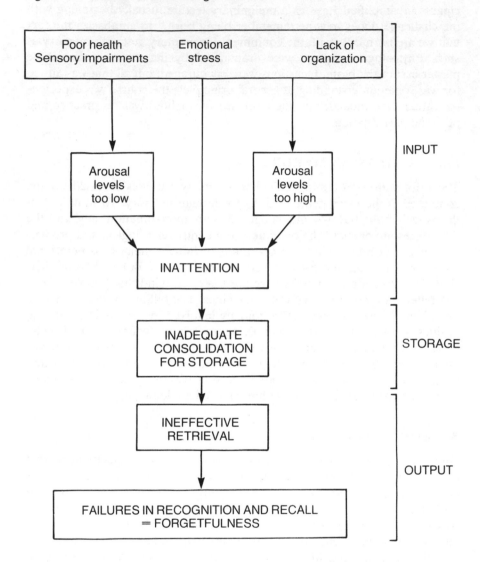

Lifestyle-related fluctuations

In addition to the biological rhythms that affect our performance in every sphere, there are also what might be called lifestyle-related fluctuations due to our state of health, the things we eat, the amount of exercise we take, the effect of medication, the effect of other drugs such as alcohol or cigarettes. The fitter we are physically – the better our diet, the more we exercise, the less we have to rely on prescribed or other drugs – the more likely we are to be fit mentally as well. Improving health is an important step in improving memory, and should include doing everything possible to overcome sensory impairments such as deafness or poor eyesight by means of modern technology. Being hard of hearing or having poor eyesight makes input into memory more of an effort, and without initial input of an effective kind there can be no long-term storage or eventual retrieval.

Emotion

Normal fluctuations in memory performance are also caused by changes in emotional state. Depression inevitably leads to a lowering of arousal levels, often below the threshold for attention. On the other hand, anxiety is likely to pitch arousal levels too high for concentration. The ideal, of course, is to be relaxed but alert, and though it is possible to cultivate that ideal, variations in mood must be expected as part of the normal human condition. Information is selected as worth remembering primarily on emotional grounds – though the emotion concerned may be no more than simple curiosity. Novelty appeals; something new tends to arouse interest, and thereby catches attention. But it must not be so new that it makes no sense at all, or it will be rejected because it will not fit comfortably into the existing information networks built up in long-term memory over a lifetime.

All these are perfectly normal fluctuations in mood and circumstances that contribute to variations in ability to remember. To keep them within optimal parameters and thereby fend off undue forgetfulness, we need to show people how to deal with stress, improve their health, and organize their lives productively. Only when these fundamentals have been attended to is it worth teaching specific skills of remembering. Zarit (1981), Poon *et al.* (1985) and others have made much the same point.

Figure 14.1 sums up these points under the heading 'General causes of forgetfulness'.

MEMORY PROBLEMS OF THE ELDERLY

Paying attention to achieve input, consolidating to achieve storage, retrieving to achieve output may all become more difficult for the old. It is important not to overemphasize the moderate loss of neurones normal to old age – a loss which, to quote from leading authorities, 'is far below the level that would cause neurological deficit symptoms' (Meier-Ruge *et al.*, 1978). Let us consider instead psychosocial factors such as the difficulty of paying attention to items in a routine so entrenched that it lacks the stimulus of novelty; and the difficulties involved in consolidating items for storage if encouragement to talk them over to reflect on them is lacking. Similarly, it is more difficult to retrieve them promptly if the stimulus to be quick on the conversational uptake is lacking: either because of living alone; or living with a partner of such longstanding that words are hardly necessary; or living in some sort of group setting in which the person is made to feel an inferior, undervalued member. All these things are quite usual accompaniments to aging. Add to them an increase in sensory impairments that hamper attention, and chronic illnesses that hamper all three stages of the memory process, and we have a better understanding of why elderly people, without any diagnosable neurological pathology, so often complain of memory loss.

The main message of the workshops was one of reassurance. It was not difficult to elicit from participants instances of lapses that were evidence of normality rather than otherwise, and these were used to build up confidence. For example, Mrs A may complain that her 'short-term memory is failing' because she can name all her companions in a 50-year-old school photograph but may forget whether or not she has put tea in the pot. But rather than demonstrating short-term memory failure, this is an example of the highly desirable process of habituation causing a perfectly normal lapse in attention. It is normal to become habituated to what we do over and over again; it loses the interest value of novelty so that it fails to reach the threshold of attention. All repetitive actions are subject to habituation, freeing the mind for more important matters. It becomes a serious problem only for those who become trapped in an inflexible routine, and the remedy is actively to seek new experiences.

Later stages in the memory process – consolidation for storage, and retrieval for recognition and recall – are subject to similar entirely normal lapses. Some participants complain that they can pick up a book and read several chapters before noticing that it is one they have already read. This is quite normal for people who do a lot of recreational reading and pile one chapter on top of another, one book on top of another, without pausing for a period of reflection on what was read. The remedy is to allow time for such reflection, so that the material can be consolidated for storage before absorbing more.

But it is in the third step, retrieval, that older people typically find most difficulty. With increasing age the slowing of reaction times may contribute to those irritating lapses when we retrieve the word or name we want several seconds, or minutes or even hours after the need has passed. This does not mean that we should accept a general slowing-down as an inevitable consequence of the passage of years; research has shown that it is very variable, both within and between individuals – some older people retain faster reaction times than are measured in the young. But doing things fast does not necessarily mean doing them better; if age teaches anything, it teaches the value of caution. In any case some people of high intelligence are inherently more cautious about committing themselves to a decision – even a decision as to what is the right word to use at a given moment – and this tendency sometimes, though not always, increases with age (Botwinick, 1978).

The sheer quantity of information accumulated over a lifetime may also slow down retrieval by complicating the sorting process and increasing the likelihood of interference from false cues. In addition, over the years people inevitably suffer sorrows and embarrassments that are instinctively blotted out from immediate consciousness, along with other information associated with it – often quite remotely associated. Nor is it only traumatic events that cause emotional blockages in memory networks – in fact, the major traumas have so much impact that they are seldom successfully forgotten. It is the minor embarrassments, the little things that make people feel foolish, that are most successfully suppressed, and these may cause those un-expected blockages when suddenly the word we want, the name we want – though we know we *know* it – refuses to come to our tongue. It is normal – indeed, it is inevitable – to suffer this kind of blockage occasionally. It is simply a part of being human, and there is no point in becoming anxious about it and thereby increasing the likelihood of lapses. For this type of blockage we can do no better than accept our fallibility as human beings, and wherever possible, to learn to laugh at ourselves.

IMPROVEMENT WITH AGE

Eliciting memory problems from participants usually establishes that the great majority, whatever the age of the sufferer, are well within the normal range. But reassurance can go further.

It should be pointed out that the detrimental changes to memory that occur with age are largely superficial, while other changes normal to old age can be rated as definite improvements. This is particularly evident among the increasing numbers of retired people who undertake courses of study, who in several respects have definite advantages over younger learners. They might not see as well, but they are more appreciative of what they see. They might not hear as well, but they are more likely to be interested enough to listen carefully. They might find it takes more conscious effort to remember things, but having made the effort, they make more sense of what they remember. Having acquired the precious gift of some humility, they are not so tempted to leave everything to the last minute; they do their work more thoroughly and get more out of it.

Changes for the better are the cumulative result of the riches of knowledge stored in long-term memory, and the ways of using them that experience has taught. There is nothing more valuable than experience, and it cannot be acquired except through years of living. Reiteration of this reassuring message had a tonic effect upon participants, especially when they were given the opportunity to demonstrate the richness of their memories and the intricate interconnections between them by a session of shared reminiscences.

SPECIFIC CURES FOR FORGETFULNESS

Much of the content of the workshops was based on ways of improving each of the three stages in the memory process, summarized in Figure 14.2

Improving attention

Attention can be improved, first of all, by bringing home the importance – frequently overlooked – of this initial step. The reasons for inattention are often quite deep-seated, and correcting them may involve a re-ordering of priorities and possibly quite drastic lifestyle changes. Depression, an unstimulating routine and preoccupation are enemies of alertness to what is going on around us; on the other hand, so is a complete lack of routine, a lifestyle so disorganized that the very narrow limits of normal short-term memory are constantly overloaded.

Effective exercises for improving attention can be based on old parlour games in which a brief message is passed, word for word, from one participant to the next, often with hilarious results when the last to receive the message reports it to the group as a whole. Paying close attention to what is said, without being diverted by planning one's reply, is a particularly important memory strategy for elderly people, for whom self-preoccupation is socially encouraged.

Improving consolidation for storage

In its preliminary stages consolidation for storage is a conscious function of short-term memory. The more we consciously work on the material we want to remember, the better it is transferred into long-term memory for permanent storage, and the more quickly and easily we can retrieve it again when needed. Initially storage strategies have to be practised consciously; they become effortless only through effort sustained over a period, just as in the acquisition of any other skill.

Six consolidation strategies were suggested in the workshops: organizing into chunks, arranging in a meaningful sequence, attending to context, making distinctions, using imagery and rehearsing with self-testing.

Organizing into chunks is, of course, a fundamental step, which to some extent we all do automatically; but it can certainly be improved if we recognize this short-term memory task and set about it with greater awareness. The technical term 'chunk' was coined by Miller (1956) in the 1950s to refer to any cluster of items organized into a unit – perhaps just by pausing, as in telephone numbers; or by similarity of meaning; or by grammatical convention; or by rhythm or rhyme; or quite arbitrarily, through haphazard associations. But we retain chunks better if the connection between the items make some logical or emotional sense – for

Figure 14.2 Some specific cures for forgetfulness

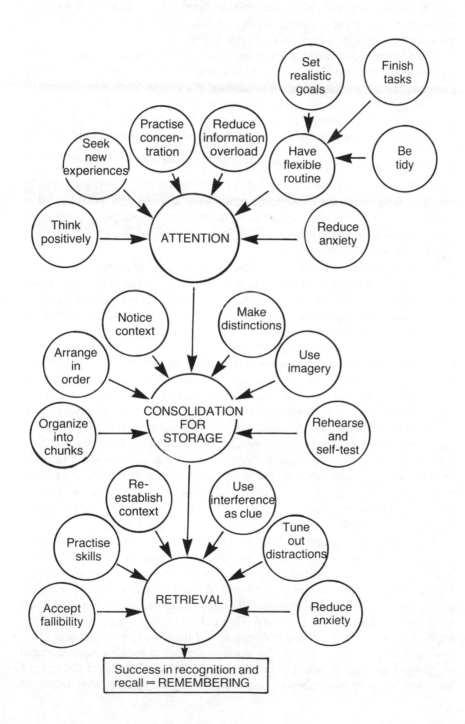

example, in a shopping list, grouping dairy food into one chunk and vegetables into another rather than mixing them up. It also helps if we keep the items comprising a chunk mostly to two or three, which short-term memory finds easiest to deal with comfortably.

The second recommended strategy is to arrange chunks in some sort of logical sequence or order, and again it does not matter what the ordering principle is – simple counting, or arranging in a hierarchy of importance, or perhaps following through some rhythmical or grammatical imperatives, or anything else that seems to fit the material, building bigger and better chunks that fit neatly into the networks of associated meanings that we carry around in our heads. Once chunking becomes a well-established habit, lists and other external aids to memory become better organized and therefore more easily remembered if for any reason they are not physically available when required. And participants were assured that leaving a list at home is a very normal lapse, best overcome by adopting deliberate checking strategies such as the 'cockpit drill' outlined in Chapter 4 of *Fending Off Forgetfulness* (Job, 1985).

Next, the importance of context was pointed out. We seem to absorb a huge variety of contextual associations with every input item; but again, becoming more aware of the process, so that we consciously tag chunks of information with appropriate contextual cues, is a strategy that is particularly effective for later retrieval.

I found it useful to distinguish three different sorts of context – semantic, situational and personal. Semantic context establishes the meaning of the item in question – for example, the fact that the word 'operation' occurs in a paragraph with military references establishes that the operation is not a medical one. Then there is the situational context: the external environment in which the message was received, its physical setting – the book it was in or the person who said it or the scene in which the event took place. Third, there is the recipient's own internal environment, the person as the receiver of the message – emotions at the time, state of health, levels of arousal, intent to learn or otherwise – in short, the personal context, which research into state-dependent learning (Swanson and Kinsbourne, 1979) has shown to have considerable bearing on consolidation for storage.

The fourth consolidation strategy recommended concerns distinctiveness. Not only do we need to slot our orderly chunks, complete with their appropriate context, into the networks of associated meanings through which memory operates; we also have to do our best to eliminate interference from other very similar material. The wrong name, Barton, can keep blocking out the right one, Barker. This is less likely to happen if we have made a habit of noting distinctive features of the people we meet and associating them in some way with the name – perhaps through a mental image of a large name tag attached to the distinctive feature. Whatever the type of information to be remembered – names or numbers or any other facts – it

certainly helps if we can distinguish them in some way, during the consolidation process, from similar material already stored in our networks of
associations.

Then there is imagery. The classic mnemonic systems – such as the
method of loci, peg-words, narrative and interactional chaining – all make
deliberate and effective use of the oft-neglected art of making images of the
material to be remembered. Whether we are naturally good visualizers or
otherwise, the mere attempt to make a mental image of the item to be
remembered is a very powerful consolidation strategy. With practice,
image-making can be improved, as in the attachment of name tags to faces
in the example given above. It is easy for most people to visualize concrete
objects such as people, but research has shown that this ability can be
extended to abstract propositions; we can turn them into Venn diagrams, or
some other self-explanatory diagram or picture (Whimbey and Ryan,
1969). The power of imagery may derive from linking right-brain pattern-
making faculties quite deliberately and specifically to left-brain verbal and
analytical functions, a liaison well worth cultivating.

Finally, there is rehearsal – in other words, repetition – especially in the
form of self-testing. They differ in that repetition can be parrot-like, especially if it is verbal, whereas self-testing requires some effort of retrieval and
usually has its own built-in psychological reward for success. It is among
the most potent of storage strategies, and rather than being threatening, it
can be enjoyable. Self-testing simply means recalling to mind new input
before going on to pile more on top of it, as we do in talking over some
experience with a friend. It helps us get more out of what we put in by
giving us the opportunity to savour it fully. The best sort of self-testing is
performed at gradually lengthening intervals: immediately after the initial
input, again within the hour, again a few hours later and perhaps next day.
Normally that is plenty, but if the material is very important occasional
testing should continue as long as necessary, especially before going to
sleep at night.

Analysing consolidation for storage into these six different steps makes
them seem more separate than they are. Actually, of course, they are
closely connected and tend to happen together. Meaningful chunking leads
naturally to orderly sequence and placing in context; making images is one
way of making distinctions; rehearsing and self-testing involve recalling to
mind these distinctive, meaningful chunks, in image form if possible. But
conversely, inefficiencies in these preliminary, conscious strategies involved
in the storage process tend to spread from one to another. Correcting them
may mean altering long-ingrained habits of thought, which is not an easy
matter. But an increased awareness of what those habits are, and how they
may be improved, is a big step on the way to overall storage improvement.

Improving retrieval

Finding the information again, its retrieval from storage, is the third and final step in remembering something, leading to the output of recognition and recall. The effectiveness of this third step depends heavily on the quality of prior input and storage – how well we attended to the material in the first place and how well it was stored. Ninety-nine times out of a hundred, alert attention and efficient storing lead to prompt and effortless retrieval of the information for recognition and recall. But sometimes, for the reasons already given, retrieval fails us.

Where retrieval failures are persistent, time and patience are required, building up self-confidence and possibly making changes in priorities and general lifestyle. Strategies adopted to improve attention are likely also to have a direct effect on retrieval abilities. Again it is essential to emphasize positives rather than negatives: for example, most participants have had the experience of going into a room for a particular purpose only to forget it until they return to the spot where the thought first occurred to them. They find it reassuring to learn that in doing so they are resorting to a normal, and very effective, retrieval strategy – the re-establishment of context. It is also reassuring to discover that interference by related material is a normal hazard due to the way memory works; when it occurs, it should be accepted as a sign that they are on the track of the correct information, which will undoubtedly become available for retrieval once anxiety has subsided.

Throughout the workshops group discussion arising from quizzes, exercises and games (see Chapter 5 in *Fending Off Forgetfulness* (Job, 1985)) encouraged participants to explore their own strengths and weaknesses and the fluctuations to be expected within the broad range of normality. The practice of effective strategies can to some extent help to compensate for a degree of brain damage (see, for example, Koch *et al.*, 1984) and at worst can do no harm.

CONCLUSION

Workshops are only a beginning. Rather than ending after one intensive burst, they should offer ongoing opportunities to improve health, reduce harmful levels of stress, and practise the degree of self-discipline necessary to organize life productively as well as to deal efficiently with the input, storage and output of information. Progress depends on persistence, and persistence probably depends on perceived success, along with a large element of enjoyment. So a memory-training programme for the elderly should be non-threatening (or people will give up in despair) and an enjoyable social occasion (or people will give up because of boredom).

Realistically, it needs to be accepted that in many respects memory training is like general fitness training, the promotion of better health. It is comparatively easy to persuade people to adopt a fitness programme; it is another matter to persuade them to continue it after the first enthusiasm has worn off. But for the elderly as for the young, physical fitness remains a worthy objective, even though many participants may drop out after a few weeks. Only a tiny minority will go on to become athletes, veteran or otherwise; but even the dropouts will have gained something from their experience. They are unlikely to slide further into indolence than before adopting the programme. They will remain aware that the benefits they gained, though temporary, could be theirs again if they wished.

Similarly, once people accept that lapses of memory are less often due to irreversible biological decline than to socially established habits that are amenable to change, they can decide for themselves whether or not they consider the effort needed is worthwhile. They feel more in control. The determination to make constructive lifestyle changes can be encouraged within the context of a memory-training programme long after a course has been completed; the learning of any skill, the pursuance of any interest, in itself improves memory.

It was pointed out at the beginning of this chapter that remembering is an emotional business, and that in helping people to remember we must take emotions into account. Negative emotions – such as fear and self-denigration – lead to negative outcomes, and there can be nothing more negative than the unfounded assumption that lapses of memory happen only to the old or to the prematurely senile, and that eventually everyone who lives long enough will suffer loss of memory. Alzheimer's disease and related disorders, despite their increasing incidence, still afflict only a minority of the old, even among the very old (Arie, 1973).* It is important to present another side to the picture besides the well-publicized 'silent epidemic' of senile dementia, so often proposed as inevitable in an aging population.

People need reassurance. They need hope. That is the one absolutely essential ingredient in any memory-training programme for the old.

NOTE

*Arie (1973) estimates that 20–25% of those aged 80 and over may be affected. Alarm at this high figure should not obscure its concomitant – that the overwhelming majority of very old people do not have this problem.

REFERENCES

Anderson, J. (1983) 'A spreading activation theory of memory', *Journal of Verbal Learning and Verbal Behavior* 22: 261–95.
Arie, T. (1973) 'Dementia in the elderly: diagnosis and assessment', *British Medical Journal* 4: 540–3.
Baddeley, A. (1983) *Your Memory: A User's Guide*, Ringwood, Victoria: Penguin.
Berger, P. and Luckmann, T. (1966) *The Social Construction of Reality: A Treatise*

in the Sociology of Knowledge, New York: Doubleday (reprinted in 1979 by Harmondsworth: Penguin).

Bergland, R. (1985) *The Fabric of Mind*, Ringwood, Victoria: Penguin.

Botwinick, J. (1978) *Aging and Behavior: A Comprehensive Integration of Research Findings*, New York: Springer.

Cermak, L. (1972) *Human Memory: Research and Theory*, New York: Ronald Press.

—— and Craik, F. (1979) (eds) *Levels of Processing in Human Memory*, Hillsdale, New Jersey: Lawrence Erlbaum.

Eccles, J. (1973) *The Understanding of the Brain*, New York: McGraw-Hill.

—— (1979) *The Human Mystery: The Gifford Lectures, University of Edinburgh, 1977–8*, Berlin: Springer Verlag.

Folkard, S. and Monk, R. (1978) 'Time of day effects in immediate and delayed memory', in M. Gruenberg, P. Morris and R. Sykes (eds) *Practical Aspects of Memory*, London: Academic Press, pp. 301–10.

Hobman, D. (1978) *The Social Challenge of Ageing*, London: Croom-Helm, p. 7.

Job, E. (1983) 'Retrospective lifespan analysis: a method for studying extreme old age', *Journal of Gerontology*, 38 (3): 369–74.

—— (1984) *Eighty Plus: Outgrowing the Myths of Old Age*, St Lucia/London/New York: University of Queensland Press.

—— (1985) *Fending Off Forgetfulness: A Practical Guide to Improving Memory*, St Lucia/London/New York: University of Queensland Press.

Karczmar, D. and Eccles, J. (1972) *Brain and Human Behaviour*, Berlin: Springer-Verlag.

Koch, C., Luscz, M., Overstreet, D. and Henschke, P. (1984) 'Transient improvement of memory in senile dementia following mnemonic training', *Australian Journal on Ageing* 3 (1): 16–20.

Loftus, E. (1980) *Memory: Surprising New Insights into How We Remember and Why We Forget*, Reading, Mass.: Wesley.

Loftus, G. and Loftus, E. (1976) *Human Memory: The Processing of Information*, Hillsdale, New Jersey: Lawrence Erlbaum.

Mark, R. (1974) *Memory and Nerve Cell Connections*, Oxford: Clarendon Press.

Meier-Ruge, W., Hunziker, O., Iwangoff, P., Reichlmeier, K. and Sandoze, P. (1978) 'Alterations of morphological and neurochemical parameters of the brain due to normal ageing', in K. Nandy (ed) *Senile Dementia: A Biomedical Approach*, vol. 3, New York: Elsevier North-Holland.

Miller, G. (1956) 'The magical number 7, plus or minus 2: some limits on our capacity for information processing', *Psychological Review* 63: 81–97.

Neisser, U. (ed.) (1982) *Memory Observed: Remembering in Natural Contexts*, San Francisco: W.H. Freeman.

Norman, D. (1976) *Memory and Attention: An Introduction to Human Information Processing*, 2nd edn, New York: Wiley.

Poon, L., Fozard, J., Cermak, L., Arenberg, D. and Thompson, L. (1985) *New Directions in Memory and Ageing: Proceedings of the George Tailland Memorial Conference*, Hillsdale, New Jersey: Lawrence Erlbaum.

Rosow, I. (1974) *Socialisation to Old Age*, Berkeley: University of California Press.

Schank, R. (1982) *Dynamic Memory: A Theory of Reminding and Learning in Computers and People*, Cambridge: Cambridge University Press.

—— and Abelson, R. (1977) *Scripts, Plans, Goals and Understanding*, Cambridge: Cambridge University Press.

Seamon, J. (1980) *Memory and Cognition: An Introduction*, Oxford: Oxford University Press.

Swanson, J. and Kinsbourne, M. (1979) 'State-dependent learning and retrieval: methodological cautions and theoretical conclusions', in J. Khilstrom and F. Evans (eds) *Functional Disorders of Human Memory*, Hillsdale, New Jersey: Lawrence Erlbaum.

Wagner, D. (1978) 'Memories of Morocco: the influence of age, schooling and environment on memory', *Cognitive Psychology* 10: 1–28.

Whimbey, A. and Ryan, S. (1969) 'Role of short-term memory and training in solving reasoning problems mentally', *Journal of Educational Psychology* 60: 361–4.

Whitehead, T. (1978) 'Ageing and the mind', in D. Hobman (ed.) *The Social Challenge of Ageing*, London: Croom-Helm, chapt. 7.

Wingfield, A. and Byrnes, D. (1981) *The Psychology of Human Memory*, New York: Academic Press.

Zarit, S. (1981) 'Memory-training strategies and subjective complaints of memory in the aged', *Gerontologist* 21 (3): 158–64.

Chapter 15

Memory training for older adults

Forrest Scogin

INTRODUCTION

Many older adults are understandably concerned about their memory functioning. Media attention to the dementing illnesses, particularly Alzheimer's disease, has alerted the public to the extraordinary effects of pathological cognitive impairment. Superimposed on this attention is the considerable evidence that there are age-related decrements in memory function that are non-pathological in nature. Thus, the older adult is left with the nettlesome question of evaluating their own memory failures and judging whether they are 'normal' or indicative of a disease process. It is no wonder that many participants in memory training programmes ask the question 'Am I going senile?' This chapter will present information on memory training for community-dwelling older adults. Given the number of elders who are concerned about their memory, this topic has wide application for the practitioner who works with older adults and presents many opportunities for the gerontological researcher. The chapter will also address through speculation the reasons for the relatively infrequent utilization of memory training for older adults, despite some accumulating evidence that such training has modest yet reliable benefits for participants.

MEMORY PERFORMANCE AND MEMORY COMPLAINTS

Despite the concerns of many persons, the actual prevalence of moderate and severe cognitive impairment among older adults is relatively low. Though figures vary considerably owing to methodological differences, most investigations report rates in the range of 1 to 15 per cent (Bayles and Kaszniak, 1987). The incidence and prevalence of mild cognitive impairment is considerably higher. It is the latter condition with which memory training has been found to be successful. The distinction between normal age-related changes and pathological changes in memory function is not only hard for the older adult to discriminate, it is also a vexing and at times agonizing distinction for the clinician and researcher. Later in this chapter, I will describe some of the screening that is conducted in our programmes to attempt to delineate these conditions.

Memory functioning does change as one ages. Deficits in secondary/ effortful functioning have been documented in a variety of studies. The reasons for these deficits have been the foci of a substantial body of research. Most pertinent to the topic of memory training have been the studies which have examined information-processing skills among older adults. The gist of this research is that elder's tend not to use the most efficient or effective memory skills (Poon *et al.*, 1980). For example, age differences on free recall tasks are usually larger than on recognition tasks. An example of a free-recall task is recalling a list of items without reference or cues, while a recognition task would be recognizing the items on the list from a series of distractor items. The differences in free recall and recognition suggest that storage of information has occurred but that retrieval strategies are not optimal. These and similar findings are the basis of the skills taught in most memory-skills training programmes for older adults.

As noted above, memory complaints by older adults are common. In a community survey, Lowenthal *et al.* (1967) found that 50 per cent of their older respondents reported having serious memory problems. Similarly, Sluss *et al.* (1980) found that 80 per cent of their sample of older men complained of memory difficulty. The magnitude of these complaints suggests that interventions directed to memory complaining older adults should strike a responsive chord. Anecdotal support for this observation comes from the author's experience of being flooded with requests for participation in a training programme after an announcement in an obscure portion of a metropolitan newspaper.

Thus, one can infer that the majority of older adults will report memory complaints yet evidence non-pathological declines in memory performance. Given this set of circumstances it is puzzling that relatively little research has been conducted on memory training for older adults. A brief review of selected memory training literature follows.

MEMORY TRAINING STUDIES

There have been several studies that have investigated the efficacy of instructing elders in the use of a specific mnemonic technique (Treat *et al.*, 1981; Smith and Winograd, 1978). For example, Robertson-Tchabo *et al.* (1976) taught subjects the method of loci, with subsequent improvements in memory functioning. The method of loci is an ancient mnemonic technique in which the subject develops a familiar path of imageable locations, for example around the interior of one's home or on a familiar journey. To-be-remembered items are then associated in imagery with each of the locations. Retrieval is facilitated by a trip through the locations in which the associated imagery is reviewed. Yesavage and his colleagues have conducted a series of similar studies in which participants were instructed in the use of interacting images for name–face recall with relaxation training (Yesavage, 1984) and with instructions to judge the pleasantness of the interacting images, a deep processing cue (Yesavage *et al.*, 1983). Older adults demonstrated improved name recall following training, with a more recent study demonstrating that specific pretraining in relaxation and deep processing cues was associated with greater preservation of training effects at 6-month follow-up (Sheikh *et al.*, 1986).

The limitation of these studies is that they are focused on the acquisition of a specific technique rather than memory skills in general. Zarit and his colleagues conducted several published investigations of more robust memory training programmes (Zarit *et al.*, 1981a; Zarit *et al.*, 1981b). In each of these studies, non-demented elders were provided group training in a variety of mnemonic techniques, including organizational strategies, imagery and rehearsal. Memory training was compared to control conditions focused on personal growth in one study and discussion of current events in the other study. Interestingly, the conclusions that can be drawn from these studies are that participation in a group experience is helpful in so far as reducing complaints about memory and that instruction in memory-enhancement techniques has the added benefit of actually improving objective memory performance. Follow-up evaluations suggested unfortunately that the training effects were short-lived. None the less, these studies by Zarit and his colleagues were instrumental in experimentally demonstrating that elders could benefit from structured intervention.

A study conducted by Zarit *et al.* (1982) is worth mentioning in the context of establishing the parameters of memory training. These investigators offered memory training to dementia patients and their care-givers. The results of this study are somewhat ironic. The patients evidenced fleeting improvements on measures of memory function, but care-givers actually felt greater distress at the conclusion of the programme. I believe the message from this study is that memory training participants should be carefully screened and only those who have the potential to achieve meaningful gains should be allowed to participate. To do otherwise is potentially a disservice to the participant and their family.

SELF-HELP EXTENSION OF MEMORY TRAINING

The studies reviewed above suggesting modest but reliable gains for older adult's participating in memory training led the author to explore alternative training modalities. A popular alternative in recent research and practice has been bibliotherapy. Bibliotherapy is the use of literary work in the treatment of emotional and physical problems. Substantial reviews by Glasgow and Rosen (1978; 1979) illustrate the diversity of problems addressed by bibliotherapeutic intervention. The extension of this modality to memory training for older adults seemed natural. Various writers have discussed the reasons for underutilization of mental health services by elders (e.g. Gatz and Pearson, 1988). These include economic, geographical, temperamental and informational issues. The nature of bibliotherapy seemed to surmount to some degree a number of these encumberances. For example, bibliotherapy is cost-efficient, tends to reduce transportation costs since fewer visits to training sites are required, and is usually readily accepted by would-be participants as a non-invasive intervention relative to group or individual training. Additionally, some research suggests that older adults tend to perform best under self-paced conditions (Treat and Reese, 1978). Certainly, bibliotherapy is a self-paced training modality, and thus capitalizes upon this advantage.

The efficacy of self-taught memory training was investigated in a study by Scogin *et al.* (1985). A 92-page manual was developed by the first author to serve as the training material. The manual was divided into 16 training sections, with material designed to take approximately one hour of work per day. The manual presented introductory material on memory and aging, followed by extensive coverage of a number of experimentally tested mnemonic techniques. The techniques presented were the method of loci, chunking, categorization and novel interacting images for name–face recall. Many exercises and applications were included in the manual in order to facilitate compliance. Sixty community-dwelling adults, 60 years of age or greater who complained of memory difficulties were randomly assigned to an immediate or a delayed training condition. Participants were contacted once per week while they were working with the manual to answer training-related questions and monitor progress. Thus the programme was not a completely self-administered one but involved a minimal-contact component. This issue will be discussed more thoroughly later in this presentation.

A variety of objective and subjective memory assessments were conducted prior to, immediately following and 1 month after training. Objective measures included immediate and delayed recall of a noun list, a shopping list and a series of names and faces. Subjective measures included the metamemory questionnaire (Zelinski *et al.*, 1980), an assessment of memory complaints, and the Zung self-rating depression scale (Zung, 1965). The results were both promising and puzzling. The promising part was that improvements were observed on a number of the objective memory performance indices; the puzzling part was that it was difficult to detect significant changes on the subjective assessments, especially the memory-complaint inventory. One-month follow-ups suggested that little slippage had occurred in the training effects. Despite the mixed findings, as a beginning piece of research this study established that elders could successfully train themselves in memory skills.

An extension of this research was conducted in a 1986 dissertation by

Flynn. She compared the efficacy of two training conditions: group memory training plus the manual versus the manual alone. Both the combination conditions and those with the manual alone were superior to the control condition in terms of memory improvement, but the combined group and manual training was superior to the manual alone. These results suggest that both group and self-administered training possess efficacious components. Many questions remain, however, as to which modalities are best suited for particular combinations of memory problems and participant characteristics. The results of the research reviewed suggest that memory training can be beneficial to older adults.

APPLICATIONS OF MEMORY TRAINING

In the following paragraphs I would like to overview some of the practical considerations involved with offering memory training programmes. These considerations include announcements concerning availability of services, practitioner preparation and qualifications, screening of participants and programme evaluation. Some problems that may be encountered will also be addressed with suggestions made for remedies.

The most logical place to begin would seem to be with the practitioner. My experience would suggest that credentials *per se* are less important to providing memory training to elders than is a solid grounding in gerontology. More specifically, one should be conversant with the literature on memory and aging, the dementing illnesses, and the relationship of mental-health/attitudinal factors to memory functioning. It is almost a guarantee that one will be asked to comment upon or address these issues in the course of training; furthermore, it is my belief that discussion and information dissemination on these issues is a central component of a well-rounded training programme. Thus, if one's training does not include exposure to these topics, then some background preparation is in order.

The next consideration is the training itself. What form and content? There are many options available. The two forms that I am most familiar with are group and self-taught modalities. Each has strengths and limitations. Group memory training is probably the more popular and certainly the more traditional of the two. The strengths of the group approach are the opportunity to share experiences, resolve difficult training issues and socialization. I believe the latter to be quite powerful, especially as concerns the mental-health and memory-perceptions link alluded to earlier. The drawbacks to groups are that they require greater trainer-time commitment, trainer experience in leading groups and multiple trips to and from the training site by participants. Another personal observation in leading groups with older adults is that the variability in participant concentration and retention skills makes didactic pacing difficult. What seems repetitive and simple-minded to participant A may be devilishly confusing to participant B. The work of Zarit and his colleagues would suggest that the effect of being in a group in and of itself is beneficial to the older adult complaining of memory difficulties. Most likely these effects are attributable to the 'common factors' described in the psychotherapy literature (Garfield, 1980), such as expectancy, trainer concern and support. It may well be that the group memory training format facilitates these common factors.

The other modality I wish to describe is self-taught memory training. My research efforts in memory training have been investigating the efficacy of this approach. Several resources exist for establishing a self-taught memory-training programme. Books and manuals have been developed by Scogin and Flynn (1986), Lorayne and Lucas (1974) and Lapp (1987). So far as I know, only the Scogin and Flynn manual has been evaluated for efficacy, though based on content I would expect these sources to be quite interchangeable. Our self-taught programmes have been run as follows. Community-dwelling elders are recruited for participation and screened for the presence of non-dementing memory impairment. We have used the mental status questionnaire (Kahn *et al.*, 1960) for this purpose, though any number of instruments exist for such screening. We also routinely screen for reading ability. This is done informally by asking the person if they read and if so, what they read. If we have any questions regarding their reading ability, we have them read a sample passage (usually our consent form). Interest in reading is so crucial to the self-taught approach that it is mandatory and common-sensical to screen on this dimension.

Though this may seem obvious, it is also useful to evaluate the individual's complaints about their memory functioning and their actual memory performance on laboratory tasks. These variables tend not to be isomorphic, that is there tends not to be a linear relationship between level of memory complaint and degree of memory impairment (Zarit, 1982; Sunderland *et al.*, 1986). Thus, for the purposes of our programmes we are interested in elders who exhibit low memory performance, high memory complaints or both. Criteria are available for evaluating these constructs in a most useful special issue of *Developmental Neuropsychology* (vol. 2, no. 4, 1986). In addition, the administration of such measures before and following training gives both the participant and trainer some sense of progress made. In our studies, we have tried to create a blend of traditional laboratory and more 'everyday' memory tasks. For example, twenty nouns in a free-recall task, as a traditional laboratory measure, and a twenty-items grocery list as an everyday analogue. We also include a validated inventory of memory complaints such as the memory functioning questionnaire (Gilewski *et al.*, 1983, August) and a measure of mental health such as the symptoms checklist (Derogatis, 1977).

Self-administered training itself consisted in our studies of supplying participants with training materials and following up with weekly telephone calls to monitor progress. Participants work at their own pace, with the training manual divided into twenty-four sections designed to take approximately 1 hour of work. The manual begins with an introduction to memory and aging, in which basic information-processing constructs are overviewed and typical changes with aging are presented. Particular attention is devoted to refutation of the 'senility myth' and the belief that 'old dogs can't learn new tricks'. The subsequent chapters are devoted to the mastery of mnemonic skills, beginning with physical reminders, followed by chunking, categorization, method of loci and novel interacting images. The manual is set up in workbook fashion so that exercises and written assignments are frequently included. Review sections are also included throughout the manual. The present manual is 117 pages in length and is available through the Behavioral Sciences Document Service (1986).

Group memory training has been offered in our studies so as to closely approximate the content of the training manual outlined previously. This is in large part a research consideration, but it is also a time consideration. Our groups meet on four consecutive weeks for 2-hour sessions. Group participation and mutual problem solving is encouraged by the group leader, and homework assignments are made after each session. We have limited group size to approximately twelve persons, so as to facilitate group cohesiveness and guard against the training becoming a classroom lecture to an assembled audience. A protocol for leading group memory training has been developed and is available (Scogin *et al.*, 1988) upon request. The protocol is an outline of suggested activities for the four group meetings. For example, the outline for group session two is broken down into six sections; (1) overview of session, (2) review of previous session, (3) chunking, (4) categorization, (5) imagery/visualization, (6) homework assignments. Within each major section of the meeting are a number of more specific activities, for example, within the 25 minutes allocated for categorization, the leader is expected to cover the following; (a) why categorization is effective, (b) examples of categorization in use, (c) exercises with categorizable lists (six lists). Thus, this protocol provides a rather detailed guide to leading a memory training group.

CONSIDERATIONS AND POTENTIAL PROBLEMS

Several factors should be considered prior to initiating a memory training programme for older adults. As alluded to earlier, some decisions as to the types of persons to whom the training will be offered must be made. By virtue of our recruitment efforts, we have largely trained non-demented, moderately to highly motivated, reasonably well-educated persons. While these characteristics are by no means necessary, common sense suggests these to portend success in the types of programmes described in this chapter. In our screening, we attempt to informally assess the motivation for training. In some cases, this takes no more than insuring that the potential trainee speak to our staff. Quite often, family members are the motivated party, while the potential trainee expresses little or no interest in the programme. Another situation that arises with some frequency is the person who wants improvements with their memory functioning, but is not interested in a skill-learning approach, preferring a more passive intervention such as medication. We feel it is crucial to properly screen on these dimensions for the sake of the potential participant as well as the success of the programme.

Two important problems that occur in any psychosocial intervention are non-compliance and attrition. Self-administered programmes are more adversely affected by the former, while group memory training is more affected by the latter. In that self-administered programmes are almost wholly dependent on the participant, non-compliance in essence means that the assigned tasks are not being completed or done with little enthusiasm. Fortunately, the manner in which our self-administered programmes have been run have resulted in rather high compliance. In the study undertaken by Scogin *et al.* (1985), compliance was assessed by reviewing manuals to see if blanks had been filled in on the chapter assignments. We found a compliance rate of 94 per cent. Though this variable has not been systematically manipulated, I believe the weekly telephone contact is the programme variable that accounts by far for most of this high compliance rate.

Attrition is a problem for both self-administered and group memory training, but is a greater concern in terms of planning for the group modality. The group-training attrition rate of 33 per cent in the Flynn (1986) study is quite comparable to that reported in the psychosocial treatment literature. Thus, if one begins with a group composed of twelve persons, typically the group will end with around eight members. If the latter number becomes too small, the group loses its cohesiveness and demoralization can result. Consequently, we attempt to begin groups with a critical mass that will withstand the effects of attrition. A final note on attrition. In both of our bibliotherapy programmes for geriatric depression (Scogin *et al.*, 1987; Scogin *et al.*, 1989), dropouts and completers were found to be significantly different in the number of years of education completed (*M*'s = 12.3 and 13.9, respectively). Though we have devised no exclusion criterion based on this finding, it does bear consideration in a comprehensive screening interview.

A final consideration is the issue of maintenance of training gains. The training studies reviewed earlier have generally included follow-up periods up to 1 month. The results of most of these follow-ups have shown maintenance of training effects. However, in the only long-range follow-up of which I am aware, we (Scogin and Bienias, 1988) found that at 3-year follow-up there was no evidence of training maintenance. Memory performance measures had returned to pre-training levels for the training participants, while an untreated control group had experienced no 'age-related' changes. In response to this finding, it seemed important to study ways to retard training losses. This led to an investigation of an additional training component: booster sessions. In a study funded by the American Association for Retired Persons, we are studying the effects of booster sessions on both self-administered and group memory training. Fifty per cent of the participants who complete training will attend booster sessions during the follow-up period. Three sessions will be conducted over the course of the 6-month follow-up. For participants who received group training, the booster sessions will be group meetings focused on review and discussion of memory aid usage. For participants in the self-administered condition, the booster sessions will involve review of written material and extended telephone contacts focused on discussion of memory aid usage. We expect that participants who receive booster training will demonstrate less training slippage at the follow-up period than those who have not received such training. If indeed our assumption about booster sessions is confirmed, this may become an important recommendation for those planning memory training programmes.

CONCLUDING REMARKS

I have pondered for sometime the following question: Why isn't memory training more popular given (1) that so many older adults have subjective memory complaints and (2) that there are actually some encouraging reports in the literature? I now have at least some speculations on the matter. First, psychosocial interventions in general tend to be less frequently targeted and extended to older adults, though this appears to be changing. Psychotherapy, counselling and training programmes rarely focus on elders. Thus, the relative lack of popularity of memory training programmes is at least in part attributable to the lack of popularity of psychosocial programmes for older adults in general.

Another reason for the relative infrequent offering of memory training has to do with shortage of gerontologically trained practitioners. I believe this is particularly true of the persons probably best equipped by training to lead such programmes – psychologists. I believe this situation is changing however, with increasing numbers of clinicians pursuing training in gerotonology. Given the frequency of memory complaints among older adults, the provision of memory programmes is a natural application of helping skills.

Two additional reasons come to mind as potential explanations for the 'memory training shortage'. The first I believe is that many service providers are simply unaware that such programmes have been designed and evaluated. In truth, there have not been that many studies done on memory training for older adults, and the results are published in rather specialized journals. The publicity that does surround memory training tends to be of the variety seen in magazine advertisements that promise 'instant memory' or 'total recall' with little or no expenditure of effort on the part of the consumer. Discerning readers can easily surmise that these claims are bogus and, unfortunately, legitimate memory training programmes suffer from the association. Until more realistic publicity is generated, individuals may shy away from memory training for fear it is quackery.

The final reason I believe that memory training is less popular than one might expect is that it truthfully is not a powerful intervention. Most people do improve as a result of training, but the changes are neither extraordinary nor permanent. Not surprisingly, I believe that further research on the enhancement of training efficacy is necessary to overcome the accurate perception of relatively weak effects for an effortful training experience. With a proven, relatively powerful training programme to offer, more older adults and more practitioners will engage themselves in memory training.

REFERENCES

Bayles, K.A. and Kaszniak, A.W. (1987) *Communication and Cognition in Normal Aging and Dementia*, Boston: College-Hill Publications.

Derogatis, L.R. (1977) *The SCL-90 Manual I: Scoring, Administration and Procedures for the SCL-90*, Baltimore, MD: Johns Hopkins University School of Medicine, Clinical Psychometrics Unit.

Flynn, T. (1986) 'Memory performance, memory complaint, and self-efficacy in older adults', unpublished doctoral dissertation, Washington University, St Louis, MO.

Garfield, S. (1980) *Psychotherapy: An Eclectic Approach*, New York: Wiley & Sons.

Gatz, M. and Pearson, C.G. (1988) 'Ageism revised and the provision of psychological services', *American Psychologist* 43: 184–8.

Gilewski, M.J., Zelinski, E.M., Schaie, K.W. and Thompson, L.W. (1983) 'Abbreviating the Metamemory Questionnaire: Factor structure and norms for adults', paper presented at the meeting of the American Psychological Association, Anaheim, CA.

Glasgow, R.E. and Rosen, G.M. (1978) 'Behavioral bibliotherapy: a review of self-help behavior therapy manuals', *Psychological Bulletin*, 85: 1–23.

—— (1979) 'Self-help behavior therapy manuals: recent developments and clinical usage', *Clinical Behavior Therapy Review* 1: 1–20.

Kahn, H.L., Goldfarb, A.I., Pollack, M. and Peck, A. (1960) 'Brief objective measures for the determination of mental status in the aged', *American Journal of Psychiatry* 117: 326–8.

Lapp, D. (1987) *Don't Forget: Easy Exercises for a Better Memory At Any Age*, New York: McGraw-Hill.

Lorayne, H. and Lucas, J. (1974) *The Memory Book*, New York: Ballentine Books.

Lowenthal, M.F., Berkman, P.C., Buehler, J.A., Pierce, R.C., Robinson, B.C. and Trier, M.L. (1967) *Aging and Mental Disorder in San Francisco*, San Francisco: Jossey-Bass.

Poon, L.W., Walsh-Sweeney, L. and Fozard, J.L. (1980) 'Memory skill training for the elderly: salient issues on the use of imagery mnemonics', in L.W. Poon, J.L. Fozard, L.S. Cermak, D. Arenberg and L.W. Thompson (eds) *New Directions in Memory and Aging: Proceedings of the George A. Talland Memorial Conference,* Hillsdale, NJ: Erlbaum, pp. 461–84.

Robertson-Tchabo, E.A., Hausman, C.P. and Arenberg, D. (1976) 'A classical mnemonic for older learners: a trip that works!' *Educational Gerontology* 1: 215–16.

Scogin, F. and Bienias, J. (1988) 'A three-year follow-up of older adult participants in a memory-skills training program', *Psychology and Aging* 3: 334–7.

—— and Flynn, T. (1986) 'Manual for memory-skills training', *Social and Behavioral Sciences Documents* 16: 14.

——, Hamblin, D. and Beutler, L. (1987) 'Bibliotherapy for depressed older adults: a self-help alternative', *Gerontologist,* 27: 383–7.

——, Jamison, C. and Gochneaur, K. (1989) 'Cognitive and behavioral bibliotherapy for mildy and moderately depressed older adults', *Journal of Consulting and Clinical Psychology* 57: 403–7.

——, Prohaska, M. and Flynn, T. (1988) 'Protocol for group memory training', unpublished manuscript, University of Alabama, Tuscaloosa, AL.

——, Storandt, M. and Lott, L. (1985) 'Memory-skills training, memory complaints, and depression in older adults', *Journal of Gerontology* 40: 562–8.

Sheikh, J.I., Hill, R.D. and Yesavage, J.A. (1986) 'Long-term efficacy of cognitive training for age associated memory impairment: a six-month follow-up study', *Developmental Neuropsychology* 2: 413–21.

Sluss, T.K., Rabins, P., Gruenberg, E.M. and Reedman, G. (1980) 'Memory complaints in community residing men', *Gerontologist* 20: 201.

Smith, A.D. and Winograd, E. (1978) 'Adult age differences in remembering faces', *Developmental Psychology* 14: 443–4.

Sunderland, A., Watts, K., Baddeley, A.D. and Harris, J.E. (1986) 'Subjective memory assessment and test performance in elderly adults', *Journal of Gerontology* 41: 376–84.

Treat, N.J. and Reese, N.W. (1978) 'Age, pacing and imagery in paired-associates learning', *Developmental Psychology* 12: 119–24.

——, Poon, L.W. and Fozard, J.L. (1981) 'Age, imagery, and practice in paired-associates learning', *Experimental Aging Research* 7: 337–42.

Yesavage, J.A. (1984) 'Relaxation and memory training in the elderly', *American Journal of Psychiatry* 141: 778–81.

——, Rose, T.L. and Bower, G.H. (1983) 'Interactive imagery and affective judgements improve face–name learning in the elderly', *Journal of Gerontology* 29: 197–203.

Zarit, S.H. (1982) 'Affective correlates of self-reports about memory of older people', *International Journal of Behavioral Geriatrics* 1: 25–34.

——, Cole, K.D. and Guider, R.L. (1981a) 'Memory training strategies and subjective complaints of memory in the aged', *Gerontologist* 21: 158–64.

——, Gallagher, D. and Kramer, N. (1981b) 'Memory training in the community aged: effects of depression, memory complaint, and memory performance', *Educational Gerontology* 6: 11–27.

——, Zarit, J.M. and Reever, K.E. (1982) 'Memory training for severe memory loss: effects on senile dementia patients and their families', *Gerontologist* 22: 373–7.

Zelinski, E.M., Gilewski, M.J. and Thompson, L.W. (1980) 'Do laboratory tests relate to self-assessment of memory ability in the young and old?' in L.W. Poon, J.L. Fozard, L.S. Cermak, D. Arenberg and L.W. Thompson (eds) *New Direc-*

tions in Memory and Aging: Proceedings of the George A. Talland Memorial Conference, Hillsdale, NJ: Erlbaum, pp. 519–44.

Zung, W.W.K. (1965) 'A self-rating depression scale', *Archives of General Psychiatry* 12: 63–70.

Chapter 16

The structured life-review process: a community approach to the aging client

Barbara Haight

SUMMARY

This chapter describes the use of a structured life-review process with three different samples of elderly people. This life-review process encourages clients to review their lives from birth to death. A therapeutic listener conducts the process using a life review and experiencing form (LREF). Three research projects using control and experimental groups tested the therapeutic efficacy of the life-review process. The LREF group showed life-satisfaction increases of approximately six points, whereas the control group, receiving only a friendly visit, had life-satisfaction score decreases of approximately one point.

INTRODUCTION

First, the life review as a useful tool for the clinical management of clients with minor cognitive impairment will be discussed. Second, a theoretical basis derived from the works of Butler and Erikson is presented as well as a review of the literature describing the history of life review in the United States. The method and recommendations for use of a structured life review are presented with supporting research results. Finally, a case study, Marjorie's story, illustrates the use and success of the life-review process with an aging client suffering transient and minor cognitive impairment.

REVIEW OF LITERATURE

Reminiscence of life review has a central position in psychological functioning during old age. Erikson, in his theory of the ages of man, proposes that the primary task of the older person is to accept his life as it has been lived in order that he may age successfully and achieve integrity. He states that integrity characterizes the individual who has adapted himself to the triumphs and disappointments of living, and represents a person who is at peace with himself and who is achieving life satisfaction (Erikson, 1950).

Butler, a proponent of the life review as a therapeutic aid, suggests there is a universal occurrence in older people of reviewing one's life. Butler believes this process is an inner experience that accounts for increased reminiscing and may also contribute to the occurrence of late-life depressions. He states that depression is particularly prevalent when an individual is fixated at a certain point or experience in his past and cannot reintegrate an event. Butler sees the life-review process as a means to successful reintegration which can give new significance and meaning to an individual's life (Butler, 1974). Butler's conclusion drawn from the comparative analysis of these two philosophies is that Erikson's eighth stage – integrity – is helped through the process of life review.

In his 1963 work, Butler postulated the universal occurrence in older people of an inner process of reviewing one's life. It was the seminal document propagating several more years of studying the concept of life review. Butler described the common stereotyped view of reminiscence in the elderly as a negative one. The stereotyped version of reminiscence depicted a wandering beyond the control of the older person that was both spontaneous and unselective. Butler further stated that one tends to consider the past most when prompted by current problems and crises. For example, one is more apt to review the past on the occasion of the death of a spouse, to remember times together, and to regret moments of misunderstanding when these instances can no longer be mended. Crises are likely to make one consider one's identity and examine one's lifestyle.

Butler (1974) postulated that endogenous depressions in the elderly may owe their existence to the inner process of the life review. He stated that the relationship of depression to the ongoing inner process of the life review needs to be studied. Along with this relationship, the roles of guilt, lack of resolution and despair need to be examined. It is possible that the quiet, depressed older person is 'stuck' at some guilty point in his or her life review and therefore regards his or her past life as useless.

The possibility of the life review occurring irrespective of the psychotherapeutic situation and causing depression and despair, suggests the need for a participant observer. A participant observer is a willing listener who can help the reviewer in coming to terms with his or her life. The listener acts as a sounding board and in this manner assists the reviewer to integrate past events and to gain satisfaction in the way his or her life has been lived. The life-review process, taking place with another individual, allows the reviewer to try out his or her ideas and, with reinforcement of these ideas, to establish a new identity. The elderly take stock of themselves as they review their lives and, if they achieve integrity, they will be able to decide what to do with the time they have left (Butler, 1978).

In 1974 Lewis and Butler wrote an article proposing the use of life review as therapy. Both stated that life review was not a process initiated by the therapist but rather a listening-in to an already ongoing self analysis.

They defined the purpose of therapeutic intervention as one which enhances the life-review process and makes it more conscious, deliberate and efficient.

Lewis and Butler further described the life review as a process which by its very nature evokes a sense of regret and sadness. However, deep depression is more likely to happen when the person makes judgements without testing or sharing them. Further, the life review is greatly enhanced by listeners. Even untrained high school students have successfully aided the elderly by listening attentively. Life review in groups is especially useful in decreasing the sense of isolation and uselessness felt by the elderly and gives older people a way to catch up with the times.

REVIEW ARTICLES

Coleman (1986) contributed an extensive piece to the literature through his book, *Aging and Reminiscence Processes*. He reported 15 years of research and clinical practice using a phenomenological perspective to examine people's own views of themselves. His book presents case studies throughout which serve to illustrate particular parts of the reminiscence process. Coleman warns us all to consider each person and the person's process of reminiscing as individually different.

Two other authors contributed significant reviews to the literature. The first, Merriam reviewed the research on reminiscence in 1982 and concluded that the idea of reminiscence and its relationship to other affective processes was not clearly delineated. Additionally, findings regarding the adaptive value of reminiscence in later adulthood were inconclusive. Very little has been done to conceptualize the phenomenon of reminiscence or to determine its function in old age. Most research studies have used small non-random samples and it has been difficult to generalize results to the elderly population as a whole. Merriam stated that researchers needed to conceptualize the phenomenon of life review and concentrate on discovering the attributes of reminiscence. This way, an exploratory inductive theory-building methodology might generate insights which can later be operationalized and tested empirically. Merriam further suggested that more descriptive data be accumulated regarding the content included in reminiscing as well as the type and the amount of reminiscing.

The concept of life review was examined again in a review of the literature by Molinari and Reichlin (1984–5). These two authors evaluated and interpreted much of the work on life review in the past twenty years. They reached interesting conclusions that may be a guide for future research on the subject. These authors proposed the following: A need for basic demographic data, a separation of life review and reminiscence in future research, a clarified process of life review, a division and clarification of intrapersonal and interpersonal reminiscence, an examination of life-review differences in community versus institutional settings, longitudinal studies to examine long-term effects of life review and last, more collaboration between the clinical and research areas. Each of these suggestions is valuable and contributes to a clarification of the issues surrounding life review.

CLINICAL STUDIES

Nurses were pioneers in observing the existence and therapeutic value of life review and in reporting their clinical impressions. Burnside (1978), a noted nurse gerontologist, discussed life review as a useful group process and technique. Ebersole contributed many articles to the nursing literature on reminiscing. Ebersole (1976) described reminiscing as promoting self-understanding and reinforcing one's coping mechanisms. Safier (1976) reported a clinical observation which attested to the observed value of the life review as a therapeutic modality.

Reminiscing may be used in other ways. Babb de Ramon (1983) offered a very comprehensive guideline for instituting life review as a final task for the dying patient and Chubon (1980) wrote of the occurrence of life review in dialysis patients who face death daily. Chubon retold the story of Annie who reviewed her life through a novel depicting a story similar to Annie's own life story.

King (1982) reported the benefits of reminiscing groups. Her group took place in an adult day-care centre and was deemed therapeutic through self-report. King mentioned that sharing past events was almost competitive between group members until they discussed life during the Second World War. After the sharing of the events of the Second World War, empathy developed between group members in the sharing of mutually experienced hardships. King saw this sharing as a turning point for her group.

Schnase (1982) reported the benefits of therapeutic reminiscence and spoke repeatedly of the value of a therapeutic listener. Schnase looked at reminiscing as an extension of the hedonistic theory of memory and saw the preoccupation with past and pleasurable memories as supporting the hedonistic tendency to talk about the good old days. He also pointed out that the older person used reminiscence to signify his or her present position and to improve his or her relationships with others. Schnase advocated dealing with negative memories and positive memories and envisioned therapeutic reminiscing as providing a structured and positive setting for a life review which might otherwise have negative results. Schnase advised nurses to take a few minutes in a busy day to be sensitive listeners and to ask reflective questions that may help the older person to review silently within.

Hausman (1980) addressed life review as therapy and a means to intervene with people who do not use reminiscence in constructive ways. She visualized the goal of life-review therapy as reviewing, reorganizing and resolving the unfinished business interfering with the achievement of ego integrity. Life review is also a means of discovering areas of unfinished business. Hausman recognized the value of reviewing troubled spots in one's life and reported on several clients who successfully completed life review with excellent therapeutic results. She stated that successful life-review therapy can have a variety of results. A person may behave in a new way, gain new insight, find places where growth is still possible or gain pride in experiences that were not previously valued. Hausman quoted Albert, a retired writer, calling life review a 'clear memory button'.

Cook (1984) reported the efficacy of reminiscing with confused nursing-home residents. She described a pilot project designed to interrupt excessive isolation and mental decline in confused nursing-centre residents. A reminiscing group met on a weekly basis 45 minutes each week. Observational reports were made of the beneficial effects of the group. Members appeared more alert and there was a dramatic increase in the length of time group members spent socializing. Cook made an excellent point concerning reminiscing with the confused elderly. She noted that reminiscing capitalizes on remote memory functions, the last to be eroded in the process of memory decline, giving an additional reason for using reminiscing with the confused elderly.

CHRONOLOGICAL DESCRIPTIVE RESEARCH

The preceding literature, consisting of reviews, case studies and observational reports, is very positive concerning the therapeutic aspects of life review. With such positive reports, researchers in the United States began to examine life review more closely. Many of the research reports were less positive when discussing the value of life review. Much of the research in the field is based on a reminiscing experience of 1 hour and perhaps this is the reason the research reports are less favourable.

McMahon and Rhudick (1964) conducted a landmark research study on reminiscence. They confirmed that reminiscence is positively correlated with successful adaptation to old age through maintaining self esteem, reaffirming a sense of identity, and mastering personal losses. Twenty-five subjects were selected from the out-patient clinic of the Boston Veterans Hospital. Each subject was interviewed for 1 hour and a tendency was discovered in the non-depressed group to reminisce more. McMahon and Rhudick reported an increase in reminiscing in the elderly as a coping behaviour which facilitated adaptation. The tendency to remember only the good was addressed by quoting Peal, 'The mind never photographs, it paints pictures.' This halo effect was illustrated by the story of a football player who only remembers and retells his glories on the playing field. This halo effect depreciates the present and glorifies the past while it enforces self-esteem and reinforces a sense of identity. This same type of reminiscing is evident in those remembering only the good things about the dead. The study was concluded with the statement that reminiscence was positively related to freedom from depression.

THE FIRST AMBIGUOUS FINDINGS OF THE VALUE OF LIFE REVIEW

The Committee on Human Development of the University of Chicago conducted research on the life review in the late 1960s. Lieberman and Falk (1971) stated that the committee's findings did not permit a clear answer regarding the worth of reminiscence information: 'We have failed to find empirical support for the proposition that it makes a difference in adaptation or adjustment whether an individual is highly involved or uninvolved in his reminiscence activity and that the aforementioned theories need re-examination.' Included in this research and under the direction of Lieberman, Gorney (1968) developed an 'experiencing scale' and examined the relationship between experiencing and age. Gorney postulated that the greatest amount of reminiscing occurred between the ages of 60 and 70 years. He looked at three age levels in 10-year increments. His research supported the hypothesis that people aged 60 to 70 were high-level reminiscers. Gorney reasoned that this was because people in this age group were just beginning to review their lives now that they had the time to do so. Gorney further proposed that the older age group, 70 to 80 years, were low-level reminiscers because they had already accomplished the life review. Gorney did not test the level of life satisfaction in his subjects. This would have added the important dimension of knowing whether the 80 to 90-year-old had in fact completed the life review and achieved integrity as compared to those who had just begun the life review.

Falk (1969), also doing her research under the direction of Lieberman, examined the correlation of adaptation and reminiscing as one portion of her dissertation. She examined data and life histories from the same population that Gorney had used in his study. Falk defined adaptation as the ability to adjust to institutionalization. Adaptation was measured by a global assessment of data collected by nursing home personnel for one year after the initial confinement. Thirteen of the subjects died within a year's time and these subjects were included in the measure of 'inability to adapt.' There was no description of the mental and physical condition of those who died to show they were different from the adapters.

A panel of judges measured reminiscing by rating written statements of life history. The life history was divided into three segments: childhood, adulthood and total life span. By counting incidents of reminiscing, low-level reminiscers were differentiated from high-level reminiscers. Falk developed and used a life-review form to categorize the reminiscence information into three portions of the life span. As a result of her data, Falk made this statement, 'The findings do not support theories postulating a universal task of life reviewing occurring with the approach of death; neither do they shed any light upon the issue of the adaptive value of reminiscence' (Falk 1969).

The first portion of Falk's statement refutes Butler's theory that life review occurs more frequently with the approach of death. She made this judgement on the basis that the older age group (80 to 90 years), did not do the most reminiscing even though they were the closest to death. The second portion of Falk's statement reveals no support for the adaptive value of reminiscence. Falk did not distinguish between her definition of adaptability and that of Butler, McMahon and Erikson. Falk measured ability to adapt to institutionalization whereas Butler's and Erikson's definition of adaptability is much broader, resulting in an invalid comparison and correlation between her findings and those of Erikson and Butler.

THE FIRST SYSTEMATIC STUDIES OF LIFE REVIEW

During this same period, Coleman (1974) conducted a methodological study examining reminiscing characteristics in a sample of elderly people living in sheltered housing in London. Coleman was one of the first researchers to differentiate life review from reminiscing when he examined those concepts as adaptive features in old age. From his research, Coleman concluded, then, that simple reminiscence was not adaptive but that life review appeared to be adaptive in people who were dissatisfied with their past lives.

Kiernat (1979) looked at reminiscing groups as a way to elicit behaviour change in confused residents. Group leaders and chief nurses evaluated behaviour change through a ward behaviour scale (WBS) and a group behaviour scale (GBS). Results showed those with the highest attendance rate showed the greatest improvement in behaviour. The scales were only partially useful and the researchers agreed that anecdotal records of each session provided the clearest picture of residents' change. Kiernat's group sessions ran for a total of 10 weeks and met twice a week for twenty sessions. Participants were those who were described as confused in the charted notes at least twice and who's confusion had been present for at least 3 months. Events were presented in chronological sequence beginning with childhood and ending with the present. Group leaders presented a particular era and asked group members to participate. Kiernat reported that one resistant resident seemed to benefit the most. She further concluded that life-review groups provided valuable therapy but admitted her results were difficult to measure. Her reports of success about the therapeutic value of life review were mostly due to observation.

Revere and Tobin (1980–81) examined reminiscence data from a middle-aged and old-aged sample. They expected the older age group to be more involved with reminiscing and this proved to be true. The results suggest that older people were more involved in their past and in mythicizing their recollections. Investment in the past decreased as people approached their sixties and seventies but reminiscing still provided a source of self-esteem. These authors state that the aged persons recast their memories to make the uniqueness of themselves vivid. Actually, the myth becomes the reality.

Ferguson (1980) tested the effect of reminiscing counselling on the psychological wellbeing of elderly females in nursing homes. A random sample of forty-five was divided into three groups: one no-treatment group, one group with relaxation training, and one group with relaxation training and reminiscing. The groups met twelve times, twice a week, for approximately 1 hour. The reminiscing modality consisted of encouraging group members to recall pleasant events and to share them with one another. Ferguson focused only on pleasant experiences and viewed positive reminiscing as having adaptive value for elderly people. Bradburn's affect–balance scale (ABS) measured the dependent variable and psychological wellbeing using the suggested scoring method of Moriyawki. Results of this study were positive for the use of reminiscing counselling to increased psychological wellbeing. The group participating in reminiscing counselling increased mean scores on the ABS from 5 to 7.8 for a gain score of 2.8, whereas the other two groups had no such increase. Prior to treatment, all groups were homogeneous with regard to psychological wellbeing.

The ability of reminiscence groups to improve cognitive functioning was examined by Hughston and Merriam (1982). They used three groups: no treatment (control), structured reminiscing and new activities. The experimental group, the structured reminiscing group, met weekly for 4 weeks. Tasks were prepared in advance for the four weekly sessions of the experimental group. For example, one week the participants in the structured reminiscing group named their first-grade teacher and children in the class, while the new activities group was called on to remember a list of current items. Women in the reminiscing group improved in cognitive functioning. Members of the activities group decreased in cognitive functioning on posttest and the no-treatment group remained the same. This study demonstrated that memories can provide sufficient raw material for improvement of cognitive skills.

Georgemiller and Maloney (1984) examined the effect of a life-review workshop on four variables. Chronbach's purpose-in-life test was used to test for meaninglessness. The second variable was tendency for religion, the third was self-esteem, and the fourth, attitude toward death. Sixty-three seniors participated in the treatment and no-treatment groups. The only change noted in the treatment groups was a decrease in denial of death. The life-review workshop consisted of seven meetings of 90 minutes each divided into sections – didactic and experiential. The authors reported that evaluations of the group experience were high and the authors were surprised that there were no greater differences between experimental and control groups. Georgemiller and Maloney critiqued their own design saying the measures were confusing. Possibly the measures of the dependent variable were inappropriate and perhaps they were not valid measures of the changes one would expect as a result of a successful life review. Additionally, the design for the life-review groups did not allow for enough independent introspection and reviewing. It is possible that review as integration did not really occur.

In 1983, Hedgepeth and Hale examined the effect of positive reminiscing on affect, expectancy and performance. The positive reminiscing intervention consisted of 1-hour-long interview discussion of past experiences as compared with a second group who discussed positive present experiences. Both groups received dependent measures after the interview. The control group received the dependent measures before the interview. Dependent measures consisted of a short form depression scale, an individual's estimate of performance on a test, and a digit symbol test, testing psychomotor performance. Results demonstrated no significant differences in mean scores between groups, concluding that reminiscing does not serve an adaptive function.

Hyland and Ackerman presented a paper at the Thirty-Seventh Annual Scientific Meeting of the Gerontological Society of America in San Antonio in 1984. They examined a subject pool of thirty-six individuals at varying age levels. Their method consisted of requiring each subject to characterize the quantity and affect of personal reminiscing and then to correlate the results with the results on the Bradburn affect–balance scale. Results demonstrated the highest percentage of negative events on the affect–balance scale was found in older subjects. Also, younger subjects had significantly higher negative scores than middle-aged or old subjects. When correlations were computed for each age and sex group, the relationship for affect–balance and reminiscence frequency was strong only for middle-aged males. These researchers concluded that subjects of all ages viewed reminiscence as an affectively pleasant event. However, expected significant correlations between frequency of reminiscence and scores for the affect–balance scales were not found.

Brennan and Steinberg (1984) examined the patterns of interrelations among measures of reminiscence, morale and activity at San Francisco State University. A group of forty female seniors, chosen from a pool of volunteers, was interviewed individually and in private for one hour. The participants received the social activities subscale and the life satisfaction index pre-test and post-test. Three interviewers, trained in the interview procedure, used two open-ended questions for three periods of life and assessed reminiscing according to the Falk model. The authors postulated that reminiscence would be positively correlated with morale and negatively correlated with activity. They were unable to prove their hypothesis and instead found that high reminiscers were more active and did not have higher morale. This research project is similar to many, where the reminiscing modality is limited in time to 1 hour. It is difficult to imagine an aged individual integrating an entire lifetime in 1 hour. This particular study demonstrates that short-form reminiscence is not positively correlated to morale.

SUMMARY OF RESEARCH FINDINGS

The research literature does not provide a clear picture of the value of reminiscing or life review. Too many authors who used an intervention of 1 hour, concluded that life review is non-adaptive. Life review needs further examination. Life review must be differentiated from reminiscing and the process of life review must be delineated. Further, the variables predicting a successful or unsuccessful life review must be identified and closely examined. In general, the research concludes that life review and/or reminiscing are positive experiences for elderly people and at times serves an adaptive function.

RESEARCH STUDY: A STRUCTURED LIFE-REVIEW PROCESS

A synthesis of the research findings led this author to develop a structured life-review process for use as a research guide and to test this structured process empirically. Since the development of the life review and experiencing form (LREF), three research projects have been conducted with three distinctly different aging populations in three different sites. The purpose of these research projects was to examine the therapeutic role of a structured life-review process as a pathway to increased life satisfaction. The following hypothesis was tested in all three studies: Those elderly people who participate in a structured life-review process with a nurse who is an attentive listener will exhibit an increase in their general state of life satisfaction.

The following concepts were explored and they are defined as follows.

Definitions

Life satisfaction: the adaptation to the triumphs and disappointments of life and eventual peace with one's self (Neugarten *et al.*, 1961).
Life review: a naturally occurring universal process characterized by the progressive return to consciousness of past experience and unsolved conflicts which are surveyed and reintegrated (Butler, 1963). Instruments used in the studies include:
Life Satisfaction Index-A (LSI-A): a scale designed to test five

components (zest, resolution, achievement of goals, positive self-concept and mood tone) which together measure life satisfaction (Neugarten *et al.*, 1961).

Life Review and Experiencing Form (LREF): the LREF was devised to facilitate the interviewing process and to assure consistency among subject interviews while conducting the life review. Questions for the LREF were drawn from the work of Gorney and Falk, along with newly devised items (Haight 1979) (see Table 16.1).

Table 16.1 Haight's life review and experiencing form (LREF)

Childhood:
1 What is the very first thing you can remember of your life? Go as far back as you can.
2 What other things can you remember about when you were very young?
3 What was life like for you as a child?
4 What were your parents like? What were their weaknesses, strengths?
5 Did you have any brothers or sisters? Tell me what each was like.
6 Did someone close to you die when you were growing up?
7 Did someone important to you go away?
8 Do you ever remember being very sick?
9 Do you remember having an accident?
10 Do you remember being in a very dangerous situation?
11 Was there anything that was important to you that was lost or destroyed?
12 Was church a large part of your life?
13 Did you enjoy being a boy/girl?

Adolescence:
1 When you think about yourself and your life as a teenager, what is the first thing you can remember about that time?
2 What other things stand out in your memory about being a teenager?
3 Who were the important people for you? Tell me about them. Parents, brothers, sisters, friends, teachers, those you were especially close to, those you admired, those you wanted to be like.
4 Did you attend church and youth groups?
5 Did you go to school? What was the meaning for you?
6 Did you work during these years?
7 Tell me of any hardships you experienced at this time.
8 Do you remember feeling that there wasn't enough food or necessities of life as a child or adolescent?
9 Do you remember feeling left alone, abandoned, not having enough love or care as a child or adolescent?
10 What were the pleasant things about your adolescence?
11 What was the most unpleasant thing about your adolescence?
12 All things considered, would you say you were happy or unhappy as a teenager?
13 Do you remember your first attraction to another person?
14 How did you feel about sexual activities and your own sexual identity?

Family and home:
1 How did your parents get along?
2 How did other people in your home get along?
3 What was the atmosphere in your home?
4 Were you punished as a child? For what? Who did the punishing? Who was 'boss'?
5 When you wanted something from your parents, how did you go about getting it?
6 What kind of person did your parents like the most? The least?
7 Who were you closest to in your family?
8 Who in your family were you most like? In what way?

Adulthood:
1 What place did religion play in your life?
2 Now I'd like to talk to you about your life as an adult, starting when you were in your twenties up to today. Tell me of the most important events that happened in your adulthood.
3 What was life like for you in your twenties and thirties?
4 What kind of person were you? What did you enjoy?
5 Tell me about your work. Did you enjoy your work? Did you earn an adequate living? Did you work hard during those years? Were you appreciated?
6 Did you form significant relationships with other people?
7 Did you marry?
     (yes) What kind of person was your spouse?
     (no) Why not?
8 Do you think marriages get better or worse over time? Were you married more than once?
9 On the whole, would you say you had a happy or unhappy marriage?
10 Was sexual intimacy important to you?
11 What were some of the main difficulties you encountered during your adult years?
     (a) Did someone close to you die? Go away?
     (b) Were you ever sick? Have an accident?
     (c) Did you move often? Change jobs?
     (d) Did you ever feel alone? Abandoned?
     (e) Did you ever feel need?

Summary:
1 On the whole, what kind of life do you think you've had?
2 If everything were to be the same would you like to live your life over again?
3 If you were going to live your life over again, what would you change? Leave unchanged?
4 We've been talking about your life for quite some time now. Let's discuss your overall feelings and ideas about your life. What would you say the main satisfactions in your life have been? *Try for three. Why were they satisfying?*
5 Everyone has had disappointments. What have been the main disappointments in your life?
6 What was the hardest thing you had to face in your life? Please describe it.
7 What was the happiest period of your life? What about it made it the happiest period? Why is your life less happy now?
8 What was the unhappiest period of your life? Why is your life more happy now?
9 What was the proudest moment in your life?

Table 16.1 continued

10 If you could stay the same age all your life, what age would you choose?
    Why?
11 How do you think you've made out in life? Better or worse than what you
    hoped for?
12 Let's talk a little about you as you are now. What are the best things about the
    age you are now?
13 What are the worst things about being the age you are now?
14 What are the most important things to you in your life today?
15 What do you hope will happen to you as you grow older?
16 What do you fear will happen to you as you grow older?
17 Have you enjoyed participating in this review of your life?

Note: Derived from new questions and two unpublished dissertations. Gorney, J. (1968)
'Experiencing and age: patterns of reminiscence among the elderly', unpublished doctoral
dissertation, University of Chicago. Falk, J. (1969) 'The organization of remembered life
experience of older people: its relation to anticipated stress, to subsequent adaptation and
to age', unpublished doctoral dissertation, University of Chicago.

Source: Barbara K. Haight, 1989, College of Nursing, Medical University of South Carolina.

Hypothesis

Older people receiving the therapeutic intervention of the life-review
process will increase levels of life satisfaction more than those who receive a
friendly visit only.

Research design

The experimental design of pre-test, post-test, utilizing experimental and
control groups with random assignment was employed. In all three studies
the experimental group received the therapeutic intervention of the life-
review process and the control group received six friendly visits. The third
study incorporated a 'no-treatment' group as well, and subjects received
pre- and post-tests only. The dependent variable, life satisfaction, was
measured by the difference between pre-test, post-test, in all groups.

Sample selection

Inclusion criteria for all studies were 50 years and older, able to communicate, and having normal cognitive abilities.

Study one

The initial study was conducted as a pilot for using the life review and
experiencing form (LREF) with a group of elderly people in good health in

the community. Two nutrition sites supplied enough volunteers for the study. After a random selection the first called was put in to the experimental group, the second in the control group. The average age of the subjects was 74. There were four males and eight females. Half the sample was black, half Caucasian. There were no dropouts in this study. Seven members were widowed, three married and two divorced.

Study two

The second study group consisted of veterans residing in a nursing home. A sample of thirty veterans started the study; twenty-one completed the study. Of those who were unable to complete the study, four died, three became too ill to complete and two transferred to another hospital. Because they were veterans, all subjects were male, average age was 74. Of these nursing home residents, eleven were married, four were widowed, four single and one divorced. These subjects were also randomly selected. Nursing students, trained and working under the direction of the author, performed the life review. Each student visited one subject in the control group and one subject in the experimental group, controlling for the possibility that one particular student may be more effective in facilitating review than another.

Study three

The third study divided subjects into three groups and tested additional variables. Only the results of the life-satisfaction index will be reported here. Sixty participants, twenty subjects to each group, were selected to participate in this study. This subject size was chosen using Cohen's power analysis based on the earlier studies. The effect size was calculated as 1.3829. Using the power tables for an α of 0.05 in Cohen's statistical power analysis, a sample size of sixteen in each group provides 95 per cent power.

All participants in this study were physically disabled in some way and depended on 'at-home services' to live independently in the community. One was a double amputee, another was a stroke victim paralysed on the right side. All had to be cognitively aware to participate in the study. There were nine dropouts in this study. Of the dropouts, one subject died, two were hospitalized and two refused to complete the study, one in the control group and one in the experimental group. Four other subjects refused to participate on the advice of their children. The children did not want their parents visited by strangers nor did they want their parents to discuss their private lives. Average age for subjects completing the study was 76. This group was predominantly female with forty females and only eleven males. Thirty of these subjects were widowed, sixteen married, three single and two divorced. Thirty-two subjects were Caucasian and nineteen were black.

Procedure

In all three studies a master list was obtained either through the council on aging or the nursing home. Names were drawn alternatively by the persons trained to conduct the life review in each study. The first subject name drawn was asked to participate in the life-review process; the second subject name drawn was asked to participate in a friendly visit. In the study with the no-treatment group the subjects in the no-treatment group were asked to fill out the questionnaire only. Data collectors were trained to use the life review and experiencing form (LREF) to conduct the life review for the experimental group.

Members of all experimental and control groups received eight, hour-long visits over an 8-week period of time. The first and last visits were used for pre-test and post-tests in all groups. The control group participated in six social visits and the experimental group participated in a structured life-review process through use of the LREF.

The structured life-review process consists of eight 1-hour visits. During the first visit, socialization takes place and the researcher presents the plan for the remaining visits. The clinician and the reviewer talk about the LREF together and form a contract whereby each agrees to seven more visits using the LREF. The reviewing individual is given a copy of the LREF to anticipate the content of the ensuing visits. At the end of the first visit the reviewer is instructed to think about the topic for next week's discussion – childhood.

Results

These three studies were conducted over a period of 6 years. As the research progressed, the investigations became more sophisticated and systematic. The investigator alone conducted the initial study. The second study used student nurses as reviewers under the direction of the investigator. The third study used three groups and four dependent variables (only the LSI-A is reported here) and was a double-blind study with the investigator and one data collector remaining ignorant of group assignment until the data was entered into the computer.

Analysis of data

Pre-test, post-test and gain scores were calculated for each subject on the dependent variable, life satisfaction, in all three studies. Analysis of covariance (ANCOVA) was chosen to statistically analyse the data in all three studies. This analysis was chosen to control for possible variances in the pre-test scores of individuals. Table 16.2 presents the gain scores from pre- to post-test for all three groups.

Table 16.2 Mean scores for three study groups

Gain scores Subjects – M	Pre-test Mean	Post-test Mean	Gain Mean	 S.D.
Study no. 1 – well elderly				
Experimental group A (n = 6)	25.8333	31.833	6.0	3.899
Control group B (n = 6)	23.667	22.833	−0.833	2.64
Study no. 2 – veterans as nursing home residents				
Experimental group A (n = 10)	19.70	25.30	5.40	4.57
Control group B (n = 11)	17.09	16.36	−0.72	2.83
Study no. 3 – homebound elderly				
Experimental group A (n = 16)	17.94	24.63	6.69	4.27
Control group B (n = 16)	21.13	19.63	−1.50	5.63
No-treatment group C (n = 16)	19.53	20.79	1.26	3.90

Despite the elaboration of the research method over time, it is interesting to note that the gain scores for all three studies were very similar. Change scores for the experimental groups were 6.0, 5.40 and 6.69 respectively. Change scores for the control groups were −0.833, −0.72 and −1.50 respectively. The positive gains for the experimental group in all studies were significant while the negative gains in the control group were not significant.

ANCOVA was chosen to statistically analyse the data using the pre-test as the covariate. The sample of nursing-home residents particularly had pre-test scores much lower than the other two samples. ANCOVA adjusts the scores on the post-tests by eliminating the effect of the covariate (pre-tests) taking into consideration the nature of the linear regression of the covariate on the dependent variable. All hypotheses were tested at the 0.05 level of significance. Table 16.3 illustrates the ANCOVA for each study.

Discussion

These studies demonstrate that a structured life-review process is an effective method of improving life satisfaction in the elderly. In these studies the life review was artificially structured and imposed upon people who gave no indication of readiness to perform life review, yet the process was effective.

The findings suggest the structured role of life review may be a therapeutic modality of great benefit to the elderly. Researchers are encouraged to use and explore this structured process of life review. This new knowledge should encourage interested researchers to explore the efficacy of the life review, to concentrate on a structured evaluative process rather than other

Table 16.3 ANCOVAs and level of significance for three study groups

Analysis of covariance Source of variation	df	Type III SS	F-value	P-value
Study no. 1 – well elderly				
Groups	1	245.000	57.57	0.0001
Covariate	1	105.171	24.87	0.0011
Group X covariate	1	18.669	4.42	0.0683
Study no. 2 – veterans as nursing home residents				
Groups	1	132.17	13.75	0.0017
Covariate	1	905.43	94.16	0.0001
Group X covariate	1	28.85	3.00	0.1013
Study no. 3 – homebound elderly				
Groups	2	489.962	11.52	0.0001
Covariate	1	23.714	1.12	0.2963
Group X covariate	2	4.340	0.10	0.9067

forms of random reminiscing. The story of the lady in apatrtment 302D serves to further illustrate this process.

Case study

This study is presented to illustrate the possible 'preventative' treatment role of life review in the community.

A community health nurse, visiting clients in a community high rise, was asked by the building manager to visit Mrs H, who had not been seen for many days. The nurse complied with this request and knocked on the door of apartment 302D. In response to the nurse's knock, a quavering voice called 'Come in.' As the nurse entered the unlocked apartment, a bent and stooped elderly woman, depending on a walker for mobility, came through the bedroom door. She was wearing a night gown, her hair was uncombed and she had a generally unkempt appeareance with a frenzied look in her eye. She motioned the nurse to sit down in a chair and did so herself while lighting a cigarette and engaging in continuous and anxious movements. As the nurse began to question the elderly woman, the nurse found the woman unable to concentrate and answer her questions. After 10 to 15 minutes of unproductive conversation, the woman asked the nurse to go to the refrigerator to get a drink. The nurse opened the refrigerator door and found the refrigerator empty, except for several cartons of cigarettes and bottles of Coca-Cola. When questioned, the woman explained that she had not left her apartment for 6 years and that those items were the only items she could remember to order from the grocery store.

In view of the woman's apparent nutritional deficits, the community health nurse began her interventions by arranging for the elderly woman's nutritional needs to be met. After providing nutritional support, each week the nurse visited the woman to provide care and to further assess the elderly woman's functional and health status. During these visits, the woman continued to be confused, belligerent and resistive to care. Despite these conditions, the nurse struggled to obtain a health history. As the health history evolved, the elderly woman addressed her own agenda and Majorie's story unfolded.

Marjorie was born in the late 1920s and grew up in the depression, experiencing poverty but enjoying a close family life. Jobs were difficult to find and Marjorie worked as a waitress for $3.75 a day. Marjorie soon met and married a young man called John. After 2 years of marriage John was drafted to serve in the Navy. John served for 5 years in the Second World War and at the same time Marjorie worked in a factory, enjoying her role as an independent and productive woman. Finally, the Second World War concluded and John returned home a changed man suffering from alcoholism. Times were hard as John and Marjorie tried to resume their marriage roles; they argued and John often beat Marjorie. One morning, after a particularly vengeful argument, Marjorie awoke in a Kansas City hospital with a broken pelvis, broken arms and legs, multiple bruises and contusions. Marjorie vowed then that she would never return to John and discharged herself to her parent's home where she began divorce proceedings.

As Marjorie's story was told she kept saying, 'I never told anyone this before', and 'I am so ashamed.' Her behaviour began to change. She became interested in her surroundings. She wanted to go to the grocery store, to the hairdresser and to communicate with her neighbours. She seemed to get clearer and younger in spirit each day. She was also able to follow and respond to conversation. Marjorie's story continued and she told of a second marriage, this one successful, to a man called Terry.

Marjorie met Terry at her parents' home while recuperating from physical abuse and her first marriage. As Majorie's divorce became final, she fell in love and married Terry. The marriage was an idyllic one until one evening Marjorie became ill. Marjorie's story progressed through a painful illness resulting in her present stooped, debilitated condition and a tale of drug addiction and chronicity which she survived because of the love and care of her second husband, Terry. Marjorie never identified the nature of her illness, but in the retelling of the event Terry's devotion and care for her were portrayed. Each weekend Terry rode the bus 200 miles to visit her in the hospital, slept in the bus station overnight and then rode 200 miles home again. When Marjorie was discharged, Terry became her sole caretaker and only contact with the outside world.

Though she was now an invalid and dependent upon Terry for all her needs, the love story continued for several more years until Terry's death.

Marjorie's story ended with details of her husband's death, resulting from lung cancer, a month prior to the community health nurse's arrival at her door. Angry at being victimized by terminal illness, her beloved husband kept details of his illness from Marjorie and rejected her care. One night he collapsed and, in desperation, Marjorie called an ambulance. As Terry was carried away he said, 'Why did you do this to me you bitch?' Marjorie never saw him or heard his voice again, and on Christmas Eve she received a call from the hospital, detailing the events of his death. This dependent woman had lost her one connection with the world and was plunged into solitude and grief with only negative disturbing memories for companions.

Marjorie repeated her tale over and over and sought reasons for Terry's comments before he died. She loved him and she was hurt by him, and now he was gone. The repetition of this tale seemed to act as catharsis for Marjorie. Each time the telling was easier, and Marjorie found it easier to rationalize reasons for Terry's anger. The community health nurse, as a therapeutic listener, assisted in this rationalization and acceptance of the event. The nurse described the difficulty some independent people experience in accepting help when ill and also described the stage of anger portrayed in Kübler-Ross's stages of illness and death (1975). Marjorie was then more able to understand and accept Terry's anger. As the life review progressed, Marjorie was also able to forgive herself for her divorce and to accept her shame of spouse abuse.

With catharsis came clarity and purpose in life and Marjorie was no longer a confused old recluse. She sought out the company of other residents within the high rise. She began to use taxis and, with the help of her walker, went to the grocery store and to the beauty parlour. As Marjorie's healing progressed, she joined the governing council at the high rise and soon worked at the desk in the high rise as a part-time receptionist, looking out for other residents. Marjorie had surpassed her despair and was reaching out for new life.

Marjorie's story of grief and confusion is a common one. The ending, however, is uncommon and demonstrates the powerful use of life review. Had Marjorie and the nurse not discovered the phenomenon of life review together, Marjorie might today be labelled as senile and relegated to the back wards of a mental hospital or nursing home.

Marjorie's story depicts the use of life review in a community setting with an individual suffering from mild and transient cognitive impairment. Cases such as Marjorie's illustrate that the use of life review as a therapeutic modality should not be left to chance. In Marjorie's case, the cognitive impairment may have been the result of poor nutrition, grief, depression or lack of human contact. Each of these causes was treated in some respect during the course of the community health nurse's visits. However, Marjorie's ability and desire to put things past in their proper place and to move on to live life more fully is attributed to the power of the life review.

REFERENCES

Babb de Ramon, P. (1983) 'The final task: life review for the dying patient', *Nursing 83* 13 (2): 44–9.

Brennan, P.L. and Steinberg, L.D. (1984) 'Is reminiscence adaptive?' *International Journal of Aging and Human Development* 18 (2): 99–110.

Burnside, I. (1978) *Working with the Elderly, Group Processes and Techniques,* California: Belmont Publishing Company.

Butler, R.N. (1963) 'The life review: an interpretation of reminiscence in the aged', *Psychiatry* 26: 65–76.

—— (1974) 'Successful aging and the role of the life review', *Journal of the American Geriatric Society* 22 (12): 529–35.

—— (1978) 'The doctor and the aged patient', *Hospital Practices* 13 (3): 99–106.

Chubon, S. (1980) 'A novel approach to the process of life review', *Journal of Gerontological Nursing* 6 (9): 543–6.

Coleman, P. (1986) *Ageing and Reminiscence Processes: Social and Clinical Implications,* Chichester: John Wiley.

Coleman, P.G. (1974) 'Measuring characteristics from reminiscence conversation as adaptive feature of old age', *International Journal of Aging and Human Development* 5 (3): 281.

Cook, J. (1984) 'Reminiscing: how it can help confused nursing home residents', *Social Casework: The Journal of Contemporary Social Work,* 65 (2): 90–3.

Ebersole, P. (1976) 'Problems of group reminiscing with the institutionalized aged', *Journal of Gerontological Nursing* 2 (6): 23–7.

Erikson E. (1950) *Childhood and Society,* New York: W.W. Norton.

Falk, J. (1969) 'Organization of remembered life experience of older people: its relation to anticipated stress, to subsequent adaptation, and to age', unpublished doctoral dissertation, Committee on Human Development, University of Chicago.

Ferguson, J. (1980) 'Reminiscence counseling to increase psychological wellbeing of elderly women in nursing home facilities', unpublished doctoral dissertation, College of Education, University of South Carolina.

Georgemiller, R. and Maloney, H. (1984) 'Life review and denial of death', *Clinical Gerontologist* 2 (4): 37–49.

Gorney, J. (1968) 'Experiencing and age: patterns of reminiscence among the elderly', unpublished doctoral dissertation, Committee on Human Development, University of Chicago.

Haight, B. (1979) 'The therapeutic role of the life review in the elderly', unpublished thesis, School of Nursing, University of Kansas.

Hausman, C.P. (1980) 'Life review therapy', *Journal of Gerontological Social Work* 3 (2): 31–7.

Hughston, G.A. and Merriam, S.B. (1982) 'Reminiscence: a non-formal technique for improving cognitive functioning in the aged', *International Journal of Aging and Human Development* 15 (2): 139–49.

Hyland, C. and Ackerman, H. (1984) 'A cross-sectional study of the correlation between reminiscing frequency and personal affective value'. Conference paper,

37th Annual Scientific meeting of the Gerontological Society of America, San Antonio, USA.

Kiernat, J. (1979) 'The use of life review activity with confused nursing home residents', *The American Journal of Occupational Therapy* 33 (5): 306–15.

King, K.S. (1982) 'Reminiscing psychotherapy with aging people', *Journal of Psychological Nursing Mental Health Services* 20 (2): 21–5.

Kübler-Ross, E. (1975) *Death the Final Stage of Growth*, New York: Touchstone.

Lewis, M. and Butler, R.N. (1974) 'Life review therapy: putting memories to work in individual and group psychotherapy', *Geriatrics* 29 (1): 165–73.

Lieberman, M.A. and Falk, J.M. (1971) 'The remembered past as a source of data for research on the life cycle', *Human Development* 14: 132–1,

McMahon, A.W. and Rhudick, P.J. (1964) 'Reminiscing: adaptional significance in the aged'. *Archives of General Psychiatry* 10: 292–8.

Merriam, S. and Cross, L. (1982) 'Adulthood and reminiscence: a descriptive study', *Educational Gerontology* 8: 275–90.

Molinari, V. and Reichlin, R.E. (1984–5) 'Life review reminiscence in the eldery: a review of the literature', *International Journal of Aging and Human Development* 20 (2): 281–92.

Neugarten, B., Havighurst, R. and Tobin, S. (1961) 'The measurement of life satisfaction', *Journal of Geronotology* 14: 134–43.

Revere, V. and Tobin S.S. (1980–1) 'Myth and reality: the older person's relationship to his past', *International Journal of Aging and Human Development* 12 (1): 15–26.

Safier, G. (1976) 'Oral life history with the elderly', *Journal of Gerontological Nursing* 2 (5): 17–23.

Schnase, R.C. (1982) 'Therapeutic reminiscence in elderly patients', *The Journal of Nursing Care* 2 15–17.

Chapter 17

Community care services for the elderly mentally infirm

Chris Gilleard

INTRODUCTION

Why care? Some underlying assumptions

Community care for the elderly mentally infirm can be discussed in both descriptive and prescriptive terms. Descriptively one can identify the types of care received by the elderly mentally infirm while living in their own or a relative's household and contrast that with the types of care provided in various institutional settings. Prescriptively one can make recommendations concerning the means by which the elderly mentally infirm currently living in the community could best be cared for. The gap between the descriptive and prescriptive models of care gives some sort of index of the need for change, innovation or improvement – in the eyes of the commentator, of course. So in this chapter I would like to both describe then prescribe community care practices. But before doing so it is helpful to examine what need there is in the first place for a community care service for the elderly mentally infirm.

Underlying most models of community care are a set of assumptions to the effect that the current circumstances under which the majority of dementia victims are living are socially unsatisfactory. A number of research-based findings seem to indicate that: (a) dementia is a condition found in much greater numbers amongst the elderly living outside of institutions, i.e. in the community; (b) care-givers for these dementing people are mostly close kin who, as a result of their care-giving, experience impairments in their mental and physical health and a greater degree of social deprivation than would otherwise occur in the absence of this care-giving responsibility; (c) institutional care is neither preferred by the caring family nor by the general public nor by the elderly themselves; and (d) institutionalization of the elderly mentally infirm results in a greater deterioration of their social, emotional and cognitive functioning than would otherwise be observed during the course of their dementia were they to continue being cared for in their own homes. In this introductory section

I would like to briefly re-examine some of the research findings concerning these assumptions.

EPIDEMIOLOGY OF DEMENTIA IN THE COMMUNITY

In 1964 two key British articles appeared based on studies in Newcastle and Edinburgh which indicated that between 5 and 10 per cent of over-65-year-olds suffered from dementia, that the majority of dementia patients were to be found not in institutions but in the community, and that these dementia victims were largely unknown to their local medical and social services (Kay et al., 1964; Williamson et al., 1964). While many reviews since have reiterated these findings (cf. Kay and Bergmann, 1980) in recent years there have been a number of epidemiological studies which at the very least cast doubt on the spatial and temporal generality of those early findings. Thus Molsa et al. (1982) observed a rate of dementia of only around 2 per cent in the over-65s of the Finnish city of Turku; Hagnell et al. (1983) observed a striking reduction in the incidence and prevalence of both senile and multi-infarct dementia over a 30-year period for the elderly population of Lundby in southern Sweden; Clarke et al. (1986), Gibbins (1986) and Jachuck et al. (1986) all reported equally low prevalence rates of moderate-to-severe cognitive impairment amongst over-70s in several English general practice surveys (rates were all below 3 per cent); while Shibayama et al. (1986) reported rates below 3 per cent of moderate and severe dementia amongst the over-65s in one Japanese province. Finally a Nigerian study of the epidemiology of neurological disorders found only one case of dementia amongst several hundred elderly people surveyed.

But it is not only a matter of revising down estimated prevalence rates. The proportion of the elderly who are found to be cognitively impaired in the community will to some significant extent depend upon the rate of institutionalization of the elderly mentally infirm in a particular locality or country. Preston (1986) has estimated that in Victoria, Australia half of the cases of moderate and severe dementia are living in some form of residential care. Adolfsson et al. (1981) considered that the majority of moderate and severely demented elderly people in Sweden were in institutional care, a point further testified by Nilsson's (1984) longitudinal study of the incidence of dementia in Gothenburg: all but two of the cases of moderate to severe dementia were institutionalized during the course of his study. Molsa et al. (1982) found ten times as many 'probable' dementia cases amongst the nursing home population in Turku compared with those on the caseloads of the city's domiciliary services. Clarke et al. (1986) in their study of over-70s in Melton Mowbray, England found almost equal numbers of moderate and severe cognitive impairment in their institutional sample as in their community sample. At the very least all these recent findings suggest that before major capital development projects are initiated to serve the needs of community-dwelling victims of dementia a preliminary requirement should be a careful and comprehensive survey of the elderly in that district – in the absence of any existing screening and/or anticipatory case recording.

THE STRAINS OF COMMUNITY CARE-GIVING

What of the circumstances of care-givers in the community? Several recent surveys have been made in Britain all of which have employed very similar measures of emotional health of relatives caring for a dementing person: the general health questionnaire (GHQ: Goldberg, 1978). Levin *et al.* (1983) found 35 per cent of her care-givers scoring in the 'distressed' range on the questionnaire. Gilleard *et al.* (1984a) observed rates of disturbance varying from 57 to 74 per cent in three different samples. Gibbins (1986) obtained a rate of 59 per cent in a similar survey while Whittick (1985) observed a rate of 65 per cent in her sample of daughters caring for a dementing parent. Research from North America confirms the high rate of emotional distress associated with caring for an elderly mentally infirm relative and in addition has indicated that social isolation and a greater consumption of psychotropic drugs are also characteristic of such care-giving family members (George, 1984; Ory *et al.*, 1985).

A feature of almost all these and other studies in this area has been the reliance upon samples of relatives who are in touch with either special voluntary organizations like the Alzheimer's Disease Society or statutory domiciliary health and social services. Such groups may be more likely to report emotional disturbance precisely because they have sought help or assistance in some way. Those caring for a dementing relative without recourse to voluntary or statutory services may not in fact find the experience of care-giving particularly burdensome. Support for this view has come from a recent survey of care-givers of cognitively impaired elderly in the northeast of Scotland. As a result of a previous survey of 1,765 elderly subjects, Eagles *et al.* (1987) were able to conduct follow up interviews with co-resident supporters of seventy-nine of these elderly people. Of the forty considered mildly, moderately or severely demented, they failed to find evidence of significantly raised psychiatric morbidity among their supporters, although there was evidence of greater stress in this sample. Although the numbers with moderate or severe dementia was rather small (n=20) their findings do suggest that non-consulting family relatives of the elderly mentally infirm may not find the experience of care-giving as distressing as those who do consult either the voluntary or statutory services. The study was conducted in a rural area of Britain and it may be that more extensive informal support systems and a degree of rural stoicism contributed to the low level of distress observed. What remains to be discovered is the relative size of the two groups of supporters – the silent copers and the consulting distressed. Since there seems little evidence that in general, users of existing formal community services are better off as a result of their contact, one question that the above study raises is whether this is because of initial differences in coping resources between consulters and non-consulters or as others have suggested because of the inability of existing services to meet effectively the needs of care-givers in the community. If both conclusions are equally accurate representations of reality, then it would suggest that our efforts would best be directed at assisting those who do consult as much as possible while leaving alone those informal care-givers who do not consult. The evidence of need reflected in surveys of care-givers of the elderly mentally infirm may thus require some qualification. Nevertheless, when matched for level of service contact it is apparent that compared with looking after elderly physically handicapped or younger mentally handicapped dependent supporters of the elderly mentally infirm consistently show greater signs of emotional disturbance (Gilleard, 1984; Whittick, 1985). This would seem to reinforce the assumption that caring for the elderly mentally infirm is a particularly stressful task for many families. The broader significance of this distress can be gauged by the fact that there is a consistent association between such distress and a greater preparedness to seek institutional care for one's dependent (Levin *et al.*, 1983; Morycz, 1985; Gilleard, 1986). Since such attitudes also predict the future breakdown of community care and subsequent institutionalization (Levin *et al.*, 1983; Gilleard, 1986) it seems a logical assumption that preventing high levels of strain among the supporting kin of the dementing elderly will sustain continuing care in the community. But this assumption also implies that expressed preferences for care of the elderly mentally infirm in the absence of distress inherently favours community over institutional care.

PUBLIC AND FAMILY CARE PREFERENCES FOR THE ELDERLY MENTALLY INFIRM

As far as the general public, young and old, are concerned British evidence suggests that such preferences are not in fact widely held. In a detailed public opinion survey of attitudes toward 'appropriate' care of various dependency groups, West *et al.* (1984) found that in sharp contrast to all other dependency groups the elderly mentally infirm were seen by an overwhelming majority of the public to be most appropriately cared for in an institutional setting. Since assisted community care was the preferred option for all the other dependency groups one cannot conclude that the findings simply reflect a general bias against community care. In a limited survey of 129 supporting relatives of newly admitted psychogeriatric day-care patients we found the majority (71 per cent) prepared to consider institutional care for their dependent if the situation worsened. The single kin group least prepared to consider this option were elderly spouses (Gilleard, 1986; see also Levin *et al.*, 1983; Gilhooly, 1986). While these latter studies indicate that a long shared life together binds fit and frail partners in a marriage into habits of interdependency, for the general public and for most other care-giving kin, institutional care is clearly perceived as a necessary component in the societal response to the problems of the elderly mentally infirm.

THE IMPACT OF INSTITUTIONALIZATION

But is it simply a necessary evil, a question of balancing the harm done to the dementing person with the benefits accruing to family and neighbours? Studies of the effects of relocation/institutionalization have generally been interpreted as showing deleterious effects arising from entry to institutional care. In a review of the impact of relocation Rowlands concluded that: 'those whose mental functioning is impaired either through psychosis or severe brain syndrome and those who are depressed ... may be particularly vulnerable to death following relocation' (Rowlands, 1977: 364). Since this review researchers have been more equivocal concerning the enhanced morbidity risk associated with relocation (Borup, 1983; Horowitz and Schulz, 1983). Often minimal and generally non-significant changes have been reported from pre- to post-institutionalization (cf. Tobin and Lieberman, 1978) although declines in social contact and feelings of control have been reported in groups of 'impaired' elderly entering residential care (Arling *et al.*, 1986). Such studies rarely restrict the sample to a wholly dementing sample and consequently it is difficult to generalize such findings to such a sample. Even within non-dementing groups of elderly there is evidence that a move to a new residential setting can be beneficial (Carp, 1967). To an important extent it depends upon what is being left behind and what sort of place one is moved to. Woods and Britton make these telling comments in their review of observational studies of long-term care settings: 'Institutions for the elderly may be characterized as places where inactivity is the norm where there is little social interaction where staff contact mainly relates to physical care and where dependence ... is positively encouraged' (Woods and Britton, 1985: 265). At home the dementing elderly are more likely to be treated as people whose behaviour is automatically interpreted within the context of a historically meaningful relationship. Such a context may enhance a sense of security and purpose that institutions fail to provide. Support for a more detrimental effect arising from institutional care may be gleaned from an interesting study described by McDonald *et al.* (1982). They compared changes in cognitive and behavioural functioning of carefully matched groups of moderately demented people in hospital, residential-home, day-hospital and day-centre settings. Over a 9-month period least deterioration was observed in the attenders at day centres, suggesting the benefits that may occur with assisted community care when contrasted with institutional care.

But against these presumed costs of institutional care one must weigh the benefits. Most relatives who place their mentally infirm dependent in care do so when they feel there is no alternative. They generally report a sense of relief for having done so and report feeling that their dependant is happy and settled in care (Adolfsson et al., 1980; Gilleard, 1986). One may compare the effect to that arising from an anticipated death – as a sad but necessary end. For the dependant who goes into care it remains to be seen whether institutionalization must indeed be a living death. A recent study by Wells and Jorm (in press) suggests it may not be so. More research and better research is needed in this area, but above all, better institutions are required before any convincing answers can be given.

COMMUNITY CARE: A DESCRIPTIVE ACCOUNT

The previous sections have tried to qualify the view that the demented elderly currently receiving services are merely the tip of an iceberg and that the coming demographic winter will usher in a further massive increase in dementing old people that will exhaust the capabilities of families to care and swamp the existing domiciliary services completely. Shadowing such demographic projections is another fear, of course, that such a scenario will produce a massive and uncontrollable increase in government expenditure that will impose intolerable burdens on the tax-paying, income-generating public. How far the relative limitations in institutional provision in such countries as Japan, the United States and Britain are currently placing members of their communities at serious risk of breakdown in either their physical or mental health is a debatable issue but one that cannot be ignored. Whether such instances of family breakdown are a reflection of the failings of existing community services and how far they reflect inherent limits to family care is one of the main issues that this second section of the chapter addresses.

Informal family care

The bulk of community care is given by members of the family of the dementing elderly person so it is appropriate to start with a description of care in this sector. Although we know a considerable amount about the problems faced by families caring for the dementing elderly we know much less about the routine round of caring that takes place within the household. The account given here is necessarily tentative.

Four components of care-giving: household maintenance; personal care; attention and supervision; effortful interaction

When the elderly mentally infirm share a household with others, many of the domestic activities carried out are parts of routine household care that would arise as tasks in any set of circumstances – dusting, cleaning, shopping, washing, preparing meals, carrying out household repairs and dealing with household bills. The same set of activities performed by a supporter who also maintains a separate household become more obviously care activities when they are performed in the dependant's household. Less easily distinguishable as care is, the gradual assimilation of responsibility for previously shared domestic tasks which may accompany the shift in relationships as the fit partner moves to do more as their frail spouse can do less.

Less ambiguity surrounds personal care activities. Helping the elderly person dress and undress, take a bath or wash, cut his or her toenails are care activities with a high level of personal intrusion which are highly visible signs of incompetence in the dependant. One result of such evident imbalance between care and cared for is that such care activities can more easily serve as triggers for misinterpretational conflicts and the activation of primitive defences by the dementing person.

Activities which draw more upon attentional resources rather than physical strength or stamina are more likely to preoccupy the carers who share the same household with their dependant since they are more likely to notice the errors and accompanying risks and dangers arising from the cognitive failings of their relative. In contrast, the supporter who maintains a separate household may fail to observe such everyday problems until some concrete evidence emerges of these errors such as a burnt pan, soiled linen or a visit from the police after an episode of wandering. Awareness of the pervasive potential for danger may depend upon personal characteristics of the carer, including factors such as gender and neuroticism, but they are rarely absent from the caring relationship. While often difficult to classify such activities as care-giving behaviour since they mostly describe covert or cognitive activity, research points to their importance in causing burden to care-givers (Gilleard *et al.*, 1984a).

Similar comments apply to the fourth category of care activities which have been termed 'effortful interaction'. These activities represent attempts by the supporter to carry out interactions which in the past would occur automatically from the history of interactions that build up in any relationship over time. They consist of a range of behaviour from attempts to jog a person's memory, correct a misinterpretation, assert a normative viewpoint or simply sustain a conversation. As Greene *et al.* (1982) have shown, apathy and lack of communication may prove singularly stressful in a domestic context precisely because of the historical meaning that spouses and parents possess for their supporters.

Trainable and exchangeable home care practices

With the above framework it is possible to see that the latter type of care-giving activity is problematic primarily for close family care-givers. On the other hand, household-maintenance activities may prove much less problematic to the family than might be perceived by an outsider. One result is that many elderly carers refuse home helps simply because they do not perceive such household maintenance as beyond their ability. What they may fail to perceive is that home helps implicitly provide a respite from the supervisory care-giving that often is a significant burden to relatives. Careful analyses of the nature of home care is needed in order to determine what aspects of the care relationship can or cannot be exchanged with existing domiciliary services and what aspects of care-giving can or cannot be improved by informal training. Of course, not all care activities are easily classifiable. Consider this aspect of personal care:

> He kept cutting himself with the razor so I thought I'd buy him a battery razor ... well he's just about driven us silly with it ... whether he doesn't understand it I don't know but he keeps on bringing it out ... he'll do one half of his face and he'll do the other half another time ... he wants it out every 5 minutes like a child with a toy ... he gets up in the middle of the night and he will try and shave then. I tell him he shouldn't do it now but he asks what time can I get up and he keeps asking.

For a professional outsider it would be just as easy to take away the razor and come in once or twice a week to give the old man a shave; there is no need to insist upon meaningful, purposive patterns of behaviour in a dementing client after all. Several other personal care activities like bathing and dressing can often be more easily handled by a home nurse or similar care-giver who is not involved in sustaining a belief in the intentionality and fundamental integrity of the dementing person. It may prove much harder to teach family care-givers to 'switch off' their personal relationships during such personal care and then 'switch on' again on other occasions. By suggesting or training family supporters to act like professional carers in order to reduce strain and increase their sense of coping one may simply accelerate the processes of distancing and disengagement with the result that care-giving is carried out with greater reluctance and less commitment. Exchanging care practices with professional workers may have unexpected consequences, too, in accelerating institutionalization and reducing further the care-giver's morale. Existing research has suggested that outside help has very different consequences for husband and wife care-givers, the former feeling better while the latter feels worse as though such outside help signifies personal failure in a lifelong career as carer (Zarit, 1982). In short, while domestic care activities may be capable of analysis and categorization to determine potential areas of exchange and/or training from professionals, family care-giving may be more of an integrated whole which demands an approach incorporating aspects of family therapy into any behavioural analysis.

Domiciliary services

While family members may have difficulty in tolerating some aspects of care for their dependant it is also true that many of the problems of the elderly infirm do not generate sympathetic responses from professional helpers themselves (Mitterness and Wood, 1986), and they may feel acutely aware of the absence of purpose and structure to their visits (Luker, 1981). The failure of insight manifested by many dementing people can make for difficulties especially for professionals used to negotiating a shared perspective of their clients' problems (cf. Crosbie, 1983; Reifler et al., 1981). In particular, domiciliary service providers such as health visitors and social workers may find their roles frustratingly limited to either linking family supporters to other services or simply screening and casefinding for primary health and social services. Reluctance to take on this kind of work often stems from the awareness that other appropriate services are simply not available. Care management and home monitoring may be more satisfying when an adequate community psychogeriatric service is operating. In contrast to care-managing services the direct care-giving roles of home helps and home nurses explain why these services have been found to be most often in touch with the dementing elderly in the community (Bond and Carstairs, 1982; Foster et al., 1976). While such services reach many though by no means all of the elderly mentally infirm living alone, they do not reach the majority of the elderly mentally infirm who live with others and by and large are simply not available to non-pensioner households in which a dementing parent may be living. Although home helps informally perform both personal care and supervisory care activities for periods of up to 3 hours a day, many tasks arise which are incidental to their main function of household maintenance. Thus the apparent and actual benefits of home helps may not be evident from their designated role in performing household tasks. Evidence of a significant stress-reducing function of the home help service in Britain (Levin et al., 1983) makes such limitations in their availability particularly unfortunate.

The home nursing service is the second most widely employed service in Britain and their contact with the elderly mentally infirm may be particularly high when there is accompanying physical disability. Although the care-giving service of the home nurse is more limited in terms of contact time and is more overtly directed toward 'medical' personal care, the potential limits of the service are by no means clear. Possible extensions of home nursing could involve incontinence management, night nursing, medication control and health checkups.

Before turning to the closely linked home or community psychiatric nursing service, mention should be made of the other domiciliary services that in scattered form exist in Britain and other European countries. Thus chiropody services, community occupational therapists, physiotherapists, hairdressing services, dieticians and incontinence laundry services all remain, on paper at least, elements of a potentially coherent service for the elderly that in practice are spread too thinly or too unevenly to achieve such an integrated service. Such services, because they are relatively specific in what they can offer the elderly may be much less disruptive to the overall balance of care provided by the family while at the same time may make a significant contribution to relieving some of the more taxing aspects of personal care.

Finally the community psychiatric nurse in Britain at least is fast becoming seen as the best form of domiciliary service for the elderly mentally infirm and considered by many to be the central resource of community psychogeriatric care. Like health visitors and social workers the community psychiatric nurse offers a care-management rather than care-providing role. But unlike the former, the role of the community psychiatric nurses is such that they can perform a pivotal task in linking family care-givers to such specialized services as psychogeriatric day care, home help, sitter services as well as inpatient psychogeriatric hospital beds. Since they may also offer counselling and advisory services to family care-givers which permit ventilation of problems without explicitly taking over from the family, they can also establish particularly close relationships to act as key workers in linking families with statutory care.

Innovatory services: respite care and family support services

The introduction of specialized services to support the impaired elderly in the community has met with demonstrable success in reducing both the rate and extent of institutional bed occupancy in controlled trials where the comparison has been with standard domiciliary services (Challis and Davis, 1980; Nocks *et al.*, 1986). While such studies demonstrate the potential of innovatory services to supplement existing community care and reduce rates of institutionalization the targeted population of such interventions has not been limited to the elderly mentally infirm. For this particular group, such controlled studies of supplementary care are lacking, although persuasive evidence exists that psychogeriatric day care can successfully reduce strain in family care-givers and thereby help sustain community care (Gibbins, 1986; Gilleard, 1987). While it would be mistaken to dismiss out of hand the potential of such innovatory services to prevent the breakdown of family care and reduce rates of institutional use, it would be equally mistaken to assume that by providing enough low-cost services these goals will inevitably be achieved. The limits to which care activities can be exchanged between informal and formal services without turning the household into a mini-hospital may seriously reduce the chances of replacing institutional care with assisted community care. Areas where training and exchange of care-giving can be of benefit probably do exist but there may well be feedback effects that restrict such benefits.

At present the principal forms of specialized support are psychogeriatric day-care centres/hospitals and less often support groups and sitter services. In Britain the voluntary sector has been strongly encouraged to play a significant role in initiating these services. Although attempts to evaluate these innovations are few, on the whole the results of such studies have generally been positive. Day-hospital services have been shown to be viewed positively by the family supporters (Jones and Munbodh, 1982: Gilleard et al., 1984b); they achieve a significant reduction in the emotional strain experienced by supporters (Gibbins, 1986; Gilleard, 1987); and they succeed in maintaining about one-half of the dementing patients who attend in the community for periods of over 6 months (Gilleard et al., 1984b). But the fact that many if not the majority eventually move into some kind of institutional setting has led some workers to conclude that day care serves not so much as an alternative to institutional care but rather as a means of shortening the time that the dementing person will eventually have to spend in hospital or nursing/residential home care. Finally, while there is no evidence that introducing psychogeriatric day care reduces the admission rates to the parent hospital services (Gilleard, 1985) some evidence suggests that prior exposure to day care increases the likelihood of discharge home following such hospital admissions (Eagles and Gilleard, 1984).

Of course psychogeriatric day care need not be seen as an antithesis to long-term care in institutions. Rather than altering the balance between community and institutional care, day-care centres/hospitals may better be seen as offering an improvement over the quality and responsivity of existing community services for the elderly mentally infirm and their families. In countries or regions where extensive institutional provisions exist for the dementing elderly, the majority of the moderately and most of the severely demented elderly population will be taken into care sooner or later. Where institutional resources are more limited, individual differences in commitment and in informal back-up care may play the more significant role in determining which dementia victims go into institutional care. While day-care services generally succeed in making the experience of care-giving less detrimental to the supporters' health and wellbeing, such services rarely transform the circumstances within which care-giving occurs. On occasions, they undoubtedly do so, but not sufficiently often as to alter the overall rate at which the demented elderly as a group are admitted into care. I feel that rather than regret such apparent lack of impact, workers in the area should recognize the challenge it poses for our current models of community care.

First it is important to understand how the improvement in care-givers' morale arises during the course of day-care provision. Foremost among the benefits reported by the supporters is the element of respite care; the fact that for a definite time period the supporter is free from their care-giving responsibilities to either relax or more often attend to social or financial matters that otherwise get crowded out of their timetable. In addition to the relief afforded by time out there is evidence that other elements of day care and the associated counselling and advisory services performed by the day-care staff are of demonstrable benefit. Information helps. Many inadequacies exist in the information typically given to relatives concerning their dependant's problem (Chenoweth and Spencer, 1986; Gilhooly, 1984). A recent study by Toner (1985) indicated that combining information in the form of a self-help booklet together with community-nursing contact reduced supporters' distress to a greater extent than that associated with community-nursing contact alone. Groups for supporters aimed at providing information and advice have been shown to be as effective as specifically problem-oriented groups (Collins, 1985; Church and Linge, 1982). As well as information, understanding helps, too. Therapeutically oriented supporter groups have been associated with significant improvements in supporter morale by a number of authors (Lazarus *et al.*, 1981; Levin *et al.*, 1984). It also seems that individually oriented counselling is rather more effective than group work (Collins, 1985; Zarit and Zarit, 1984), while therapeutic work with the day-hospital attenders themselves has also been found to have spin-off benefits on supporters' morale (Greene *et al.*, 1983). Much of this work suggests general ways in which community care can be made less stressful for the supporters, but it would be wrong to assume that these beneficial elements combat a need for institutionalization.

Second, attention should be paid to the failures within the service, however difficult that may be for a relatively new and proselytizing service. Why do some patients refuse to attend? Why do relatives decline the offer of attendance at a supporters' group meeting? Why do voluntary sitter services obtain hardly any clients to take up their facilities? As the first section of the chapter indicated, need may have been exaggerated, and locality may play a role in determining differences in 'consulting' behaviour. But as the present section has tried to point out there is the need to understand the individual dynamics of a particular care-giver/dependant relationship, and the consequent interpretations that may be made of a particular service. The motives behind using or not using a service may not be easily discernible, and it would be useful to know whether those refusing or not taking up a community-based service are also the same relatives who are unlikely to seek institutional care either for their dependant. What is interesting about Eagles' research in Aberdeen is that his sample of 'non-distressed' supporters had been coping with their cognitively impaired dependent for some 2 years or so. One wonders whether they had been offered, and had refused, services during that period. Whatever may be the determinants of acceptance and rejection of community and institutional services, working with families in the community is itself a valuable training for staff to accept that sharing the care means that the professionals do not always have their own way.

COMMUNITY CARE – A PRESCRIPTIVE MODEL

The Leicestershire model

A recent paper prepared by members of the Leicestershire health-care planning team for the elderly severely mentally infirm has outlined a proposal for a community service for the elderly mentally infirm that consists of six basic elements (Arrowsmith *et al.*, 1986). These are: (1) a community dementia team, (2) a home monitoring service, (3) day centres, (4) relatives' support groups, (5) standard generic non-specialist home services, and (6) local beds. Implicit in their model is a seventh element: an inpatient psychogeriatric unit in a local district hospital. The team proposes a parallel process whereby the development of these services is accompanied by the progressive dismantling of long-stay psychiatric hospital beds. Most noteworthy amongst their proposals is the inclusion of what they call 'local beds' within the framework of a community service. The Leicestershire model thereby recognizes that a prescriptive model for giving a service to the community does not mean that such care must inevitably take place chiefly in private households. While a descriptive account of community care simply reports on care provided outside of institutions, a prescriptive model addresses the issue of how best to give care to the community without preconceptions about the form that care should take. The very act of taking responsibility for the care of the elderly mentally infirm by issuing policy guidelines, providing community services or financially priming and supporting voluntary agencies must at some point involve a preparedness to take responsibility for the bed of the elderly mentally infirm. Rather than viewing institutional beds as morally bad as well as financially extravagant they need to be considered as an inseparable part of the services offered to the community providing a positive step in the continuing care and management of this group of people. Transfer to alternative care settings need not be viewed as a failure of care but as an extension of a service that originates at the point when the family or the elderly person first makes contact with their doctor or social services. Including local beds confirms the continuity of the service.

The Leicestershire model does not, of course, make the mistake of elevating institutional provisions to the centre of the psychogeriatric service. Rather it seems to endorse a model first clearly enunciated by Whitehead (1974) where the centre of the psychogeriatric service is occupied by the day-hospital unit. Certainly this is the kind of model that I would like to prescribe in this section.

Psychogeriatric day care: centre of a community service

In order for the psychogeriatric day unit to fulfil such a central role within a community, psychogeriatric service, several transformations could usefully be made in the way such units operate. Most importantly they need to expand their role as a resource and training centre serving not only to the mentally impaired who attend the unit but extending their services to the patients' families, the existing statutory and voluntary domiciliary services and to the residential sector of care as well. The overall range of functions is illustrated in Figure 17.1.

In relation to primary health care and social services teams, the unit should encourage what Williams and others have referred to as 'anticipatory care' (Williams, 1984) by: (1) Increasing the awareness of dementia amongst health visitors, social workers and home helps so that they will be more alert to the possibility of mental infirmity amongst their elderly clients. (2) Supporting health centres and local social service teams in their efforts to develop registers of mentally frail elderly in their catchment area together with information concerning a principal support. (3) Continually reinforcing the message that an identifiable and responsive community psychogeriatric service exists in their area so that case registration and household monitoring result in actions of measurable benefit to the community.

Visits by family doctors and other members of the domiciliary services to the day unit may be one useful way to demonstrate what is available. Workshops or seminars could be held for home helps and other groups whose training may not be so extensive to discuss some of the issues surrounding care of the elderly mentally infirm. Members of the primary health-care teams could be encouraged to periodically attend the supporters' group meetings at the day unit. Training in awareness and sensitivity to the needs of the elderly mentally infirm and their families may in turn lead to more satisfactory relationships between doctors and relatives which at present may often be problematic for both parties (Smits, 1982; Chenoweth and Spencer, 1986).

In relation to the voluntary sector, it seems desirable for the psychogeriatric day unit to act as a co-ordinating centre identifying gaps in the statutory services within a particular district which the voluntary service could usefully be encouraged to fill. While many novel and helpful services have developed as a result of initiatives from the voluntary sector in Britain (Age Concern, 1983; Scottish Action on Dementia (Arrowsmith *et al.*, 1986)), there is an unfortunate tendency for such ventures to be poorly integrated into existing structures and to have uncertain futures which may limit their

Figure 17.1 Outline of the centralizing functions proposed for psychogeriatric day care

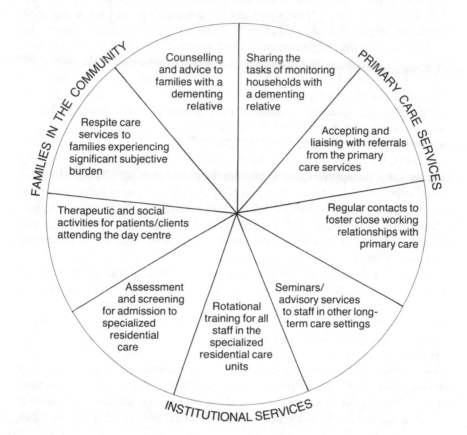

usefulness within the overall framework of available care (Osborn, 1985). There are obvious benefits to accrue in community psychogeriatric services if the voluntary sector can make flexible sitter services and transport and escort facilties available. Satellite day centres and support groups run by volunteers could link up with the central psychogeriatric day unit thereby both strengthening their own services and extending the range of families that could be reached, especially in areas with a low density of population. By ensuring a close co-ordination with existing resources the day-unit team can help ensure a more efficient use of the voluntary services in a particular district.

The psychogeriatric day unit itself offers both respite care, support and counselling services to family carers as well as specialized therapeutic acti-vities for the dementing elderly themselves. The value of support groups

that help inform and provide understanding to relatives who may themselves feel uncertain and anxious about their dependant's care has already
been noted. By liaising with voluntary services it may be possible to provide
sitter services so that relatives can attend counselling sessions while their
dependant is not left alone at home. This may also be useful when the
elderly mentally infirm person cannot be persuaded to attend the day unit
itself.

If appropriate and desired by the relatives, the day unit can supply an
ideal environment for family carers to improve some of their own care-
giving strategies. Through modelling and rehearsal, staff may be able to
teach some of the more difficult personal care tasks such as listing and
transferring a heavy and disabled person. However, as pointed out earlier,
there may be important limits to the extent to which such care-giving
training may be appropriate. On other matters such as advice on home
safety, practical aids and welfare benefits, the relatives may be able to pick
up useful ideas that may facilitate their care-giving. The importance of individual counselling suggests that attempts to introduce key workers to work
with individual families would be another valuable strategy in providing
personal counsel.

The day unit can be an innovatory centre for therapeutic work with the
elderly mentally infirm themselves; using and providing training in reality
orientation and reminiscence therapy; offering computer-assisted recreation and cognitive training; recruiting volunteers to run hobby and leisure
groups; making available physiotherapy services; as well as the more
customary opportunities to sit and socialize or join in games and singsongs.
Creative use of the environment can be encouraged such as developing
'alerting' devices for wandering patients, recreating a cosy pub/cafe corner
for socialization purposes or opening the unit in the evenings to recreate a
club atmosphere for those dementing elderly used to a social night out once
a week.

Finally, the day unit should relate closely to residential care. Day units
linked both operationally and physically to residential care units have
considerable advantages in breaking down the distinction between intra-
mural and community care. Not only should there be serious attempts to
operate a psychogeriatric service as a sector of care shared between health
and social services but equally rigid distinctions between community and
institutional workers need to be eliminated. Encouraging a key-worker
approach to ensure continuity of care requires a focus outwards to the
community not inwards to one's own line of management. Rotation of staff
between the residential sector and the day unit/community team can
prevent a narrow institutionalizing approach within residential care besides
accustoming staff to see their patients within the historical context of their
family. Linking day unit and residential unit together can also ensure some
familiarity with the residential site arising from prior attendance at the day

unit. Knowing that some, at least, of the staff will be familiar faces also may help ensure that the relationship between carer and dependant is maintained with less potential for disruption if institutional care begins.

Integrated care

Much current evidence suggests that the existing non-specialist services fail to address the needs of the elderly mentally infirm and their relatives. The development of a psychogeriatric service, based in a day unit which serves both patient, family and the existing domiciliary health and social services and which has access to and decision-making capacity over long-term residential care seems to offer the most comprehensive response to the changing needs of the dementing elderly and their families. While at present there seems little justification for early case finding of unrecognized dementia, there is clearly much scope for better exploitation of the potential for anticipatory care available from the regular contacts of the existing health and social services. Adequate communication and integration of service responses may, however, be less than adequate if left solely in the hands of general practitioners or social-work team leaders. Monitoring of households containing an elderly mentally frail person should not be a task that is separated off in the hands of a specialized community nurse or health visitor. Rather, such household monitoring should fall within the function of the psychogeriatric community team, a role which all professionals within the day unit/residential unit can and should undertake. Members of staff would each be able to serve as key workers to some families, able to develop a relationship with both supporter and their dependant which will allow them to grasp the significance that the elderly person's mental infirmity has on the relationship with their supporter(s). Staff who have learned to be open, to listen and to be responsive to the needs of the family caring in the community are less likely to permit their work in residential care to follow traditional patterns of institutionalized care-giving. Knowing the staff as a visitor to their own homes will enable family members to be more assertive of their right to continue to care after their dependant's bed has moved out of their hands. The result of such a policy of open and integrated care should help ensure a more personal response to the dementing individual at all stages of their disability.

CONCLUDING SUMMARY

In this chapter I have tried to draw attention to some of the assumptions regarding the needs of a community care service for the elderly mentally infirm and to show that while the size of the problem may well have been exaggerated as a result of overreliance upon epidemiological research conducted over two decades ago, and the selection biasses of supporter surveys, there remains sufficient reason to believe that existing community services do not adequately meet the needs for many families looking after a dementing relative. Admission to institutional care may represent one of a complex of losses experienced by the dementing person which enhances morbidity and mortality and reduces the personal security of their life. The development of specialized services similar to that envisioned in the Leicestershire model centring upon a specialized psychogeriatric day unit and linked to small-scale residential units is proposed as offering a significant improvement over existing services, making family care less burdensome and institutional care less of a failure of care. Continuity of care has been emphasized recognizing that such continuity means crossing both interdisciplinary boundaries and management demarcation lines, and learning to balance a medico-technological response to dementia with a social and personal perspective. It is not difficult to perceive care for the dementing as representing one of the greatest challenges to the development of welfare services throughout the western world. While a plurality of models may be the healthiest prospect for the immediate future, I hope that the model presented here will form one of the options that care may follow in the future.

ACKNOWLEDGEMENT

I would like to thank Jan Killeen, of Scottish Action on Dementia, for keeping me up to date with developments in Britain in the care of the elderly mentally infirm.

REFERENCES

Adolfsson, R., Gottfries, C., Nystrom, L. and Winblad, B. (1981) 'Prevalence of dementia disorders in institutionalised Swedish old people', *Acta Psychiatrica Scandinavica* 63: 225–44.
——— , Kajsajunti, G., Larsson, N., Myrstener, A., Nystrom, L., Olafsson, B., Sandman, P. and Winber, J. (1980) 'Anhorigas synpunkter pa amhandertaget av alderdementa', *Lakartindningen* 77: 2519–25.
Age Concern (1983) *Mental Health in Old Age: A Collection of Projects*, Age Concern, Mitcham, Surrey.
Arling, G., Harkins, E.B. and Capitman, J.A. (1986) 'Institutionalization and personal control: a panel study of impaired older people', *Research on Aging* 8: 38–56.
Arrowsmith, D., Lodge, B., Sequeira, E., Sherrin, B. and Sivewright, G. (1986) 'The implementation of care in the community for people with dementia', paper reproduced for the Scottish Action on Dementia symposium: *Dementia: Planning Innovative Services in the Community*, Crieff Hydro, Scotland, October.
Bond, J. and Carstairs, V. (1982) *Services for the Elderly*, Scottish Health Services Study no. 42, Scottish Home and Health Department, Edinburgh, Scotland.
Borup, J.H. (1983) 'Relocation mortality research: assessment, reply and the need to refocus on the issues', *Gerontologist* 23: 235–42.

Carp, F.M. (1967) 'The impact of environment on old people', *Gerontologist* 7: 106–9.

Challis, D.J. and Davis, B. (1980) 'A new approach to community care of the elderly', *British Journal of Social Work* 10: 1–18.

Chenoweth, B. and Spencer, B. (1986) 'Dementia: the experience of family caregivers', *Gerontologist* 26: 267–72.

Church, M. and Linge, K. (1982) 'Dealing with dementia in the community', *Community Care* pp. 20–1, 25 November.

Clarke, M., Lowry, R. and Clarke, S. (1986) 'Cognitive impairment in the elderly: a survey', *Age and Ageing* 15: 278–84.

Collins, P. (1985) 'Caring for the Confused Elderly', unpublished PhD thesis, University of Birmingham (cited in Woods and Britton, 1985).

Crosbie, D. (1983) 'A role for anyone? A description of social work with the elderly in two area offices', *British Journal of Social Work* 13: 123–48.

Eagles, J.M. and Gilleard, C.J. (1984) 'The function and effectiveness of a day hospital for the demented elderly', *Health Bulletin (Edinburgh)* 42: 87–91.

—— , Craig, A., Rawlinson, F., Restall, D.B., Beattie, J.A.G. and Besson, J.A.O. (1987) 'The psychological well-being of supporters of the demented elderly', *British Journal of Psychiatry* 150: 293–8.

Foster, E.M., Kay, D.W.K. and Bergmann, K. (1976) 'The characteristics of old people receiving and needing domiciliary services', *Age and Ageing* 5: 245–51.

George, L.K. (1984) 'The burden of caregiving: How much? What kinds? For Whom? *Center Reports on Advances in Research*, no. 8, New York: Duke University Center for the Study of Aging and Human Development.

Gibbins, R. (1986) *Oundle Community Care Unit: An evaluation of an initiative in the care of the elderly mentally infirm*, research report no. 10, Northampton: Central Policy and Research Unit, Northampton County Council.

Gilhooly, M.L.M. (1984) 'The social dimensions of dementia', in I. Hanley and J. Hodge (eds) *Psychological Approaches to the Care of the Elderly*, Beckenham: Croom Helm, 88–135.

—— , (1986) 'Senile dementia: factors associated with caregivers' preferences for institutional care', *British Journal of Medical Psychology* 59: 165–71.

Gilleard, C.J. (1984) 'Problems posed for supporting relatives of geriatric and psychogeriatric day patients', *Acta Psychiatrica Scandinavica* 70: 198–208.

—— , (1985) 'Evaluating psychogeriatric day hospitals', in C. Tilquin (ed.) *System 83: Systems Science in Health/Social Services for the Elderly and the Disabled*, Montreal: Science des Systemes.

—— , (1986) 'Family attitudes to caring for the elderly mentally infirm at home', *Family Practice* 3: 31–6.

—— , (1987) 'Influence of emotional distress among supporters on the outcome of psychogeriatric daycare', *British Journal of Psychiatry* 150: 219–23.

—— , Gilleard, E. and Whittick, J.E. (1984b) 'The impact of psychogeriatric day hospital care on the patient's family', *British Journal of Psychiatry* 145: 487–92.

—— , Belford, H., Gilleard, E., Gledhill, K. and Whittick, J.E. (1984a) 'Emotional distress amongst the supporters of the elderly infirm', *British Journal of Psychiatry* 145: 172–7.

Goldberg, D.P. (1978) *Manual for the General Health Questionnaire*, Windsor, Berks, NFER-Nelson.

Greene, J.G., Smith, R., Gardiner, M. and Timbury, G.C. (1982) 'Measuring behavioural disturbance of elderly demented patients in the community and its effects on relatives: a factor analytic study', *Age and Ageing* 11: 121–6.

—— , Timbury, G.C., Smith, R. and Gardiner, M. (1983) 'Reality orientation with elderly patients in the community: an empirical evaluation', *Age and Ageing* 12: 38–43.

Hagnell, O., Lanke, J., Rursman, B., Ohman, R. and Ojesjo, L. (1983) 'Current trends in the incidence of senile and multi-infarct dementia', *Archives of Psychiatry and Neurological Sciences* 233: 423–38.

Horowitz, M.J. and Schulz, R. (1983) 'The relocation controversy: criticism and commentary on five recent studies', *Gerontologist* 23: 229–34.

Jachuck, S.J., Stobo, S.A. and Sahgal, A. (1986) 'Evaluation of the mental function of the elderly in a general practice', *Journal of the Royal College of General Practitioners* 36: 123–4.

Jones, I.G. and Munbodh, R. (1982) 'An evaluation of a day hospital for the demented elderly', *Health Bulletin (Edinburgh)* 40: 10–15.

Kay, D.W.K., Beamish, P. and Roth, M. (1964) 'Old age mental disorders in Newcastle-upon-Tyne. Part 1. A study of prevalence', *British Journal of Psychiatry* 110: 146–58.

—— and Bergmann, K. (1980) 'Epidemiology of mental disorders amongst the aged in the community' in J.E. Birren and R.B. Sloane (eds) *Handbook of Mental Health and Aging*, Englewood Cliffs, New Jersey: Prentice Hall.

Lazarus, L.W., Stafford, B., Cooper, K., Cohler, B. and Dyksen, M. (1981) 'A pilot study of an Alzheimer's patients' relatives discussion group', *Gerontologist* 21: 253–8.

Levin, E., Sinclair, I. and Gorbach, P. (1983) *The Supporters of Confused Elderly Persons at Home*, Final Report to the DHSS (3 vols), London: National Institute for Social Work Research Unit.

Luker, K.A. (1981) 'The role of the health visitor', in J. Kinnaird, J. Brotheston and J. Williamson (eds) *The Provision of Care for the Elderly*, Edinburgh: Churchill Livingstone.

McDonald, A.J.D., Mann, A.H., Jenkins, R., Godlove, C. and Rodwell, G. (1982) 'An attempt to determine the impact of four types of care upon the elderly', *Psychological Medicine* 12: 193–200.

Mitterness, L.S. and Wood, S.J. (1986) 'Social workers responses to incontinence, confusion and mobility impairments in frail elderly clients', *Journal of Gerontological Social Work* 9: 63–70.

Molsa, P.K., Martila, A.R.J. and Rinne, U.K. (1982) 'Epidemiology of dementia in a Finnish population', *Acta Neurologica Scandinavica* 65: 541–52.

Morycz, R.K. (1985) 'Caregiving strain and the desire to institutionalize family members with Alzheimer's disease', *Research on Aging* 7: 329–62.

Nilsson, L. (1984) 'Incidence of severe dementia in an urban sample followed from 70 to 79 years of age', *Acta Psychiatrica Scandinavica* 70: 478–86.

Nocks, B.C., Learner, R.M., Blackman, D. and Brown, T.E. (1986) 'The effects of a community based long term care project on nursing home utilization', *Gerontologist* 26: 150–7.

Ory, M.G., Williams, T.F., Emir, M. *et al.* (1985) 'Families, informal supports and Alzheimer's disease: Current research and future agendas', *Research on Aging* 7: 623–44.

Osborn, A. (1985) 'Short term funded projects: a creative response to an ageing population?', in A. Butler (ed.) *Ageing: Recent Advances and Creative Responses*, Beckenham: Croom Helm, 125–36.

Preston, G.A.N. (1986) 'Dementia in elderly adults: prevalence and institutionalization', *Journal of Gerontology* 41: 261–7.

Reifler, R.V., Cox, G.B. and Hanley, R.S. (1981) 'Problems of the mentally ill elderly as perceived by patients, family and clinicians', *Gerontologist* 21: 165–70.

Rowlands, K.F. (1977) 'Environmental events predicting death for the elderly', *Psychological Bulletin* 84: 349–72.

Shibayama, H., Kasahara, Y., Kobayashi, H. *et al.* (1986) 'Prevalence of dementia in a Japanese elderly population', *Acta Psychiatrica Scandinavica* 74: 144–51.

Smits, C. (1982) 'General practioners' attitudes towards old versus young vignettes and their view of psychogeriatric problems in their practices', unpublished candidatus thesis, Catholic University of Nijmegen.

Tobin, S. and Lieberman, M.A. (1978) *Last Home for the Aged,* San Francisco: Jossey Bass.

Toner, H. (1985) 'A handbook for carers of dementia sufferers: does it really work?' paper presented at PSIGE meeting, Glasgow, May.

Wells, Y. and Jorm, A.F. (in press) 'Evaluation of a special nursing home unit for dementia sufferers: A randomized controlled comparison with community care', *Australian and New Zealand Journal of Psychiatry.*

West, P., Illsley, R. and Kelman, H. (1984) 'Public preferences for the care of dependency groups', *Social Science and Medicine* 18: 287–95.

Whitehead, J.A. (1974) 'Community Hospital Services in Brighton', *Nursing Times* 70: 1340.

Whittick, J.E. (1985) 'A comparison of the attitudes to caregiving of adult daughters and mothers of the elderly mentally infirm and the mentally handicapped', unpublished M Phil thesis, University of Edinburgh.

Williams, E.I. (1984) 'Characteristics of patients aged over 75 not seen during one year in general practice', *British Medical Journal* 288: 119–21.

Williamson, J., Stokoe, I.H., Gray, S. *et al.* (1964) 'Old people at home: their unreported needs', *Lancet* i: 1117–20.

Woods, R.T. and Britton, P.G. (1985) *Clinical Psychology with the Elderly,* Beckenham: Croom Helm.

Zarit, J.M. (1982) 'Family roles, social supports and their relation to caregivers' burden', paper presented at the Western Psychological Association, annual meeting, Sacramento, California, July.

Zarit, S.H. and Zarit, J.M. (1984) 'Behavioral intervention with caregivers of dementia patients', paper presented at the meeting of the Association for the Advancement of Behavior Therapy, Philadelphia, November.

Chapter 18

Day care and dementia

Han Diesfeldt

SUMMARY

Since 1977 it has been possible for nursing homes in the Netherlands to treat psychogeriatric patients on a day-care basis. By now 116 day-care centres all over the country serve more than 2,600 cognitively impaired elderly clients. The three main objectives of day care are to enhance the patients' physical, cognitive and social abilities, to help the care-givers in looking after the patient and to prevent or defer institutionalization. Studies into the impact of day care on patients and family care-givers have demonstrated that most elderly and their families perceive day care as offering positive benefits. A longitudinal study that followed sixty-six day-care visitors until they died, showed that long-term institutionalization could be avoided for 30 per cent of them.

INTRODUCTION

This chapter will provide an overview of the role day care has in the Dutch long-term care system, give data concerning the methods and use of day care and present some findings from evaluations of day care.

Psychogeriatric day care has a relatively short history in the Netherlands. Only in 1977 the Dutch government decided that nursing homes which provided skilled nursing care and round-the-clock custodial care for elderly people were allowed to deliver day care too. Psychogeriatric day-care centres provide a setting to which functionally impaired elderly come for comprehensive assessment, care, activities or therapeutic treatment. These services are provided by an interdisciplinary team. Patients visit the day-care centre two to three times per week returning to their own homes each evening. The programme of services include nursing, social activities, personal care, nutrition services, meals and transportation.

Table 18.1 Elderly population in the Netherlands by sex and 5-year age group on
1 January 1989

age	males × 1000	females × 1000
65–69	277.0	335.4
70–74	198.8	272.2
75–79	142.6	232.8
80–84	81.2	164.1
85–89	36.0	86.3
90–94	11.1	30.0
95+	2.6	6.7

Source: Netherlands Central Bureau of Statistics, 1989.

LONG-TERM CARE FOR THE ELDERLY IN THE NETHERLANDS

In the population of 14.8 million people 1.88 million (12.7 per cent) are 65 years or older (See Table 18.1). Long-term institutional care is provided by 321 nursing homes with 50,130 beds (Bartels, 1988). Governmental planning norms allow 245 beds in nursing homes for every 10,000 elderly of 65 and over. In addition to these places so-called homes for the aged provide a residential setting with mainly domestic care and nursing care, if necessary, to 7 per cent of the elderly population.

The nursing homes provide skilled nursing care for elderly people in need of recuperative care or rehabilitation. Nursing homes also provide custodial care to those in need of long-term maintenance care as a result of disabling chronic conditions. Besides these services, many nursing homes offer day care.

The facilities for cognitively impaired elderly people are separate from departments for those who are physically frail, and cognitively well. The reasons for this segregation are partially historical as 30 years ago demented elderly people were mainly admitted to psychiatric hospitals. Nursing homes were in existence in that time, but admitted only physically impaired patients. Since 1960 nursing homes, specifically designed for demented elderly people have been built or psychogeriatric departments have been added to nursing homes for physically impaired patients. At present there are 78 psychogeriatric nursing homes, 120 nursing homes for physically impaired elderly and 123 so-called combined homes which have separate departments for demented and cognitively intact patients (Bartels, 1988). Of course, there are many patients that combine physical and mental impairments, and there may be advantages in integrated facilities for patients who are and who are not cognitively impaired, but the current opinion of policy makers and care professionals favours segregated care for the two client groups (Cicirelli and Brown, 1986; Cherry and Rafkin, 1988). This applies also to day care where separate facilities are prescribed and planned for psychogeriatric and physically impaired patients.

A typical day-care centre has about twenty-five places and offers services to about sixty patients. It is located in and associated with a skilled nursing facility. Staff includes three professional recreation workers, a full-time nurse and nursing aid and part-time: a domestic help, administrative help, a physician, a psychologist, a physiotherapist, an occupational therapist, a speech therapist and a social worker. According to governmental planning norms 75 places for psychogeriatric day care are allowed for 100,000 inhabitants of 65 years or older. In 1979 only 150 places were available for psychogeriatric day care. Growth continued rapidly through the next decade and, in 1988, 116 day-care centres (divided over 58 per cent of all institutions all over the country) served more than 2,600 cognitively impaired elderly clients on almost 1,300 places. For physically impaired elderly there are 1,500 extra places (Bartels, 1988).

The day-care centres are financed by the revenues from a scheme set up under the Exceptional Medical Expenses (Compensation) Act and from the fees charged to patients on the basis of their income (including unearned income). Day care cost in 1988 about 120 DFL per diem and per client. These costs include staffing, overheads and transportation, and are fully paid through the reimbursement system. For nursing-home entrants the expenditures were about 200 DFL per diem and per patient. Budgets, admission procedures, residents' rights and quality of care are all subject to government control (Boekholdt, 1987).

CLIENTS SERVED BY PSYCHOGERIATRIC DAY CARE

Eligible clients are elderly people who are having difficulty coping in their home setting. Clients will be considered for day care if the burden of care on other family members can be decreased, if patient quality of life can be improved, early discharge from hospital facilitated or institutionalization delayed or avoided. From a national survey it could be concluded that most clients are women (62 per cent). The mean age of the clients was 78 years. Most of them were living at home (78 per cent), and 21 per cent in residential homes for the aged (SIG Informatiecentrum voor de Gezondheidszorg, 1988).

Table 18.2 shows the five most frequent mental disorders of 2,163 patients admitted in 1987. Table 18.2 shows that a large majority of clients carried a diagnosis of senile-onset dementia, though day care can also serve those with other psychiatric disorders and those who are socially isolated. A survey of behaviour and mental impairments in 104 patients in psychogeriatric day care whose symptoms of mental deterioration had started 4 to 5 years before admission showed that the following symptoms were most

Table 18.2 Diagnoses of mental disorders on first admission for 2163 patients referred for psychogeriatric day care

Diagnosis judged most relevant to patient disabilities	%
1 Dementia (all causes)	74.6
2 Amnestic syndrome	11.3
3 Mild memory disturbance	3.3
4 Depression	2.3
5 Neurotic and personality disorders	1.4

Source: SIG Informatiecentrum voor de Gezondheidszorg, 1988.

frequent: unable to remember names of staff (91 per cent), unable to occupy themselves (85 per cent), sitting around, doing nothing (82 per cent), not safe if outside alone (81 per cent), disoriented (77 per cent), unhelpful (67 per cent), unable to dress without help (64 per cent) and lose their way in the home (58 per cent). The mood of 60 per cent of the clients was judged as depressed. Many clients showed language impairments such as expressive difficulties (39 per cent) and comprehension disturbances (31 per cent). Thirty-three per cent of the clients wandered at night and so disturbed the sleep of their care-giving partners. Urinary incontinence occurred more or less often in 33 per cent of female and in 17 per cent of male patients (Diesfeldt and Van Houte, 1985).

Most day-care centres do not admit patients who display active psychosis or violent and disruptive behaviour or those with uncontrolled wandering. However, severe dementia in itself does not warrant exclusion if the problem behaviour can be managed.

THE DAY-CARE PROGRAMME

Patients are referred by primary health care agencies or by general practitioners. A social worker visits the patient at home to explain the purpose and facilities of the day-care centre. An intake is performed which includes the gathering of a health history, a list of current medications, information on activity of daily-living skills, on the quality of the social-support network, domiciliary services and on any special characteristics of the potential client such as personality characteristics, dietary needs and special activity preferences. A comprehensive medical and psychological examination follows after admission, during the first few weeks of day care. The aims of the physical examination are to reach a diagnosis of the patient's illnesses and to detect any coexisting abnormalities that may exacerbate the patient's disability. The examination includes the nutritional status, use of medication, joint flexibility and functional abilities, mental status, speech and eye and ear examination. All patients with new onset of dementia are referred to hospital for basic and standard diagnostic studies, including laboratory tests and examinations by a neurologist or psychiatrist. The results of the examination are communicated with the general practitioner who continues to be the primary health care physician of the patient.

The neuropsychological examinations are done by the staff clinical psychologist of the day-care centre. The psychological examination includes the assessment of mood, attention, memory and learning abilities, language and speech, calculation, perception and visuospatial abilities. During the last decade several tests with adequate normative data have been developed specifically for elderly subjects (Munnichs and Diesfeldt, 1987).

The results of the psychological examination help us to understand the patient's difficulties and his or her strengths, so that a rational programme of activities and therapy can be developed. Every 3 months the nursing staff reviews the behavioural and functional status of each client by means of a standardized rating scale (Van der Kam *et al.*, 1971; Diesfeldt, 1981). The results of the examinations are discussed with the primary health care workers during regular multidisciplinary weekly meetings where all professionals discuss progress and plan future care of patients attending the day-care centre.

For the visitors a typical day in the programme starts between 9.00 and 10.00 a.m. when a staff member meets the client at home to accompany her or him in the van that drives the visitors to the day-care centre. Coffee is served on arrival and a hot meal is served at 12 o'clock. The van starts to bring the visitors home from around 4 o'clock in the afternoon. The clients participate in activities either individually or in groups. Groups consist of about eight visitors and are supported by professional and inventive recreation workers. They assist the clients during arts and crafts or interactive games. A kitchen belongs to the day-care centre's facilities so that clients can be encouraged to participate in housekeeping and preparing the meal. The staff reinforce appropriate social interaction throughout the day. In particular, communication and conversation skills and appropriate table behaviour are encouraged during lunch. Often competencies are identified that the care-giver at home supposed to be absent as a consequence of the patient's impairments. Of course the staff passes information about tasks that can be done by the client on to the care-giving family members at home.

Many social activities are planned for the clients, such as singsongs and dance sessions, slide shows, group discussions, reminiscence groups and sessions for memory training. The day centre has a room for woodwork. Clients can visit a hairdresser or have a pedicure. Clients who have difficulty taking a bath can use the bathroom and get assistance. If the day centre has a garden, participation in horticulture is encouraged, the flower boxes are easy to reach, there are plenty of seats and smooth footpaths. Favourite outings are the visits to the weekly market or trips to local museums. The municipal swimming baths have special opening hours for disabled people so that some patients can go swimming if one-on-one assistance is offered, which depends on the availability of helping volunteers. Many clients participate in a course of mobility and strengthening exercises that are offered by the physiotherapists belonging to the staff of the day centre or the adjacent nursing home.

EVALUATING DAY CARE

The three main objectives of day care are to improve the patients' physical, cognitive and emotional function, to help the care-givers in looking after the patients and to decrease institutionalization. The effectiveness of the day-care programme in attaining these objectives must be established.

The impact of day care on patients

Systematic studies with random assignment of subjects to day care or control conditions have so far not been done in the Netherlands. A few descriptive studies have shown that the clients appreciate the social contact with other clients and staff, and that the programme relieves the monotony of their daily life. Some patients receive specific treatment (physiotherapy, speech therapy, occupational therapy) which they would not have received if they had stayed at home. For other patients, especially for those living alone, day care can be a matter of life or death because of the regular monitoring of their health, nutritional status and hygiene.

Psychological treatment is mostly offered in the form of emotional support and cognitive rehabilitation. A controlled study in this respect was carried out by Allewijn (1986) who demonstrated that a course of twenty reality-orientation sessions over a period of 3 months resulted in a slight improvement of verbal orientation and free recall performance on a standardized test of memory function. There was, however, no evidence for more generalized behaviour change.

Not every patient can tolerate an entire day of day care. Some become agitated when fatigued or cannot stand the company of other clients. A retrospective study compared thirty-two patients who responded well to the day-care programme and had participated in the programme for at least 12 months, with thirty-six patients who had participated for at least one month but did not complete a full year of treatment because they were discharged to a psychogeriatric nursing home (Diesfeldt and Van Houte, 1985). All patients carried a diagnosis of senile dementia of the Alzheimer type and were still alive for a period of at least 12 months after their admission into the day-care programme. Univariate analysis of variance with outcome (still in day care after 12 months or discharged) as the dependent variable and thirty-one variables as predictors revealed that women, and cognitively and behaviourally more impaired patients carried a slightly higher risk of being institutionalized within the 1-year study period. Other variables in the analysis, such as age, widowhood, quality of domiciliary care and duration of illness did not discriminate between favourable and unfavourable outcome. Outcome studies such as these, if they can be carried out on a larger scale, will help to define selection criteria to distinguish between clients who will respond well to day care from those who cannot be helped with this kind of treatment.

Effects on family care-givers

A major objective of psychogeriatric day care is to provide respite and support to the home care-giver. The intake procedure often is the first intervention with the care-giver. Part of the day-care programme are regular meetings organized by the staff, as an opportunity for educating care-givers about the dementia or other problems of their family member. These support groups further allow the exchange of the care-givers' ideas on behaviour management, and can help to reduce the care-givers' feelings of guilt and ambivalence if they cannot cope with the demands made upon them by the need of providing continuous care. In many instances, positive experiences, including successful problem solving, are shared and reinforced which encourages feelings of solidarity and social connectedness.

A few descriptive studies tried to elucidate the effects of day care on the family members (Jacobs and Van der Schoot, 1982; Van der Kam and Miggelbrink, 1984). Eighty per cent of fifty primary-care providers felt that day care lightened the burden of care-giving, 74 per cent gave it as their view that day care helped them to delay or to avoid institutionalization of their family member. Two out of three reported that they had more time to rest and to relax. The same percentage felt that the information given by the staff was useful to their care-giving role.

According to a majority of these care-givers (68 per cent), the patients themselves did not show much change in their mental or functional status. Some care-givers reported that the patient was in a better mood (18 per cent), more active at home (12 per cent) or slept better at night (8 per cent). A few care-givers reported positive effects on the physical health of their family member (6 per cent). The most favourable effects were found in the patients with lesser cognitive impairment.

Asked for their opinion on the feelings of the patients themselves, 62 per cent of the care-givers thought that the patient was happy in day care, 38 per cent thought that the patient did not appreciate the programme. Taking the severe disability of the patients into account, one cannot be surprised that not all care-givers experienced sufficient reduction in stress caused by their care-giving roles and responsibilities. However, most elderly and their families perceive day care as offering positive benefits for them.

Long-term outcome and risk of institutionalization

According to a national survey over 2,253 psychogeriatric patients for whom day care was terminated for any reasons except death, the median length of attendance was 9 to 10 months (SIG Informatiecentrum voor de Gezondheidszorg, 1988). The most common reasons for discharge are deterioration of the patient's condition, disintegration of the support network or burnout of the care-giver so that the patient is placed into a nursing home.

In an unpublished longitudinal study I followed all 167 patients who had been admitted into psychogeriatric day care in a centre with 25 places during the period 1982–4. Outcome for these 167 new admissions was assessed 1 year, 2 years and 3 years after their first attendance. Outcome was classified into four categories: still living in the community and attending day care, living in the community without day care, institutionalized and dead. Table 18.3 shows the results.

One year after first attendance two out of three clients were discharged. This corresponds with the median length of attendance of less than one year that appeared from cross-sectional surveys. Only very few patients attend day care for longer than three years (5.4 per cent in our sample). Nearly half of the day-centre patients (47.3 per cent) remained in the community (supported by day care or not) after 12 months, which comes very close to the results reported by Bell and Gilleard (1986). The 2-year outcome was less favourable. The percentage of visitors still residing in the community fell down to 21.0 per cent with a further reduction to 11.4 per cent after 3 years since first attendance. Roughly, the number of clients residing in the community reduces by half, each year.

After 2 years since first attendance half of the clients was institutionalized in a nursing home for chronic long-term care. The mean length of survival was slightly more than 3 years for this group of elderly psychogeriatric patients, most of them carrying a diagnosis of Alzheimer-type dementia. The risk to end up in a nursing home was 71.3 per cent

Table 18.3 Outcome after 1, 2 or 3 years since initial attendance for 167 patients in psychogeriatric day care (percentages)

| Outcome | Years since first attendance | | |
	1 year	2 years	3 years
In day care	35.3	15.0	5.4
Community (no day care)	12.0	6.0	6.0
Institutionalized	41.3	50.9	44.3
Dead	11.4	28.1	44.3
Total	100.0	100.0	100.0

(including patients who died in a nursing home) after 3 years, and 76.9 per cent after 4 years. The latter percentage could be computed by following 104 patients who were admitted in 1982-3.

It is difficult to determine from these figures to what extent institutionalization was delayed or avoided by the day-care programme. From sixty-six day-care patents who were dead after 4 years since initial attendance, 30 per cent were never admitted into a nursing home which represents a fair number of patients for whom long-term institutionalization was avoided.

Future experience will show if psychogeriatric day care is an alternative to institutional placement. So far, it can be concluded that the day-care programme has been well received by many elderly patients and is much appreciated by their families.

REFERENCES

Allewijn, M. (1986) 'Oefening baart kunst', unpublished M Psychology thesis, University of Utrecht.

Bartels, L.P. (1988) *Instellingen van intramurale gezondheidszorg. Basisgegevens 1-1-1988*, Utrecht: Nationaal Ziekenhuisinstituut.

Bell, J.S. and Gilleard, C.J. (1986) 'Psychometric prediction of psychogeriatric day care outcome', *British Journal of Clinical Psychology* 25: 195-200.

Boekholdt, M. (1987) 'Supporting nursing homes in the Netherlands: profile of a program', *Danish Medical Bulletin Gerontology Special Supplement Series* 5: 44-8.

Cherry, D.L. and Rafkin, M.J. (1988) 'Adapting day care to the needs of adults with dementia', *Gerontologist* 28: 116-20.

Cicirelli, V.G. and Brown, E. (1986) 'Psychological considerations in the day care of elderly people', in I. Hanley and M. Gilhooly (eds) *Psychological Therapies for the Elderly*, Beckenham: Croom Helm.

Diesfeldt, H.F.A. (1981) 'De BOP tien jaar (The BOP, a report on ten years' experience with a Dutch Geriatric Rating Scale)', *Gerontologie* 12: 139-47.

—— , and Van Houte, L.R. (1985) *Dagbehandeling in de Larikshof te Laren. Een jaar follow-up van 104 patiënten opgenomen in 1982 en 1983*, Laren: Stichting Verpleeghuizen Nederland.

Jacobs, M. and Van der Schoot, M. (1982) 'Mantelzorgers van ouderen in dagbehandeling', unpublished thesis, University of Utrecht.

Munnichs, J.M.A. and Diesfeldt, H.F.A. (1987) 'Psychology of ageing. An overview of research in the Netherlands', *Tijdschrift voor Gerontologie en Geriatrie* 18: 117-29.

Netherlands Central Bureau of Statistics (1989) *Monthly Bulletin of Population Statistics* 37: 31.

SIG Informatiecentrum voor de Gezondheidszorg (1988) *SIVIS Jaarboek 1987*, Utrecht.

Van der Kam, P. and Miggelbrink, D.W. (1984) *Enkele onderzoeksgegevens na een jaar dagbehandeling in Lisidunahof te Leusden*, Leusden: Stichting Verpleeghuizen Nederland.

—— , Mol, F. and Wimmers, M.F.H.G. (1971) *Beoordelingsschaal voor Oudere Patiënten*, Deventer: Van Loghum Slaterus.

EDITORS' NOTE FOR CHAPTER 19

As yet, there are no special models for providing care in the community to elderly persons with dementia. We were very impressed with the COPA model and can see how it could provide a useful starting point for community care planners interested in developing a model specifically for dementia. This seems particularly pertinent given the tendency to keep persons with dementia at home as long as possible.

One of the most attractive features of the COPA approach is that it has the scope for combining both voluntary and professional services in a structured way.

Dementia, like alcoholism, is often a hidden problem with many accompanying complications; the denial of memory loss and of the inability to cope are especially problematic. In the type of approach that COPA uses, persons would not need to be directly confronted with their limitations any more than their denial/coping mechanisms allowed, yet they would still benefit from covert assessment, regular friendly visits and acute or community services when required.

Chapter 19

The COPA project as a model for the management of early dementia in the community

Sarah Saunders, Kathryn Graham, Margaret Flower and Marilyn White-Campbell

INTRODUCTION

The Community Older Persons Alcohol Program (COPA) was established in Toronto, Canada in an effort to identify a means to provide effective treatment services for elderly substance abusers, while at the same time enabling these people to remain in their homes if at all possible. These people have multiple problems and are considered to be difficult to treat.

This chapter will look briefly at the problems of older alcohol abusers, the rationale for developing a specialized treatment programme, and, in detail, the programme itself. Because the problems experienced by the elderly are multiple, and encompass all areas of the person's lifestyle, the treatment programme is comprehensive. Consequently, no single component of the programme will be discussed in detail. Rather, emphasis will be placed on the fact that, unless all problem areas are addressed, the chances of positive treatment outcome are poor. For the sake of clarity, reference will be made to alcohol abuse only. However, COPA also treats persons experiencing other forms of drug abuse.

RATIONALE FOR THE DEVELOPMENT OF COPA

Before the mid-1970s, the older person with an alcohol problem was poorly recognized. In fact the literature suggested that the problem was rare. Certainly the existing alcohol treatment programmes saw few persons over the age of 60–65.

When other non-alcohol-related services for the elderly encountered an alcoholic, this person rapidly became unacceptable because of actual, or fear of, inappropriate behaviour. If a service was provided at all, it was rapidly terminated as intoxicated or acting-out behaviour occurred. The service provider was left feeling helpless, frustrated and even hopeless about the possibility of working effectively with the actively drinking alcohol abuser.

The extensive denial of the alcohol problem by both the alcoholic, and often family members, compounded the problem.

In a closer look at existing alcohol-treatment programmes it becomes evident that they may be quite inappropriate for the older person, usually dealing with the issues of the young person rather than the older person. While some of the needs of the older substance abuser are similar to those of a younger one, many are not. Addressing the needs specific to the elderly becomes fundamental to the effectiveness of any treatment programme.

The overall goal of this programme was to provide an outreach (home-visiting) service to older persons experiencing an alcohol problem, that was designed to assist the individual to:

- identify lifestyle problems
- receive assistance of identified problems
- reduce or eliminate problem use of alcohol
- develop healthy alternatives to alcohol.

HIDDEN PROBLEMS

The extent of the problem of alcohol abuse among the elderly is difficult to assess. It is commonly denied by both the elderly and their families for the stigma attached to the label 'alcoholic' is great.

The diagnosis is often missed. Signs and symptoms that would flag a younger person as an alcoholic, are interpreted as common problems of the elderly (e.g. early dementia, unsteady gait, malnutrition, loss of friends, increased incidence of trauma). Physicians have generally not been trained to identify the problem, or even to acknowledge that it may exist. Commonly, the problem is not identified unless the person presents in an intoxicated state, usually during home visits and not office visits, or in a state of crisis while intoxicated.

GENERAL CLIENT DESCRIPTION

It is understandable that the older person with an alcohol problem is perceived to be untreatable or unmanageable. This person often presents experiencing multiple problems, very isolated and often depressed. Commonly, grossly inappropriate behaviour obviously related to alcohol consumption is demonstrated, while at the same time the client is either completely denying an alcohol problem, minimizing, or even defending, the use of alcohol with great defiance. These responses are not conducive to traditional alcoholism treatment. Accompanying this may be the fact that all significant components of life except alcohol have been lost. Thus, while the use of alcohol is creating havoc, it may also be a coping mechanism or even perceived as the last remaining pleasure.

TRADITIONAL ALCOHOLISM TREATMENT PROGRAMMES

The older person may not even meet the admission criteria of a traditional programme. Such programmes require that the alcoholic acknowledge a problem with the use of alcohol, have the desire to change the lifestyle so that use of alcohol no longer is involved, and be totally abstinent throughout the treatment process. The person who is either using denial or defiance about drinking behaviour has no reason to meet these criteria.

Even if the admission criteria are met, the programme content may be inappropriate, focusing on the younger person in terms of motivational factors, feelings and young person's problems. Intensive inpatient/day treatment programmes may not consider chronic disabilities such as hearing loss, the slowed pace of the older person, problems unique to the elderly (e.g. difficulties with activities of daily living) or the reluctance of the older person to discuss feelings in depth. Finally, these programmes are always conducted outside of the home. Commonly the older person either cannot or will not leave the home – certainly not for something labelled with the stigma of 'alcoholism treatment'.

TREATMENT OUTCOME

Traditionally, alcoholism treatment programmes have considered total abstinence to be the only acceptable treatment goal. However, because the older person uses such extensive denial or defiance about drinking behaviour, it may be impossible using a traditional approach, to ever begin to work with the client, never mind attempt to achieve a goal of total abstinence.

Because the use of alcohol may be perceived as the last remaining pleasure, and certainly may be the last significant component in life, it becomes crucial in any treatment regime to replace the alcohol with something else of importance to the person. Rather than expecting total abstinence, it may be more relevant to work towards the development of a healthier lifestyle. The use of alcohol is intricately intertwined with lifestyle. Assisting the client to reduce alcohol consumption as part of the means of resolving problems, will enhance treatment outcome.

For older persons who perceive themselves to be at the end of life, total abstinence makes no sense whatsoever and reduced consumption may be a more acceptable goal. Of course, total abstinence should be encouraged whenever possible, but refusal of abstinence by the elderly should never become a reason to not treat the person.

COPA PROGRAM DESCRIPTION

Location

The COPA program is housed in a large, chronic-care hospital. This site was deliberately chosen over that of a traditional alcoholism treatment programme in order to avoid as much of the societal stigma associated with alcohol abuse as possible. While the service provided is primarily home visiting, the office may be used for family counselling, groupwork or as a stepping stone in enabling the client to become involved in the community.

Referral

A client may be referred to COPA by any means. Commonly, family members, hospitals, community professionals or providers of services to the elderly make the referral. However, self-referrals are not uncommon, as are referrals from any concerned person. These have included cab drivers, bank tellers and the local librarian! These people may call expressing concern for, and frustration about, an individual whom they recognize as having an alcohol problem, while the person is using complete denial and refusing any assistance whatsoever. In this instance, counselling designed to encourage the alcoholic to accept intervention of any sort is provided, often for several weeks, to those referring the client.

Initial contact

Initial contact with the client is greatly facilitated when the worker is accompanied and introduced by the person making the referral. The older alcoholic has, by hard experience, often become wary of unknown people and may refuse admittance to anyone not introduced by a trusted friend.

If the referral is made by a hospital, it is invaluable to make contact as early in the hospital stay as possible. The more visits that are made in hospital, the more likely is the link to be maintained following discharge. Making use of the crisis-precipitating hospital admission can be useful. This may be the only time when the patient is able to make the link between the use of alcohol and the resulting problem. Use of denial is often lower immediately following the fracture of a hip while intoxicated, but will be back in place within a few days.

The primary goal of the initial visit is to develop enough rapport with the client to ensure acceptance of future visits. While the outreach worker always acknowledges representing the COPA Program, the major emphasis of the visit is placed on making the client feel comfortable. Immediate crises are of course identified, but following this, emphasis is placed on identifying the client's concerns with the expectation of quickly rectifying as many of these as possible within the first 2 to 3 visits. While these may not bear much resemblance to alcohol-related issues, they are none the less of concern to the client. Taking the time to listen and then actively remedy as many as possible, quickly lets the client know that you are concerned about them as a human being in need.

Assessment

Careful and detailed assessment is the backbone of effective treatment planning. Both problem areas and client strengths must be identified. Present use of existing agencies and services or lack of use, must also be addressed.

Looking into every aspect of the person's life is crucial. The older person with an alcohol problem is a classic multiproblem individual. Commonly only a minimum of these problems has been identified or addressed. However, almost without exception all the lifestyle problems are inter-woven with the use of alcohol and unless all the problems are addressed the chances of helping the client to significantly lower or discontinue alcohol consumption are remote.

This means that the quantity of information to be obtained during the assessment is great. Trying to achieve this in one or two visits would probably serve only to alienate the client. Consequently COPA staff complete an assessment over several visits. Similarly treatment planning and implementation occurs, not at the completion of a formal assessment, but in a stepwise fashion as the clients' needs are identified.

While a detailed assessment tool has been developed, it serves to ensure that the worker covers all life areas, rather than it be painfully and individu-ally filled in by the client. Such a form is threatening to most clients and would only serve to lose the client if actually used at an interview. However, from time to time a client expresses interest in this kind of detail, and the form may be used in part or its entirety.

The headings included in the form include:

Activities of daily living	Prescription drug use
Nutritional status	Accommodation
Physical health	Marital relationships
Emotional health	Family relationships
Social contacts	Financial status
Leisure time activities	Employment
Use of nicotine, caffeine	Legal status
Use of over-the-counter drugs	Psychoactive drug use
Alcohol use	

While every effort is made to cover all these life areas as early as possible in the counselling relationship, new information is constantly being unearthed and consequently the treatment plan is, of necessity, frequently revised.

Treatment plan

The treatment plan must be developed *with* the client and not *for* the client. It must include, wherever possible, the client's recognized problems as well as those identified by the counsellor, even when the counsellor feels the client's concerns are irrelevant. They may not be particularly relevant to treating the alcohol problem, but they are of the greatest relevance to the client. Resolving these will go a long way towards co-operation in implementing the counsellor's goals.

Because of the unique mixture of multiple problems for each client, the treatment plan itself must be individualized to each person. While the underlying treatment philosophy and use of various resources will remain constant, the treatment plan for each client must address the individual's unique set of problems, and be based on the unique strengths of the client.

While the problems are relatively simple to recognize, the strengths seem more difficult to find. COPA staff define a strength as anything for which one can give approval to the client. As long as a strength is considered to be a large, indefinable item such as 'courage' or 'will power', no strengths are identified. When one identifies and acknowledges the ability to grow beautiful African violets, or always to be well groomed, all sorts of strengths appear. Even with the most withdrawn, dishevelled, intoxicated individual, it is possible to find something, perhaps only after some searching! A picture of a dog, a smile after four visits of stony glumness, a cup of tea offered for the first time, all constitute strengths upon which an improved relationship and ultimately the successful treatment plan can be developed.

Because of the usual multiplicity and wide range of problems each individual experiences, it is rarely possible for the COPA worker alone to implement the treatment plan. Other helping resources are usually needed and referral to these resources becomes part of the implementation of the treatment plan.

Recognition and acceptance of any negative attitudes by counsellors directed towards elderly alcoholics, is helpful in enabling the intervention to be non-judgemental.

Treatment goals

At the onset of COPA, suggested client treatment goals were outlined and after four years they remain unchanged. They are to:

- stop or reduce alcohol consumption
- receive appropriate medical care
- follow prescribed medication routine
- develop adequate nutrition
- ability to conduct activities of daily living
- develop/improve marital/family relationships if possible

- develop/improve non-alcohol-related social and leisure skills and activities
- remain in one's own home or general community non-institutionalized setting.

Involvement with other resources for the elderly

Referral is made to an outside resource whenever the client need cannot be met by the outreach worker. Most commonly this would include medical, dental, housing, financial or housekeeping resources. Well over fifty separate services are used regularly. Other services include lawyers, friendly visitors, seniors' volunteer groups or seniors' centres, librarians, clergy, occupational therapists, etc.

In each instance the resource is requested to provide only that service which it already provides in the community, and nothing more. When service provision has previously been refused by an agency, it is usually on the grounds that the person with an alcohol problem will become intoxicated and unmanageable. The agency tends to feel it either cannot cope with the individual or refer elsewhere because of the general unacceptability of an alcoholic client.

The service provider is reassured that COPA staff will always be available for consultation or assistance should a problem related to alcohol consumption arise. When this difficulty is actively resolved by COPA staff, outside agencies accept COPA clients and treat them appropriately.

In order for this arrangement to run smoothly the outreach worker provides several functions including:

- co-ordination of the services being used by the client
- monitoring overlaps or gaps in service and resolving these
- acting as client advocate
- remaining in close contact with, and providing active support to, the agencies involved
- in a difficult situation to call a case conference involving all the agencies and sometimes include the family and/or the client as well
- provision of ongoing contact with the client as necessary.

Working with the alcohol problem itself

The outreach worker starts where the client is, in terms of recognition of the alcohol problem, or the desire to resolve it. Denial or defiance are the usual starting points – always in the face of obvious and serious problems associated with the use of alcohol.

Development of rapport and trust are more important initially than reducing the alcohol consumption. This may take several weeks but once it is established the client will begin to recognize far more readily the problems associated with the use of alcohol.

Gradually as lifestyle problems emerge, the link with the use of alcohol is identified with the client. A crisis at this time can be invaluable (e.g. eviction because of intoxicated behaviour). The link must be made at the time of the crisis or immediately following or the wall of denial is quickly rebuilt. However, resolution of the crisis by itself, can be an excellent means of developing rapport, whether or not the client makes the link with alcohol use.

Once even a minimal link is accepted, the client can be encouraged to reduce or discontinue use of alcohol as a means of attempting to improve the problem. This can sometimes be accomplished even when alcohol use is not acknowledged to be excessive. A quasi-behavioural approach can be used here with reinforcement of any behaviour directed towards problem resolution with decreased alcohol consumption, while at the same time downplaying any unacceptable drinking behaviours.

Improvement in lifestyle problems and reduction in alcohol consumption tend to go hand in hand. For some clients there may never be any overt acknowledgement of an alcohol problem even when the consumption has been significantly reduced as life improved. While this is not recognized as success in the more traditional alcoholism treatment programmes, the end result of a happier, healthier person represents improvement to the staff of COPA.

Individual life areas – problems and resolution

Issues that need to be resolved can arise in any aspect of life and frequently the complexity and multiplicity of these difficulties needs to be seen to be believed! Because it is vital to resolve all of them if one hopes to be successful, each area will be addressed briefly:

Activities of daily living

Fundamental to maintaining the person in the home is the ability to carry out necessary functions for day-to-day living. Too often, in an effort to treat the alcohol problem, these activities are overlooked completely, or are considered to be unimportant. However, nothing else is important if one cannot dress, or have a means of daily meals.

It is crucial to look at personal hygiene, food preparation, shopping, care of clothing, care of living quarters, transportation, use of telephone and physical mobility. These need to be addressed in the context of physical, mental and emotional limitations. There may be other limitations as well, related to language or cultural barriers or simple lack of experience (the widower who has never cooked).

Resolution of these problems is generally simple. Common sense suffices in most instances. For more complex issues, an occupational therapist may be helpful, or use of one or more home support services (visiting home-makers or meals on wheels).

Medical/dental

Medical problems are probably the most common of problems for the older alcohol abuser. Almost any part of the body can be affected by the use of alcohol. Along with this is the fact that heavy use of alcohol can complicate existing disease entities. Even though the disease is receiving treatment, it may be responding poorly because of the associated use of alcohol. It is not uncommon to find that the alcoholic has either not seen a physician for years, or is not following the physician's instructions even if contact has been made.

Dental problems are also common and may be severe enough to inter-fere significantly with adequate nutrition.

These problems may present as a state of crisis and be the factor pushing the client into treatment. However, whether or not they do so, it is important to help the patient achieve the optimal physical wellbeing possible. Unless one feels reasonably well physically, it is hard to work towards any other lifestyle goals.

Helping the client to make and maintain the link with a physician is important. This may necessitate ensuring that the client is accompanied to the doctor's office for the first few visits.

Nutritional status

Nutritional status is often poor in the older alcoholic for many reasons. Alcohol may be more important than food. The person may be unable to shop for or prepare the food. Even minimal memory loss or confusion can play havoc with one's food intake. Depression, common in the older alco-holic, may eliminate any interest in food. Medical/dental problems may create loss of appetite or inability to eat.

Resolution of the underlying disorder, whether it be assistance with shopping or treatment of depression, will usually lead to improved eating habits. Provision of one meal a day by a friend, family member or meals on wheels, or in a setting outside the home or with someone else may be all that is needed.

Emotional health

While any emotional disorder can accompany alcoholism, depression is by far the most common. It may be difficult to identify whether the heavy drinking is in response to the depression or the depression is resulting from the drinking. In either case both problems need to be treated. If the depression is severe it may need to be treated very early in the process, since it can be almost totally debilitating, preventing any other form of effective intervention.

While the presence of a significant anxiety state may also occur, one needs to treat this with caution. Short-term use of depressant drugs such as the benzodiazepines may be invaluable for the prevention of delerium tremens or to alleviate acute anxiety at the time of alcohol withdrawal. Use for longer than 4 to 6 weeks may serve only to produce a benzodiazepine dependency leaving the patient with both an alcohol and a drug dependency to be treated. Wherever possible the underlying cause of the anxiety should be addressed rather than the symptom alone.

Marital/family

Where a marriage is still intact, there are likely to be many problems in the relationship requiring some form of counselling. Not uncommonly the spouse may also be a heavy alcohol user, although this may be difficult to detect.

Frequently, the alcoholic is living in complete isolation with no family contact at all, or at best, only at birthday and Christmas. The family members have left, out of frustration when all offers to help the alcohol abuser have been refused, and the unacceptable drinking behaviour continues unabated.

However, once treatment has been established, and the family realizes that the COPA staff member is actively involved, it is often possible to re-establish positive family contact. This may be accomplished by working with the client and the family together, or by providing separate family counselling, designed to support the family members as they work through the negative and complicated feelings about the alcoholic.

Housing

Housing problems are common. Threat of – or actual – eviction may occur following inappropriate, unacceptable verbal or physical behaviour while intoxicated, or by virtue of being a fire hazard. Regular non-payment of rent is also common.

Once it is known that the client has an active drinking problem, placement in any new housing setting becomes difficult. No-one wants this person. However, if there is reassurance by an involved counsellor that support will be provided for both the alcoholic and the landlord, and that the client will be removed if problems arise, the alcoholic is accepted much more readily. Similarly a threat of eviction may be withdrawn if the client's behaviour improves with treatment.

An interim step of living in some form of sheltered housing may be necessary before the client can become completely self-sufficient. An appropriate boarding home might be useful for this purpose.

Financial status

The problem identified most frequently at COPA is the client who is not receiving all the financial benefits to which he or she is entitled. A close second is mismanagement of existing money. This may result from spending all money on alcohol, but more commonly it is related to lack of knowledge about money management or inability to manage due to physical or mental disabilities. From time to time family members or friends are found to be mismanaging, primarily deliberately removing money from the client's bank account into their own. This, of course, requires immediate legal attention.

It may be necessary to provide formal assistance with financial management, at least on a temporary basis. However, as the client's lifestyle improves and stabilizes, he or she can often become able to manage his own funds.

Socializing skills and use of leisure time

The ability to relate to others has generally become poor, unless conducted through the medium of alcohol, in which case it may be inappropriate. Any activities involving other people tend to be alcohol related. Any leisure activities, whether with others or in isolation, become alcohol related as well. All other relationships, interests or activities tend to be dropped completely. Socializing difficulties may be compounded by long-term inappropriate behaviour which has alienated any potential social contact. Alcohol consumption and television tend to become the sum total of life.

Resolution of social and leisure problems is difficult and long term. A well-trained volunteer can be invaluable as non-alcohol-related interests and activities are explored. This is both time-consuming and frustrating as the counsellor searches for possible interests. The tendency is to try to impose one's own interests or ideas, a situation which may quickly bring the relationship to an end. The key here is to explore possibilities *with* and not *for* the client. The client must make the final decision – not the counsellor. The client has not thought in these terms for many years and ideas will come slowly.

Involvement in any social activity not involving alcohol is threatening to the client. Consequently, the client needs to be accompanied the first few times such involvement is proposed, or he or she simply will not go, even after expressing interest.

Alcohol-related issues

These thread through all aspects of life and need to be explored in the context of each identified problem area. Wherever possible the client is encouraged to recognize the link between problems and use of alcohol, followed by reduction of alcohol consumption to help alleviate the problem.

Use of therapeutic groups

Group process tends to be threatening to the older person experiencing an alcohol-related problem. Even the use of groups for a socializing experience is difficult. However, if a group is possible, it can become an effective means of developing socializing skills. Once a group is established and the members are comfortable attending regularly, it may be possible to add in some discussion of problem areas. However this may need to be handled judiciously by the therapist, recognizing any development of discomfort by the other group members. It may be necessary, at least initially, to curtail the discussion rather than lose the group members. Socializing groups, especially if conducted by a familiar outreach worker, can be a useful first step in helping the client leave the home.

Use of groups can be invaluable in providing support for family members or other care-givers. Both self-help groups and those conducted by trained therapists are important. For the family or other care-givers, the mere recognition that others are experiencing the same apparently insoluble difficulties is powerfully supportive. This is reinforced as they then begin to work together to identify new means of resolution of these difficulties.

Family involvement

Families may be involved both before or during client contact. In fact, families alone may be involved without client contact at any time. This latter would occur when the alcoholic is refusing any sort of assistance. Family members may receive anything from advice and consultation over the telephone, to full family counselling, to involvement in group process.

Through family involvement the members are provided with support when they are at their 'wits' end', a sounding board to discuss their problems with the alcoholic, and some possible suggestions as to how to proceed with assisting the alcoholic to accept treatment.

When COPA is already involved with the alcohol abuser, the family may be a source of more accurate information than the client is able to give. This information is not to be used as a club to hold over the client, rather it provides a more accurate client profile so that there is increased chance of effective treatment planning.

The issue of confidentiality becomes important with the necessity of maintaining the confidentiality of both parties unless there is specific permission to break it. This may occur naturally as the treatment goal of improved family relationship is achieved.

Length of client involvement

This varies widely from person to person. Initially the client is seen by the outreach worker on weekly visits unless a crisis demands more frequency. Other agencies, services and care-givers are involved as soon as appropriate needs are identified. As the client becomes more involved with other people, the frequency of visits by the outreach worker will become less. However, the client's progress continues to be monitored by the outreach worker through the involvement of others. If any difficulty with these services seems to arise, the outreach worker will attempt to correct it before it becomes severe.

While in many instances it is possible, as a strong community support system is developed around the client, to discontinue any client involvement with COPA, in other situations this is not possible. While ongoing involvement by COPA may be necessary, it is rarely intensive. Once the client has stabilized, a visit every 3 months or the occasional telephone call is usually all that is necessary. This simply tells the clients that you have not forgotten them and are there to help with any developing problems. Where there is no family involvement, a simple birthday or Christmas card is a powerful reminder of someone who cares.

Consultation outside of the catchment area

The majority of client involvement occurs in the client's home. This is extensive and time consuming, at least early in the treatment process. With a small staff this precludes active client intervention outside of a limited urban catchment area of approximately 175,000 persons. Consequently, only a small portion of metropolitan Toronto can be provided with direct service at the present time.

COPA staff attempt to provide a consultation service to any care-giver or family member outside the catchment area who contacts COPA about management of an older person experiencing alcohol-related problems. Consultation is provided primarily on a one-to-one basis, and is also time-consuming. At the present time there are no other resources available to provide this supportive service.

In an effort to improve this, COPA also provides regular educational workshops for health care professionals in general, and inservice training for specific agencies and services (e.g. community health nurses), whenever possible.

By these means COPA is able to provide some service to the rest of metropolitan Toronto.

Role of COPA outreach worker

While the role will vary depending on the individualized client needs, it includes:

- supporting family or other referring person until client will accept a COPA worker
- development of rapport with client
- assessment and development of treatment plan
- crisis management
- implementation of treatment plan including making appropriate referrals
- support of client, using problem solving, practical counselling techniques (usually provided in the home on a weekly basis)
- support of agencies after referrals have been made
- support of other family members.

Care for the care-giver

Because of the demanding nature of this involvement, it is vital that these activities be interspersed with non-client-oriented ones such as providing or attending educational events, or participating in the general planning process of the programme, in order to provide a change of pace or focus for the outreach worker.

Use of volunteers

A well trained, caring volunteer may be able to achieve goals with the client that are impossible for the outreach worker alone. Because the volunteer has more time, it is possible to encourage improved personal hygiene (a trip to the hairdresser does wonders!), and teach shopping skills, meal preparation or how to use the public transport system. The volunteer can gradually assist the development of social and leisure skills that are relevant to the client. This usually entails actual involvement in the activities until the client is able to do it alone.

However, in order for this to happen, there are a few requirements for an effective volunteer programme. The candidates for the programme need to be caring, empathic people, not easily stressed by difficult and painful life situations. Commitment needs to be for at least 6 months and preferably longer. Older alcohol abusers do not trust other people quickly or without testing. Developing the relationship between volunteer and client may be slow and painstaking. If the volunteer withdraws after a few visits, the client simply has his or her mistrust of the human race reinforced.

The prospective volunteer needs considerable training before client involvement, and steady ongoing support after involvement. COPA staff provide individual support after each volunteer visit, and monthly group meetings of all the volunteers.

This means that matching and placing a volunteer with a client is no less time-consuming for the worker than actually seeing the client. However, it provides for a level of practical and social involvement that the outreach worker cannot give.

When this model is inappropriate

It seems obvious to point out that this model is inappropriate for anyone experiencing medical, mental or emotional disabilities that are severe enough to prevent even partial self-care. Furthermore, the person who is a danger to self or others does not belong in this programme.

This would seem to preclude many persons with alcohol abuse. In actual fact, once a person is established in treatment and begins to respond, the majority of the disabilities improve remarkably. Providing the client becomes totally abstinent, this may even include a lessening of a mild-to-moderate dementia that is alcohol-related.

Consequently, even when the patient seems completely unable to survive in the community, it is worth a short-term institutional admission to assess possible changes with total abstinence and comprehensive therapy. Not uncommonly, the person improves enough to manage well in a semi-sheltered setting and eventually may even be able to return to the original home. If nothing else, this may serve to lengthen the time the person is able to manage on his or her own before permanent institutional care is necessary.

Further identified needs

It would be helpful to have a halfway house specifically for the older alcohol-dependent person who is making the transition from a life where alcohol is all important to one where physical, mental and emotional wellbeing is all important without the use of alcohol. However, it is often possible to find a homelike setting for this person in many communities.

Both the care-giver and the client will need to be monitored carefully, and if there are several clients to monitor in different settings, the monitoring becomes enormously time-consuming. A separate home could resolve some of this.

For the patient who is willing to leave the home but experiencing a wide range of problems, a day-hospital programme would be very useful. Such a programme could not only provide improved medical, nutritional and ther-

apeutic care, but also act as a sheltered centre for the beginning development of social and leisure activities which could proceed at a pace
compatible with the client. It could also provide basic teaching in any of the
life areas. At the present time those few patients who are appropriate are
placed in an existing day-hospital programme conducted within a chronic-
care hospital. Some do well but others do not. The alcohol-specific
problems may intrude into other components of treatment upsetting both
staff and other patients. The staff who are busy with other patients do not
have the time or the knowledge to work with the alcoholic, and he or she
may be discharged as being uncooperative, which in that setting, he or she
was! A day-hospital programme designed to include management specific
to alcoholism, would alleviate this difficulty.

EVALUATION OF THE COPA PROGRAM

Background

Evaluation of the COPA program has been, and still is, a slow and complex
process. The COPA project is a new experimental multi-goal programme
for elderly people with alcohol problems. Evaluation of any treatment
programme for substance abuse has not been without controversy. In particular, there are a number of features of alcoholism that make treatment
evaluation particularly difficult, such as appropriate goals (abstinence?
higher quality of life?), the validity of self-report measures of consumption,
high loss to follow-up, sampling problems, and a host of other methodological pitfalls. Evaluation of COPA has all the evaluation problems of any
addictions treatment programme *plus* a number of unique programme
features that makes it a particularly challenging evaluation project. These
features include the following:

1   *Clients typically enter the programme for help with other problems (e.g.
    accommodation) and not for addictions treatment.* Although clients are
    aware that the programme is for alcohol abuse, the programme itself
    focuses on the immediate problems of the client, dealing directly with
    alcohol use only when allowed by the client. Many clients entering the
    programme are not ready to admit that they have a substance problem.
    They have been referred by someone who has identified alcohol is part
    of the client's problems, but the client may not be at a stage of
    perceiving an alcohol problem, or admitting a problem if one is
    perceived.
        When clients enter the programme and are treated for problems
    other than alcohol abuse, it is not appropriate to focus evaluation
    exclusively on changes in alcohol use or abuse. Moreover, other life

areas besides alcohol use might be as important or even more important in determining programme success with any particular client. In fact, for some clients, modest stabilizing housing arrangements might be all the programme can be expected to accomplish; for others more ambitious outcomes may be possible.

Given that the evaluation must focus on changes in many life areas, measuring improved status in certain life areas can be problematic because of this initial denial of alcohol problems by the client. Programme staff have indicated that initial data gathered from the clients are very likely to be inaccurate especially concerning alcohol abuse, but also concerning life areas where alcohol is strongly related to the problems. One is faced with the alarming possibility that because of early denial and later acceptance of problems, clients will appear to become worse rather than better as a consequence of the programme intervention.

2   *Goals for the client are individualized and constantly changing depending on the client's status and other factors.* For example, when a client enters a programme the first goal may be to meet emergency housing needs. Next, the client and worker may set goals concerning nutrition. Many clients are very isolated and social and leisure activities may be the next focus. At this point, the groundwork is usually established to bring to the client's awareness the common role of alcohol in many problem areas and it may be possible to begin working on reducing or eliminating alcohol use.

Thus, not only is the programme an omnibus one, but the focus can vary over time as well as vary from one client to another. For example, while a pre-post-treatment approach may show the resolution of the client's housing crisis, intervening crises in other areas that emerged and were resolved during treatment would not be apparent. Clearly, outcome measures and intervention measures for the programme need to be sufficiently flexible to describe a variety of problems treated in a variety of ways. In addition, the long-term responsive nature of the programme requires that measures monitor client progress and worker interventions on a continuous basis – that is, that the programme does not fit the model of a single problem identified and resolved by a single intervention.

3   *There is no set intervention.* The programme is intended to help clients as required and the workers will and have done a wide range of tasks from supportive counselling to feeding a client's cats while she was in the hospital, to appearing in court as a witness for a client, to intervening on a client's behalf with health or social service agencies. Evaluation procedures must be able to describe the variety of efforts required from those who work with substance abusing elderly and, in the long run, relate specific types of interventions to specific outcomes.

4   *The clients are elderly.* Certain attributes of the elderly population can make evaluation more difficult. Measures standardized on a younger population may not necessarily be valid for the elderly. Furthermore, regardless of the efficacy of the programme some clients are likely to withdraw or be unavailable for follow-up because of death, institutionalization and so on. In addition, some elderly clients may be unwilling or unable to participate in the extensive questionnaire testing common to some programme-evaluation designs. Evaluation measures must be valid and suitable for this specific population.

CURRENT APPROACHES OF THE EVALUATION OF THE COPA PROJECT

While the evaluation of the COPA project presented a multitude of methodological problems, addictions treatment programming for the elderly is an important area of concern and this innovative project had the potential to serve as a model programme. Therefore, it was important that evaluation research be conducted on the project and be as rigorous as possible, given the limitations.

Because of the lack of appropriate outcome measures for this population and the variability in implementation, it was apparent that an experimental study of programme effectiveness could not be conducted immediately. Instead, the current evaluation efforts focus on: (a) development and validation of instrumentation, (b) monitoring programme implementation and (c) monitoring client changes during the programme.

The specific components of the evaluation include the following:

1   *A comprehensive description of client status in all life areas at the time of admission to the programme.* In order to ensure that all life areas could be assessed adequately (especially, high-risk areas such as medical problems and use of medication), a detailed assessment booklet was developed (Saunders *et al.*, 1985). The assessment contains questions and approaches developed specifically for this target population. For example, because clients can be admitted to the programme who deny their alcohol use, the assessment procedures include recording information concerning alcohol use from other sources who have knowledge of the client.

2   *The development and validation of objective forms for measuring client status and worker interventions at every client contact.* A monitoring system was developed to measure programme implementation and changes in the client's status in each life area. In order to estimate the reliability of the monitoring procedures, the COPA workers were accompanied by an observer during sixty-two client contacts. Following the contact, the worker and the observer independently completed the

Table 19.1 Percentage of contacts during which each type of action occurred in each life area, averaged over all contacts

Type of worker action	Alcohol n of clients = 79 n of contacts = 490	Physical health n of clients = 78 n of contacts = 901	Emotional health n of clients = 85 n of contacts = 914	Activities of daily living n of clients = 73 n of contacts = 616	Accommodation n of clients = 43 n of contacts = 198
Monitoring monitoring seeking information seeking clarification listening	85%	73%	78%	56%	82%
Advice advice education explanation	29%	21%	13%	11%	51%
Encouragement encouragement reinforcement empathy	73%	68%	78%	23%	83%
Goal setting goal setting problem solving	14%	12%	10%	8%	43%
Confrontation	34%	7%	5%	3%	13%
Practical help	0%	2%	1%	4%	10%

Source: Graham and Birchmore Timney, 1987.

Figure 19.1 Interim summary data for a progress report on the COPA scheme

ECONOMIC	ACCOMMODATION

CURRENT ECONOMIC PROBLEMS:
(Check all that apply)
☐ change in economic status
  (e.g., change in income or expenses)
☐ poor money management
  (e.g., debts, spending, not paying bills)
☐ needs help in coping with very low
  income
☐ may not be receiving all income that he/
  she is eligible for
☐ involved in economic dispute with
  person or agency
☐ job search
☐ other _____

SEVERITY OF CURRENT INCOME PROBLEMS: *(Check one)*
☐^{1} very severe — client's basic needs
  unlikely to be met
☐^{2} somewhat severe — basic needs met
  but some economic hardship
☐^{3} slight — problems temporary or unlikely
  to cause hardship
☐^{4} problems resolved/no problems

EMOTIONAL IMPACT OF CURRENT ECONOMIC PROBLEMS: *(Check one)*
☐^{1} client extremely upset
☐^{2} client moderately upset
☐^{3} client slightly bothered
☐^{4} client perceives problem as
  unimportant
☐^{5} problem resolved/no problems

ARE CURRENT ECONOMIC PROBLEMS DUE TO *RECENT* ALCOHOL CONSUMPTION? *(Check one)*
☐^{1} yes ☐^{2} partly ☐^{3} no ☐^{0} uncertain

WORKER ACTION DURING CONTACT CONCERNING CLIENT'S ECONOMIC PROBLEMS:
_____ (Code #s)

PLANS *BEFORE* NEXT CONTACT CONCERNING CLIENT'S ECONOMIC PROBLEMS:
_____ (Code #s)

PLANS *FOR* NEXT CONTACT CONCERNING CLIENT'S ECONOMIC PROBLEMS:
_____ (Code #s)

DETAILS:

CURRENT ACCOMMODATION PROBLEMS: *(Check all that apply)*
☐ cost of present accommodation
  unsatisfactory
☐ physical characteristics of present
  accommodation unsatisfactory *(e.g.,
  size, need for repairs, furniture)*
☐ cohabitants at present accommodation
  unsatisfactory
☐ geographic location of present
  accommodation unsatisfactory
☐ being evicted or forced to move
☐ in the process of moving by own choice
☐ cannot live alone
☐ other _____

SEVERITY OF CURRENT ACCOMMODATION PROBLEMS: *(Check one)*
☐^{1} very severe — a move from present
  accommodation necessary
☐^{2} somewhat severe — some changes
  needed in accommodation
☐^{3} slight — problems tolerable for client
☐^{4} problems resolved/no problems

EMOTIONAL IMPACT OF CURRENT ACCOMMODATION PROBLEMS: *(Check one)*
☐^{1} client extremely upset
☐^{2} client moderately upset
☐^{3} client slightly bothered
☐^{4} client perceives problem as
  unimportant
☐^{5} problem resolved/no problems

ARE CURRENT ACCOMMODATION PROBLEMS DUE TO *RECENT* ALCOHOL CONSUMPTION? *(Check one)*
☐^{1} yes ☐^{2} partly ☐^{3} no ☐^{0} uncertain

WORKER ACTION DURING CONTACT CONCERNING CLIENT'S ACCOMMODATION PROBLEMS:
_____ (Code #s)

PLANS *BEFORE* NEXT CONTACT CONCERNING CLIENT'S ACCOMMODATION PROBLEMS:
_____ (Code #s)

PLANS *FOR* NEXT CONTACT CONCERNING CLIENT'S ACCOMMODATION PROBLEMS:
_____ (Code #s)

DETAILS:

DRUG USE

CURRENT PRESCRIPTION DRUG USE:
(Check all that apply)
- [ ] sleeping pills/barbiturates
- [ ] benzodiazepines
- [ ] analgesics
- [ ] diuretic/beta blocker
- [ ] heart medicine
- [ ] anticonvulsant
- [ ] antidepressants
- [ ] respiratory-allergy
- [ ] prescribed vitamins
- [ ] major tranquillizers
- [ ] other _____

CURRENT OVER-THE-COUNTER DRUG USE: *(Check all that apply)*
- [ ] ASA/Acetominophen
- [ ] laxative
- [ ] antacid
- [ ] non-prescription vitamins
- [ ] non-prescription sleeping pills
- [ ] other _____

CURRENT DRUG PROBLEMS:
- [ ] no problem/or *(Check all that apply)*
- [ ] poor compliance with prescribed drug regimen

SPOUSE/SIGNIFICANT OTHER/ COHABITANT

CURRENT STATUS:
- [ ] no major problems/or *(Check all that apply)*
- [ ] marital/family discord
- [ ] illness/death of spouse/significant other/ cohabitant
- [ ] alcohol/drug problem of spouse/ significant other/cohabitant
- [ ] other _____

RELATIONSHIP TO CLIENT:
- [ ] spouse (including common-law)
- [ ] family member (living with client)
- [ ] cohabitant (not spouse or family)
- [ ] other _____

ARE PROBLEMS RELATED TO CLIENT'S RECENT ALCOHOL CONSUMPTION?
[ ]^1 yes [ ]^2 partly [ ]^3 no [ ]^0 uncertain

WORKER ACTION DURING CONTACT:
_____ (Code #s)

PLANS BEFORE NEXT CONTACT:
_____ (Code #s)

PLANS FOR NEXT CONTACT:
_____ (Code #s)

DETAILS:

LEISURE/SOCIAL CONTACTS

PROBLEMS WITH USE OF LEISURE TIME:
- [ ] no problems/or *(Check all that apply)*
- [ ] little or no activity
- [ ] insufficient physical activity
- [ ] insufficient social contact
- [ ] leisure time not enjoyable
- [ ] activities always involve alcohol
- [ ] other _____

RATING OF CLIENT'S USE OF LEISURE TIME:
[ ]^1 client strength   [ ]^2 no problems
[ ]^3 slight problems   [ ]^4 moderate problems
[ ]^5 major problems

OVERALL STATUS OF SOCIAL RELATIONSHIPS:

	VERY NEGATIVE	SOMEWHAT NEGATIVE	NEUTRAL/ MIXED	SOMEWHAT POSITIVE	VERY POSITIVE	NO CONTACTS
COPA worker	[ ]^1	[ ]^2	[ ]^3	[ ]^4	[ ]^5	[ ]^0
COPA volunteer	[ ]^1	[ ]^2	[ ]^3	[ ]^4	[ ]^5	[ ]^0
Other agencies (including PHN, MD, COTA, etc.)	[ ]^1	[ ]^2	[ ]^3	[ ]^4	[ ]^5	[ ]^0
Casual social contacts (incl. church, seniors club, legion, etc)	[ ]^1	[ ]^2	[ ]^3		[ ]^5	[ ]^0

☐ drugs not having desired effect
☐ drugs having side effects
☐ drug addiction
☐ cost
☐ other
_____

HAS RECENT ALCOHOL CONSUMPTION
INTERACTED WITH DRUG CONSUMPTION
OR ADVERSELY AFFECTED
PRESCRIPTION DRUG COMPLIANCE?
(Check all that apply)

☐ alcohol–drug interactions
☐ not taking drugs as prescribed because of
   alcohol use or effects
☐ uncertain

WORKER ACTION DURING CONTACT
CONCERNING CLIENT'S DRUG USE:
_____ (Code #s)

PLANS *BEFORE* NEXT CONTACT
CONCERNING CLIENT'S DRUG USE:
_____ (Code #s)

PLANS *FOR* NEXT CONTACT
CONCERNING CLIENT'S DRUG USE:
_____ (Code #s)

DETAILS:

LEGAL

ARE LEGAL PROBLEMS RELATED TO
CLIENT'S RECENT ALCOHOL
CONSUMPTION?
☐¹ yes   ☐² partly   ☐³ no   ☐⁰ uncertain

WORKER ACTION DURING CONTACT
CONCERNING CLIENT'S LEGAL
PROBLEMS:
_____ (Code #s)

PLANS *BEFORE* NEXT CONTACT:
_____ (Code #s)

PLANS *FOR* NEXT CONTACT:
_____ (Code #s)

DETAILS:

Friends/close
friends   ☐¹ ☐² ☐³ ☐⁴ ☐⁵ ☐⁰
Family   ☐¹ ☐² ☐³ ☐⁴ ☐⁵ ☐⁰

ALCOHOL INVOLVEMENT IN SOCIAL
CONTACTS: *(Check rating where relevant)*

	NEVER	SOME-TIMES	USUALLY	ALWAYS
casual social	☐¹	☐²	☐³	☐⁴
close friends	☐¹	☐²	☐³	☐⁴
family	☐¹	☐²	☐³	☐⁴

RATING OF CLIENT'S SOCIAL
RELATIONSHIPS:
☐¹ client strength   ☐² no problems
☐³ slight problems   ☐⁴ moderate problems
☐⁵ major problems

ARE SOCIAL/LEISURE PROBLEMS DUE TO
CLIENT'S RECENT ALCOHOL CONSUMPTION?
☐¹ yes   ☐² partly   ☐³ no   ☐⁰ uncertain

WORKER ACTION DURING CONTACT
CONCERNING SOCIAL/LEISURE PROBLEMS:
_____ (Code #s)

PLANS *BEFORE* NEXT CONTACT
CONCERNING SOCIAL/LEISURE PROBLEMS:
_____ (Code #s)

PLANS *FOR* NEXT CONTACT CONCERNING
SOCIAL/LEISURE PROBLEMS:
_____ (Code #s)

DETAILS:

ALCOHOL

ADL

CURRENT STATUS — ADL:

	POOR	FAIR	ADEQUATE	GOOD	EXCELLENT
cooking/food preparation	1	2	3	4	5
use of telephone	1	2	3	4	5
shopping	1	2	3	4	5
banking	1	2	3	4	5
transportation	1	2	3	4	5
other	1	2	3	4	5

ARE ADL PROBLEMS DUE TO *RECENT* ALCOHOL CONSUMPTION?
☐¹ yes   ☐² partly   ☐³ no   ☐⁰ uncertain

WORKER ACTION DURING CONTACT CONCERNING CLIENT'S ADL:
_____ (Code #s)

PLANS *BEFORE* NEXT CONTACT CONCERNING CLIENT'S ADL:
_____ (Code #s)

PLANS *FOR* NEXT CONTACT CONCERNING CLIENT'S ADL:
_____ (Code #s)

DETAILS:

CURRENT ALCOHOL STATUS:

(Please answer the following questions as reported by client and according to other source [other person, worker's opinion] as relevant)

Problem rating:
CLIENT OTHER
☐¹ ☐¹ no problem
☐² ☐² slight problem
☐³ ☐³ major problem

Drinking since last contact:
CLIENT OTHER
☐¹ ☐¹ client has been abstaining
☐² ☐² client has reduced drinking
☐³ ☐³ client is drinking as usual
☐⁴ ☐⁴ client has increased drinking

Drinking pattern since last contact:
CLIENT OTHER
☐¹ ☐¹ none
☐² ☐² occasional
☐³ ☐³ frequent (but not daily)
☐⁴ ☐⁴ daily
☐⁵ ☐⁵ some drinking but frequency unknown

Daily consumption since last contact:
CLIENT OTHER
__ __ standard drinks per heavy drinking day

SIGNS OF ALCOHOL CONSUMPTION DURING CONTACT:
(Check all that apply)

- ☐ no signs of alcohol consumption
- ☐ alcohol on client's breath
- ☐ client consuming alcoholic beverage/ probable alcoholic beverage
- ☐ empties visible
- ☐ client's mood suggests prior drinking
- ☐ client has hangover symptoms/tremors
- ☐ client's behaviour or mental status indicates probable drinking
- ☐ client's gait or balance indicates probable drinking
- ☐ client's speech indicates probable drinking
- ☐ client clearly intoxicated/passed out
- ☐ client exhibiting physical or emotional problems related to recent drinking
- ☐ client's appearance suggests prior drinking
- ☐ other

WORKER ACTION DURING CONTACT CONCERNING CLIENT'S ALCOHOL PROBLEMS:
_____ (Code #s)

PLANS *BEFORE* NEXT CONTACT CONCERNING CLIENT'S ALCOHOL PROBLEMS:
_____ (Code #s)

NUTRITION – OTHER SUBSTANCES:

Eating pattern since last visit:
- □¹ eating too much
- □² eating right amount
- □³ eating too little

Does client consume the following regularly?
(Check all that apply)
- □ tobacco □ coffee □ tea
- □ junk food □ antacids □ laxatives

Do any of the following apply to client?
(Check all that apply)
- □ meals provided (e.g., MOW, boarding)
- □ on special diet
- □ physical health problems affect eating

ARE NUTRITIONAL PROBLEMS DUE TO *RECENT* ALCOHOL CONSUMPTION?
□¹ yes □² partly □³ no □⁰ uncertain

WORKER ACTION DURING CONTACT CONCERNING CLIENT'S NUTRITION:
_____ (Code #s)

PLANS *BEFORE* NEXT CONTACT CONCERNING CLIENT'S NUTRITION:
_____ (Code #s)

PLANS *FOR* NEXT CONTACT CONCERNING CLIENT'S NUTRITION:
_____ (Code #s)

DETAILS:

— — standard drinks per usual drinking day
— — standard drinks per light drinking day

SOURCE OF INFORMATION CONCERNING CLIENT'S ALCOHOL CONSUMPTION:
- □¹ opinion of worker
- □² COPA volunteer
- □³ Spouse
- □⁴ PHN/RN/VON/MD/other medical
- □⁵ landlady/landlord/bldg.superintend.
- □⁶ friend
- □⁷ family member
- □⁸ other _____

CLIENT'S ATTITUDE DURING THIS CONTACT TOWARD DISCUSSION OF:

OWN ALCOHOL CONSUMPTION	OWN ALCOHOL PROBLEM	
□¹	□¹	complete denial
□²	□²	avoids topic
□³	□³	willing to discuss, but guarded
□⁴	□⁴	talks freely
□⁵	□⁵	other

LEVEL OF INSIGHT/MOTIVATION SHOWN DURING THIS CONTACT:
- □¹ shows insight into alcohol problem
- □² partial recognition of alcohol problem
- □³ does not recognize or accept that problems caused by alcohol
- □⁴ feels alcohol makes things better
- □⁵ other _____

PLANS *FOR* NEXT CONTACT CONCERNING CLIENT'S ALCOHOL PROBLEMS:
_____ (Code #s)

DETAILS:

RATINGS

Very Poor 0–20	Poor 21–40	Some Major 41–60	Minor 61–80	Good to Ideal 81–100
Inpatient care required	Major problems requiring extensive help or treatment	Problems requiring help or treatment	Problems but functioning adequately	No problems

PHYSICAL

RATING _____ (0–100)

TYPE OF PHYSICAL HEALTH PROBLEMS:
□ [1] short-term
□ [2] chronic
□ [3] both short-term and chronic

OVERALL, IN TERMS OF PHYSICAL HEALTH, CLIENT IS:
□ [1] very well
□ [2] well
□ [3] stable
□ [4] sick
□ [5] very sick

CLIENT'S PERCEPTION OF PHYSICAL HEALTH PROBLEMS:
□ [1] no problems
□ [2] problems don't bother client
□ [3] slightly bothered
□ [4] moderately bothered
□ [5] extremely bothered

EMOTIONAL

RATING _____ (0–100)

TO WHAT EXTENT ARE THE FOLLOWING PART OF THE CLIENT'S EMOTIONAL HEALTH PROBLEMS?
(Circle appropriate number)

	NOT AT ALL				VERY MUCH
anger/aggression	1	2	3	4	5
anxiety	1	2	3	4	5
depression	1	2	3	4	5
feeling tired/weak	1	2	3	4	5
frustration	1	2	3	4	5
grief	1	2	3	4	5
loneliness	1	2	3	4	5
sleeplessness	1	2	3	4	5
worry	1	2	3	4	5

ARE EMOTIONAL HEALTH PROBLEMS DUE TO RECENT ALCOHOL CONSUMPTION?
□ [1] yes □ [2] partly □ [3] no □ [0] uncertain

MENTAL

RATING _____ (0–100)

TO WHAT EXTENT ARE THE FOLLOWING PART OF THE CLIENT'S MENTAL HEALTH PROBLEMS?
(Circle appropriate number)

	NOT AT ALL				VERY MUCH
confusion	1	2	3	4	5
difficulty concentrating	1	2	3	4	5
disoriented	1	2	3	4	5
hallucinations	1	2	3	4	5
altered speech patterns	1	2	3	4	5
irrationality	1	2	3	4	5
paranoia	1	2	3	4	5
poor memory	1	2	3	4	5
slowness	1	2	3	4	5

ARE MENTAL HEALTH PROBLEMS DUE TO RECENT ALCOHOL CONSUMPTION?
□ [1] yes □ [2] partly □ [3] no □ [0] uncertain

ARE PHYSICAL HEALTH PROBLEMS DUE TO *RECENT* ALCOHOL CONSUMPTION?

☐¹ yes ☐² partly ☐³ no ☐⁰ uncertain

WORKER ACTION DURING CONTACT CONCERNING CLIENT'S PHYSICAL HEALTH:

_____(Code #s)

PLANS *BEFORE* NEXT CONTACT CONCERNING CLIENT'S PHYSICAL HEALTH:

_____(Code #s)

PLANS *FOR* NEXT CONTACT CONCERNING CLIENT'S PHSYICAL HEALTH:

_____(Code #s)

DETAILS:

WORKER ACTION DURING CONTACT CONCERNING CLIENT'S EMOTIONAL HEALTH:

_____(Code #s)

PLANS *BEFORE* NEXT CONTACT CONCERNING CLIENT'S EMOTIONAL HEALTH:

_____(Code #s)

PLANS *FOR* NEXT CONTACT CONCERNING CLIENT'S EMOTIONAL HEALTH:

_____(Code #s)

DETAILS:

WORKER ACTION DURING CONTACT CONCERNING CLIENT'S MENTAL HEALTH:

_____(Code #s)

PLANS *BEFORE* NEXT CONTACT CONCERNING CLIENT'S MENTAL HEALTH

_____(Code #s)

PLANS *FOR* NEXT CONTACT CONCERNING CLIENT'S MENTAL HEALTH:

_____(Code #s)

DETAILS:

CLIENT CONTACT RECORD

FILE No. _____

WORKER: _____

OBSERVER: |___|___|___|
DAY MONTH YEAR

SUMMARY OF CLIENT STATUS:

Health rating

(0–20 very poor, 21–40 poor, 41–60 major problems, 61–80 minor problems, 81–100 good to ideal)

____ physical   ____ emotional   ____ mental

(If rating is less than 81 or if more details required, complete Health Form)

Alcohol consumption since last contact:

(Check one)
- [ ]¹ abstinent
- [ ]² light
- [ ]³ heavy or problem drinking
- [ ]⁸ not applicable
- [ ]⁹ no information
  (Details on Alcohol Form)

Frequency of drinking according to client:

(Check one)
- [ ]⁰ none
- [ ]¹ occasional
- [ ]² frequent (but not daily)
- [ ]³ daily
- [ ]⁴ some drinking (frequency unknown)
- [ ]⁸ not applicable
- [ ]⁹ no information
- |___| average number of standard drinks per day

Current economic status and accommodation status:

ECONOMIC   ACCOMMODATION
(Check one)   *(Check one)*

- [ ]¹   [ ]¹ no problems
- [ ]²   [ ]² slight problems but tolerable
- [ ]³   [ ]³ somewhat severe
- [ ]⁴   [ ]⁴ very severe
- [ ]⁸   [ ]⁸ not applicable
- [ ]⁹   [ ]⁹ no information

(Details on Economic and/or Accommodation Forms)

Status of current drug use:

(Check one)
- [ ]¹ no problems with drug use
- [ ]² slight problems with drug use
- [ ]³ moderate problems
- [ ]⁴ severe problems
- [ ]⁸ not applicable
- [ ]⁹ no information
  (Details on Drug Form)

LOCATION OF VISIT:

- [ ][ ] Key Code #
- [ ]⁶ Other _____ *(specify)*

DURATION OF VISIT:

|___|___| Minutes

REASON FOR VISIT:

- [ ]¹ Regular, or
- [ ][ ] Key Code #, or
- [ ]¹¹ Other _____ *(specify)*

VISIT INITIATED BY:

- [ ][ ] Key Code #, or
- [ ]⁵ Other _____ *(specify)*

OTHERS PRESENT AT VISIT:

(Key Code # and specify where appropriate for each person present)

_____
_____
_____
_____
_____

[ ][ ] [ ][ ] [ ][ ] [ ][ ] [ ][ ]

OTHER AGENCY INVOLVEMENT WITH CLIENT SINCE LAST CONTACT:

(Key Code # and specify where appropriate for each person present)

☐ ☐ ☐ ☐ ☐

SALIENT FEATURES OF CLIENT DURING CONTACT:

MOOD

anxious	1 2 3 4 5	relaxed
tired	1 2 3 4 5	well-rested
unhappy	1 2 3 4 5	happy
angry	1 2 3 4 5	not angry
frustrated/upset	1 2 3 4 5	at peace
uncertain	1 2 3 4 5	confident
other:		

ATTITUDE TO COPA WORKER

uncooperative	1 2 3 4 5	co-operative
indifferent	1 2 3 4 5	enthusiastic
passive	1 2 3 4 5	active
defensive	1 2 3 4 5	open

Worker's opinion of client's accuracy in reporting frequency and standard drinks:

FREQUENCY *(Check one)*   STANDARD DRINKS *(Check one)*

FREQUENCY	STANDARD DRINKS	
☐¹	☐¹	accurate report
☐²	☐²	under-report
☐³	☐³	over-report
☐⁹	☐⁹	no information

Social contacts
☐¹ no social contacts
☐² contacts with volunteer/agency only
☐³ limited contacts
☐⁴ satisfying social contacts
☐⁹ no information
(Details on Social Contacts Form)

Leisure activities
☐¹ very inactive
☐² some activity
☐³ satisfying recreation
☐⁹ no information
(Details on Leisure Form)

ADL/Nutrition:

	POOR	FAIR	ADE-QUATE	GOOD	EXCEL-LENT	NO INFO
personal hygiene	☐¹	☐²	☐³	☐⁴	☐⁵	☐⁹
care of clothing	☐¹	☐²	☐³	☐⁴	☐⁵	☐⁹
care of living quarters	☐¹	☐²	☐³	☐⁴	☐⁵	☐⁹
adequacy of diet	☐¹	☐²	☐³	☐⁴	☐⁵	☐⁹
appetite	☐¹	☐²	☐³	☐⁴	☐⁵	☐⁹

(Details on ADL/Nutrition Form)

Spouse/Significant Other/Cohabitant: *(Check one)*

☐⁸ Not applicable, or
☐¹ source of client strength
☐² no problems
☐³ slight problems
☐⁴ moderate problems
☐⁵ major problems
☐⁹ no information
(Details on Spouse Form)

Current Legal Status:

☐¹ no problems
☐² problems ➧ *(Details on Legal Form)*

SUMMARY OF MAJOR FEATURES OF CONTACT: *(Check all that apply)*

☐¹ focus on specific life areas
☐² general discussion and chit chat
☐³ focus on accomplishing specific tasks with client
☐⁴ other _____ *(specify)*

Preliminary summary data

REASON FOR VISIT

REGULAR	CRISIS	REQUEST BY FAM OR AGENCY	TRANSPORT OR ACCOMPANY	SPECIAL OCCASION	NON-REGULAR SPECIFIC PURPOSE	HOSPITAL VISIT ETC.	DROP IN	BRIEF INFO EXCHANGE	OTHER
522	29	3	12	12	7	15	20	20	0

LOCATION OF CONTACT

HOME	OFFICE	TELEPHONE	MEDICAL	IN TRANSIT	OTHER
420	110	52	49	4	7

CONTACT INITIATED BY

CLIENT	WORKER	FAMILY MEMBER, SPOUSE	AGENCY, GP, ETC.	OTHER
25	91	3	1	0

OTHERS PRESENT AT THE CONTACT

SPOUSE	FAMILY MEMBER	FRIEND	ROOMMATE, LANDLADY-LORD	COPA VOLUNTEER	MEDICAL	COTA	OTHER AGENCY	OTHER NON-AGENCY
106	10	8	13	3	13	2	21	0

OTHER AGENCY INVOLVEMENT WITH CLIENT

MEDICAL	COTA	HOME SERVICE, MOW	PSYCHIATRIC	DAY HOSPITAL	METRO HOUSING	SENIORS GROUP	AA, ADDICTIONS PROG.	SOCIAL SERVICES	OTHER
43	19	27	7	2	3	2	0	5	8

monitoring forms describing what occurred during the contact and the client's wellbeing in relevant life areas. A report on the inter-rater reliability of the monitoring instruments (based on comparing the workers' forms to the observers' forms) is currently being prepared (Graham, in preparation). Preliminary analyses have found fairly high correspondence on most client status variables and somewhat lower inter-rater reliability for descriptions of worker actions and for a small number of specific client-status variables.

3   *A description of programme implementation.* Using the measures completed at every contact, a description of the different types of interventions used in each life area has been developed (see, for example, Table 19.1 (Graham and Birchmore Timney, 1987)).

In addition, the monitoring forms contain basic data concerning the nature of the client contacts and other relevant programme information (see Figure 19.1 from an interim report to the programme).

4   *A description of client change during the course of the programme.* The client monitoring approach was chosen to measure client change rather than a pre-test–post-test evaluation design. The monitoring strategy offers a number of advantages, especially being able to examine the process of change for individual clients. As an example, Figure 19.2 shows the change in emotional health status of one client during the course of that client's involvement with the COPA program. It is also possible to estimate the number of clients who improved, remained the same, and deteriorated by using predetermined criteria to classify the pattern of ratings for each client in each life area. Additionally, one can examine changes in client status using standard pre-test–post-test designs (e.g, ANOVA), but based on average scores rather than single pre-and post-scores (thus overcoming some of the unreliability and regression to the mean artifacts associated with analyses of change scores).

5   *A description of exploratory analyses aimed at identifying variables that seem to be associated with program impact.* These analyses will include both the identification of the types of clients who seem to benefit most from the programme (e.g. analyses by age, sex, problem type and so on), as well as the identification of those types of interventions that appear to be most effective.

The present approach to the evaluation is intended to accomplish two major steps towards measuring the effectiveness of this type of addiction treatment programme for the elderly: (1) a process evaluation of programme implementation and client change; and (2) the development of valid and reliable measures and strategies on which to base future evaluation of the effectiveness of particular programme strategies using rigorous experimental methods.

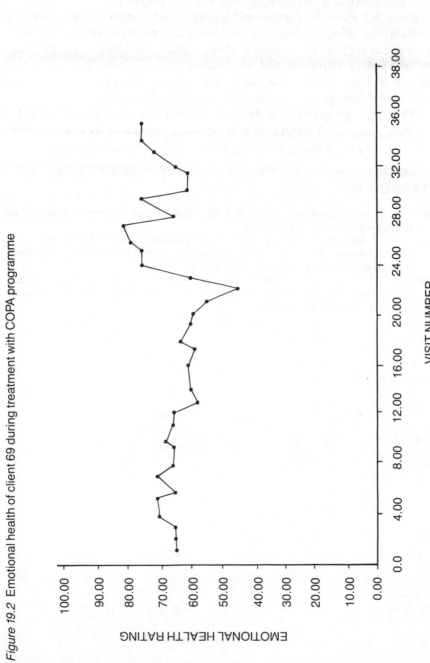

Figure 19.2 Emotional health of client 69 during treatment with COPA programme

CONCLUSION

This chapter has described a programme which has been designed to meet a need that previously has been ignored and not addressed.

The older alcoholic experiences multiple and complex biopsychosocial problems including inability or unwillingness to leave the home. With appropriate support this person is able to remain at home as the problems are resolved or improved and life becomes more worthwhile. Support is imperative not only for the client, but also for the family, friends and professional care-givers also involved with care of the client.

While this programme is involved with older persons with alcohol problems, the model could probably be made applicable to anyone experiencing multiple problems including mild to moderate dementia.

REFERENCES

Graham, K. (in preparation) 'Inter-rater reliability of data collection measures for the evaluation of the COPA project'.
——— , and Birchmore Timney, C. (1987) 'Interviews with elderly who have substance abuse problems', paper presented at the Ontario Psychogeriatric Association Conference, Toronto, Ontario, 24–26 May.
Saunders, S.J., Graham, K., Flower, M.C. and Shea, J.P. (1985) 'Community older persons alcohol project: assessment form' (internal document no. 58), Toronto: Addiction Research Foundation.

Part IV

Interventions for family

Chapter 20

Caring for a demented family member at home: objective observation and subjective evaluation of the burden

Mia Duijnstee

SUMMARY

Family members play a leading part in homecare for the demented elderly. Support for family members by people who render professional care will only have an effect if the help offered is in accordance with the need for support by these family members. This requires insight into the burden of family members. To estimate the family carer's burden, health care professionals cannot make evaluations based only on their personal assessment of the situation. The opinion, that family members themselves, have of the situation will also have to contribute to this assessment. This idea of a dual evaluation of burden is the basis for the conceptual framework governing the research described in this chapter. The objective burden can be mapped out into specific aspects, and is distinguishable from the subjective burden.

This qualitative study examines how and why this distinction between objective and subjective 'burden' arises and illustrates this distinction by giving a detailed case example.

INTRODUCTION

This chapter starts with a discussion showing that family members play a leading part in the home care for the demented elderly. Then, an outline of the various components of burden examined in this study of family members is given. Next, the way in which the burden is examined in this study is described, and illustrated with a case study. Finally, the possible relevance of this study for professionals in the field of home care is explored.

FAMILY MEMBERS IN THE LEAD

The central role played by family members

The increase in the number of elderly people, and, in the number of elderly people who need care, coincides with a decrease of the number of family members who are able to take on the care. Factors that influence this unequal development of supply and demand are, among others, the increasing longevity of people, the decreasing number of children per family, the reduction of the number of three-generation families that share a joint household, a wider geographic distribution of family members and a development towards equal opportunities for men and women, as a result of which more women are engaged in the labour force.

Yet, despite these facts, the conclusion cannot be drawn, that family members only play a small part in the care for the elderly who live at home. The research done by Shanas (1979), Cantor (1983) and Johnson (1983) among others indicates that help from the informal network (partners, children, followed by other relatives, friends and neighbours), is, the most important source of support in spite of the changes mentioned above. In relation to this, Brody (1981) points out that neither the myth of professionals delivering the main share of help in the care for the elderly is justified, nor is it true that the offer of help by professionals results in a reduction in the share family members have in the care for the elderly.

In the Netherlands likewise, the help provided by children, partners and other family members is, with regard to quantity, the most important contribution to care (STG scenario-rapport, 1985). It may be assumed that family members play a central role in the care rendered to patients with dementia. This is related to the ambulant nature of professional care in home care. This kind of care is usually not in accordance with the care that is needed. The very nature of the disease makes it necessary for most patients to receive continuous supervision and they have to be supported in many aspects of their functioning as a human being. The result of this is that their need for help cannot be put into a scheme, nor can it be relegated to certain parts of the day.

The primary care-giver

Within a given family, one person usually plays the most important part (Cantor 1983; Johnson 1983). Because of the key role they have in the home care of their demented partner or parent, this person is called the primary care-giver. In the case where the elderly person needing care still has a partner, this partner usually serves as the primary care-giver. This is true, regardless of the sex of the partner, or, the experience the partner has had in housekeeping or in the personal care for others (Shanas, 1979). If the demented person no longer has a partner, one of the children often acts as primary care-giver. Which one of the children will take this part is not a matter which is decided on exclusively between the dementia patient and the primary care-giver. The other children also play a part in this. In this way, according to the research by Bevers (1982), the children indicate that:

the child who lives nearest to the parent in need of help, and who has the fewest other, competing obligations (such as for instance a family or a job) is best suited to render care. In the selection process which take place among the children for the care-giver, as a rule, daughters are considered to better suited to care-giving than sons.

More women than men assume the lead care-giving role

Although in situations in which partners are taking care of partners, there are both men and women, in general, there are more women who act as primary care-givers (see Horowitz, 1985). This unequality between the sexes is caused in part by the fact that women marry older men, and on average live longer. As a result of this, more male dementia patients have a spouse to fall back on for care, than the other way around. The fact that more daughters than sons act as primary care-givers has to do in part with the socio-economical position of women, and a socialization process that lasted for centuries. Therefore, parents who are in need of that kind of help will probably sooner turn to their daughters rather than to their sons, and daughters will place themselves in a caring role much sooner than sons will (see Bevers, 1982). Because of this, a pattern arises of older women taking care of their husbands, and middle-aged women taking care of their mothers (-in-law) or fathers (-in-law).

THE BURDEN OF THE PRIMARY CARE-GIVER

Taking care of a family member with dementia

Taking care of a family member with dementia usually radically changes the life of a primary care-giver. In this paragraph, in order to outline the extent of this change, the responsibilities involved in taking care of a patient with dementia are compared to those of taking care of a child. In both situations the relationship between the person rendering care and the person receiving care is unequal, the care-giver always has to be present in order to supervise. He or she has the ultimate responsibility for all the decisions and offers support and help with regard to nearly all activities of daily living. These actions are usually not recognized by the person receiving care so that questions and problems cannot be shared. However, taking care of a child is usually not considered a burden. This is in contrast to taking care of a demented person. One of the reasons for this is the fact that society prepares us for the care for a child. When you seriously apply yourself to this task, you will receive appreciation and admiration from your surroundings. If problems should occur you can count on the support of others because the members of the social network as well as the people who render care professionally are acquainted with the problems of childrearing. Besides, taking care of children usually is the result of a voluntary choice, and lasts only for a limited period of time. Taking care of an elderly person with dementia is usually a task you are not prepared for, you do not choose, of which no-one knows how long it will last and about which questions and problems will arise which most people in the social surroundings will not recognize and which professional care-givers may not be able to solve either. Because others are not acquainted with the strain involved in taking care of a demented elderly person at home, the appreciation, admiration or actual support are usually not forthcoming.

Another essential difference between caring for a child and for a demented elderly person, concerns the results that are achieved by providing care. One sees a baby grow and develop. As a parent, one can be proud of the share one had in the development from dependence to independence. This is in direct contrast to caring for a demented patient, where the efforts of the primary care-giver never lead to such a stimulating result. The demented elderly person will get worse, the need for help will grow and he or she will become increasingly dependent on his or her surroundings.

Differences in the burdens of primary care-givers

My interest in the burden of primary care-givers of demented elderly persons has to do with the leading part they play in the care for the demented elderly at home. These family members literally and figuratively perform invaluable services in home health care. To keep the emotional and physical costs of these family members – and simultaneously the financial costs of health care – within acceptable levels, family care-givers will have to be adequately supported by professional care-givers. Giving this support is not a simple matter, as is evident from interviews with primary care-givers (see Duijnstee, 1985; Duijnstee *et al.*, 1987). Although all of them indicated that they experienced the task of caring, more or less, as a burden, it became clear that this burden differed greatly with regard to its cause and extent among the care-givers. From this the conclusion can be drawn that professional help offered to these family members must never be standardized, but has to be adjusted to the particular burden that an individual primary care-giver experiences at a certain moment. This immediately gives rise to the question how, and as a result of which causes, do differences in feeling burdened arise? From interviews, it can be deduced that variation in perceiving burden results in part from actual differences in the care situation. For instance, in one situation the patient was incontinent while in the other situation the patient was not incontinent at all. Other actual differences concerning the health of the primary care-giver, or, for example, the degree to which the other members of the family participate in the caring, are also important. Besides this, there appears to be variations in the burden on the primary care-giver resulting from the different way that carers perceive similar events. For instance, one care-giver considered having a job in addition to the caring as a source of strength, in which diversion and understanding could be experienced, while other primary care-givers said that having a job doubled the burden. What poses a problem to one care-giver is not necessarily a problem for the other, or, what is more, some even gain strength from extra-household events and responsibilities.

It is evident, then, that differences in the perceived burden in care-giving are not only related to actual differences in the care-giving situation, as for instance the difference in care needs of the demented person, or the degree in which the care-giver enjoys good health. Differences in perceived burden are also caused by the different meanings which primary care-givers attach to aspects of the care situation that are seemingly similar.

Therefore, the care-giver himself plays an important part in the kind, and in the intensity, of the burden that is experienced as a result of caring for a demented family member.

RESEARCH INTO BURDENING

The first studies about the burden on family members of mentally disturbed patients staying at home, relate to families of psychiatric patients (Grad and Sainsbury, 1963; Hoenig and Hamilton, 1966). In the 1970s this field of study was broadened with research into the burdening by family members of patients with dementia; a survey can be found in Niederehe and Frugé (1984) and Horowitz (1985).

These studies about the burden on family members of mentally infirm patients, among which demented patients can be placed, can be divided according to:

the particular aspects of burden which the study focuses on,
the extent of to which it is researched and
the way in which the term burden is defined.

Different aspects of studying burden

Niederehe and Frugé (1984) categorize the studies of burden as follows:

Studies in which the main focus of attention is on the identification of factors potentially burdening the family members (for instance the symptoms of the demented patient),
Studies which examine the influence of mediating factors in the burdening of family members (for instance, additional care given by the informal network),

Studies focusing mainly on the burdening of family members as a result of actually caring for a demented family member.

Difference in extent

Studies about the burden of family members of patients with dementia, have identified three variables. These are: the demented person, the primary care-giver and the surroundings. Studies vary as to the extent in which these three variables have been incorporated into the research, and with regard to the number of components identified within the variables. Some researchers for instance, concentrate mainly on the burdening of family members as a result of the symptoms of a patient (e.g. Greene, *et al.*, 1982; Gilleard *et al.*, 1982), while others emphasize the interaction between aspects of both the patients, the primary care-giver and the surroundings (Morycz, 1985).

Different definitions of the term burden

Studies differ as to how burden is measured; ranging from summary scores to a multidimensional concept. In the latter case the burden of the primary care-giver, whether related or not to certain causes, is measured for various dimensions, for instance the physical, psychological and social wellbeing (see among others, George and Gwyther, 1986).

Studies also differ according to what is meant by the term burden (Poulshock and Deimling, 1984). The result of this is that burden is a kind of 'umbrella term' that can apply to a variety of matters (emotional burden, financial burden, etc.). Also, the term burden is used to refer to objective facts as well as to the perception of these facts by the primary care-giver. In other studies however the objective burden-related aspects of a care-giving situation, are distinguished from the subjective burden the family members experience.

Since, in this study, a similar distinction is made; this distinction between objective and subjective burden is further considered. The following diagram gives a summary of the conceptualization of the objective and the subjective burden in various studies. Although the overall distinctions made in terminology in these studies correspond reasonably well, in many cases the contents of these terms do not. In looking at the items mentioned under objective and subjective burden respectively, it turns out that similar terms often indicate dissimilar contents. It is also obvious that objective burden sometimes concerns the disfunctioning of the patient and the results from this, and at other times it only concerns these results. Subjective burden is sometimes defined as the intensity of the burden experienced (Hoenig and Hamilton, 1966; Pai and Kapur, 1981) whereas elsewhere it is

Table 20.1 The conceptualization of objective and subjective burden in various studies

	Conceptualization objective burden	Conceptualization subjective burden

Hoenig and Hamilton, 1966	Disturbing behaviour a.o.[1]
	    noisy or wandering at night
	    dangerous to themselves or
	    to others
	    requiring nursing or physical
	    care
	Adverse effects on household a.o.[1]
	    financial status of patient or
	    household has suffered
	    physical strain caused by
	    patient's illness to any
	    member of the family
		'What the relatives felt and to what extent they considered the patient's illness had been a burden to them'

Pai and Kapur, 1981	Items belonging to 6 categories of burden
	    effect on family routine
	    effect on family leisure
	    effect on family interaction
	    effect on physical health of
	    other family members
	    effect on mental health of
	    other family members
	    financial burden
		'How much would you say you have suffered owing to the patient's illness – severely, a little or not at all?'

Herz *et al.*, 1976	a.o.[1]
	Patient contributes less money
	    than if well
	Family had to assume patient's
	    responsibilities
	Patient is irritable or angry
	Patient is noisy at night
	Patient needs help with
	    everything (dressing, etc.)
	Patient gets into fights
		a.o.[1]
		Subjective distress in one or more family members due to the patient:
		    worrying about financial
		    problems
		    worry about the future
		    feel embarrassed or
		    ashamed
		    sad, depressed

Thompson and Doll, 1982	Objective component:
	Social costs
	    financial burden
	    role strains
	    disrupts everyday routine
	    requires much supervision
	    problems with neighbours
		Subjective component:
		Emotional costs
		    feelings of embarrassment
		    feelings of overload
		    feelings of entrapment
		    feelings of resentment
		    feelings of exclusion

[1]a.o. = among others.

subdivided according to different kinds of burden (Herz *et al.*, 1976; Thompson and Doll, 1982). (See Table 20.1).

Hoenig and Hamilton (1966) were, as far as the author can establish, the first researchers to introduce the terms 'objective' and 'subjective' burden, explicitly. In their study of the burdening of family members as a result of the presence of a family member with psychiatric disturbances, the subjective burden reported during the period of the investigation did not always coincide with the expectations that could be derived on the basis of objective burden.

In developing a measurement instrument with which to establish the burden of family members, Pai and Kapur (1981) distinguished between subjective and objective burden. Their operationalization of subjective burden is somewhat similar to that of Hoenig and Hamilton. In order to test the validity of their instrument they compared the subjective burden reported by every family member, with the total objective burden as established by the professionals. The correlation coefficient between the average total scores on each item, as reported by family members, and by professionals, was 0.72. Although this result was reasonably high, it is clear that objective burden did not in all cases coincide with the subjective burden. Another type of distinction between objective and subjective burden can be found in the research by Herz *et al.* (1976). In this study, in which the influence of the duration of the hospitalization on the burdening of family members is examined, both objective and subjective burden were further subdivided. Indicators of the objective burden mainly concerned patient characteristics, while indicators of the subjective burden referred mainly to emotional problems of family members, and problems regarding affection.

Thompson and Doll (1982) in their study of the burden of family members of psychiatric patients, made further distinctions about subjective burden. The objective burden in this study, is subdivided into a number of 'social costs'. The subjective burden concerns the various aspects of 'emotional costs'. The total objective and subjective burden, subdivided into 'no', 'average' and 'heavy' burden, showed the following differences in objective and subjective burden. The number of family members with an average objective burden was smaller than the number of family members with an average subjective burden. The number of family members with a heavy objective burden, however, was nearly twice as large as those who experienced a heavy subjective burden. Furthermore, it became obvious that, although a statistically significant connection was found between the objective and the subjective burden, the components of the objective burden explain less than 10 per cent of the variation in subjective burden. It has to be mentioned that there may be additional factors which influence the burden family members experience. (Thompson and Doll tentatively refer to 'the adaptive tolerance' of family members.) In the study presented in this chapter this idea is developed further.

Figure 20.1 A preliminary conceptual framework

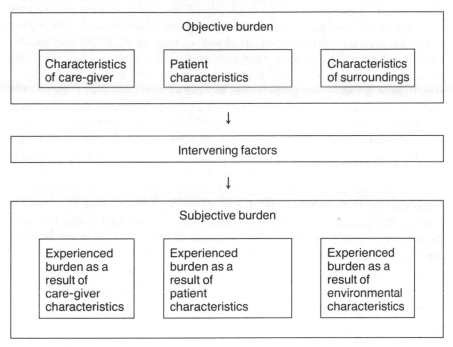

THE RESEARCH FRAMEWORK

The question this study asks is 'Why and how can the subjective burden differ from the objective burden of the primary care-giver?' The way in which this study tried to answer this question is discussed next. Figure 20.1 shows the conceptual framework used for this study.

This conceptual framework shows the objective and subjective burden of a primary care-giver at a particular moment in time. In the present investigation this is the period of time during which the interviews were held. (This did not prevent people from looking back in the interviews, however.) What this framework does not show, however, is the change in burden experienced by the primary care-giver over time. In that sense, this is not a process model.

With regard to basic concepts, this study shares with previously mentioned studies, the concept of objective burden (as assessed by an objective outsider) as opposed to subjective burden (as experienced by the primary care-giver). In the elaboration of this concept at least four developments have been made. In order to arrive at an outline that was as complete as possible, the study takes into consideration three variables. These are the patient with dementia, the primary care-giver and the environment. Next, based on literature studies and on clinical experience, the relevant components within these variables were identified. Because primary care-givers were asked to indicate the subjective burden they experienced with regard to the individual components of the objective burden, no additional indicators of subjective burdening were determined prior to carrying out this investigation. Subjective burden therefore, is defined in this study as the significance a care-giver gives to the individual variables and components that are recognized within the objective burden. Third, in this study the emphasis is not exclusively on the possible differences between objective and subjective burden. Also the question is emphasized because of what, and in what way, the subjective burden differs from the burden, such as it might be assumed to be, based on the components present in the objective burden. A fourth aspect is that the term burden is considered to consist of elements that both increase and decrease 'burden'. In this way, in a consideration of the objective burden of care-giver X, the fact that ample financial means are available, would be considered to decrease the objective burden, whereas incontinence in the patient with dementia would increase the objective burden.

HOW THE RESEARCH WAS CARRIED OUT

A qualitative research strategy

A qualitative research strategy was chosen for this study of the burdening of family members of demented elderly persons. Given the large scope of this topic, the method, and the principal questions have only partly been explored. For instance, until now a uniform definition of subjective and objective burden is notably lacking and it is not clear which aspects play a part in differences between subjective and objective burden. As a method for gathering data, interviewing primary care-givers was chosen. Two private interviews lasting approximately 3 hours were held with them in the home environment. Information about the objective burden was collected by means of an interview scheme using open and closed questions. Information about the subjective burden was collected by means of qualitative interviews (Kvale, 1983). The interviews were recorded on tape. The processing of the data started with typing out the entire interviews. The information was then coded as to entry number and theme. Analyses per care-giver were made, and the situation analyses were compared to each other. Forty primary care-givers were involved in the examination. They comprise both male and female partners, daughters (-in-law) and sons. Some are living with the demented person, others are not.

The objective burden

The objective burden involve a number of factual aspects about the care-giving situation which objectively increase or decrease the burden of the primary care-giver. In this treatment of objective burden, the significance that the primary care-giver attaches to the burden is not considered. In order to arrive at a description of the objective burden, based on literature studies and experience, a list with relevant components per variable was compiled. To give a picture of the collection of data, this paragraph appoints the main components per variable, and some of the items that belong to them.

Patient characteristics

The following list of main components was compiled to describe the functioning of the demented person, and, ensuing from this, the help that this person receives form the primary care-giver:

General daily life functions e.g. mobility, eating habits, incontinence;
Personal care e.g. washing, toiletting, dressing;
Relations with others e.g. is it possible to have a conversation with the demented person;
Deviating behaviour e.g. reversal of day–night rhythm, hallucinations;
Need for support e.g. how much and what kind of support is offered by the primary care-giver.

Characteristics of the care-giver

With regard to the care-giver, two main components are recognized which can either increase or decrease the objective burden:

Functional validity of the primary care-giver. With this, a person's physical ability to perform the care is meant;
Competing fields of attention, such as a family or a job that besides the care-giving, require time and effort.

Environmental characteristics

Circumstances in the surroundings which could decrease or increase the objective burden:

Financial situation, e.g. available means, extra expenses;
Housing situation, e.g. situation of the toilet, bedrooms, presence of a staircase;
Contributions from the social network, e.g. from whom and how often

occur positive contributions (emotional and practical support) or negative contributions (e.g. arguments about money);
Professional care, e.g. what kind of care, by whom and how much?

The subjective burden

Next, the subjective burden is examined per primary care-giver. The significance the care-giver attaches to the various components of the objective
burden is discussed. Based on this information it can be investigated to
what extent the subjective burden coincides with that which the objective
burden may lead us to expect. If, for instance, the primary care-giver
suffers from rheumatism and moves with difficulty as a result of this, this
fact is considered to increase the objective burden. With regard to the
burden experienced the following varieties are possible. Either the primary
care-giver him- or herself experiences the rheumatism as a handicap in the
care-giving (objective and subjective burden are equal in this respect) or the
care-giver in no way experiences this objective handicap as a burden
(objective and subjective burden are not equal in this respect). This leads us
to the question of which factors play a part in a possible difference between
objective and subjective burden. In the example given just now, this can
coincide, for example, with the acceptance of the handicap by the primary
care-giver, who in the course of time has learned to live with it.

Intervening factors

In the study the primary care-giver is considered to function as the translation centre through which a personal colouring of the objective burden may
occur. Intervening factors are considered as personal factors because they
can explain why the primary care-giver attaches another significance to the
separate components of the objective burden than expected. For instance,
the relationship the care-giver had with the demented person before they
fell ill, and the level of knowledge of the care-giver can play a part in that.

This study assumes that the data derived from the interviews have to
clarify which aspects play a part in a possible difference between subjective
and objective burden.

CASE ILLUSTRATION

This chapter was written while the research was still in progress. A first
analysis of the results so far, indicate that objective and subjective burden
often diverge in an unpredictable way, and that very different factors play a
part in this. In order to gain some insight into this, this paragraph describes
the first case in the research. This concerns a 64-year-old primary care-

giver Mrs W who takes care of her 71-year-old husband who has dementia.
In the description of the case, the following order is adhered to. First the
objective burden is described, then the subjective burden and the intervening factors that play a part in the difference between subjective and
objective burden are gone into. The structure of the paragraph is in confor-
mity with the variables, components and items as mentioned on p. 369 up
to and including p. 370.

The objective burden

Patient characteristics

Eating, getting dressed, washing and going to the toilet is done by her
husband himself under her supervision, when she reminds him of it. Her
husband is docile in the sense that he follows her indications and advice.
What is most prominent with regard to the possibilities of social contact
is the fact that the demented partner is forgetful and is only able to have
a superficial conversation.
Deviations in behaviour mainly concern the fact that he is suspicious,
has sudden emotional outbursts and is garrulous.
As for the need for support: Mrs W cannot leave her husband alone too
long as he needs constant supervision. She can never go out for the day
and cannot go on holiday. She has to take care of everything in the
house.

Characteristics of the care-giver

Mrs W sometimes walks with difficulty and has a broken coccyx.
There are no other matters besides the care for her husband that take up
her attention. She has no more children living at home and no job.

Environmental characteristics

Mrs W and her husband live on an old age pension. There are no financial reserves and no additional pension.
They live in an old house with a large garden. They sleep upstairs. Her
husband has difficulty climbing the stairs. There is no toilet upstairs.
Mrs W has a son and a daughter-in-law who seldom visit or seek contact
by telephone; an agreement has been made that she will ask their help
when necessary. Her son is irritated by his father's behaviour and the
daughter-in-law thinks Mrs W is spineless because she gives in too much
to her husband's behaviour.

Mrs W receives hardly any visits from old acquaintances, but she does have regular contact with her sisters who live nearby. She does not discuss her husband's situation with them.

The general practitioner has promised that her husband will be hospitalized if it becomes impossible to care for him at home. He does not make house calls that are not asked for, and he has given her no information about the illness. She takes her husband to visit the GP or a specialist if necessary. Mrs W does not receive help from a district nurse, a home help or other help organizations.

Objectively speaking it can be said that nearly all components of her situation are influenced by variables which increase her burden. Her husband continually demands her presence, needs encouragement with nearly all activities of daily living. She herself has difficulty walking, and sitting is painful; the financial means are minimal, the housing situation is impractical in some respects, and, there is no actual help from a social network or from the professional care-giving organizations.

Subjective burden and intervening factors (what and why)

Patient characteristics

Mrs W has no problems with regard to her husband's present level of functioning. She regularly stresses the fact that she is happy her husband is continent. She does not think she can cope with incontinence, and she says that if Mr W becomes incontinent she will probably have to have him hospitalized, which she does not want. In the course of time she has learned to deal with the functional disorders of her husband. Her total range of coping mechanisms is large and varied. A few examples include: checking to see to what extent problematic situations with her husband result from her own behaviour, realizing that for her husband, too, it is a nasty situation and he cannot help it, not doing each and everything for her husband, not entering into arguments with her husband, making a joke rather than a fuss about a situation, praising her husband and emphasizing what he still can do, giving him the feeling that he is not useless, continually adjusting her expectations of her husband to fit his abilities.

What she sometimes regards as an increase in her burden is the fact that she can no longer go on holiday. Taking care of her husband is a continuous job. She misses the holidays as a period of rest and intermission in which she has time to herself. About this she says 'There are days when I think it would be wonderful just to have my rest, not to have to pay any attention to anyone else, just to do nothing and just be occupied with myself.'

Characteristics of care-giver

She does not pay any attention to the fact that she sometimes walks with difficulty and that she has a broken coccyx. When asked what she thinks of this, it becomes clear that she accepts this handicap as a fact of life: 'You have to make do with what you've got. One day I'm better able to do some things than the next, that is just a fact.'

Environmental factors

Mrs W clearly regards her limited financial status as increasing her subjective burden. She regularly comes back to this in the interviews. Not having more financial means at her disposal makes her angry. 'Money sweetens much', she says, and more money would make things easier for her. She has to do a lot of figuring out now. She only uses the car when absolutely necessary, and never for fun. Furthermore, she cancelled her newspaper in order to be able to afford the car. The possibility of the car breaking down and her not being able to buy a new one is a terror to her. Then her world will become very small. She would want DFL 100 more per month. Then she could 'buy' private help, she could renew things in the house, or she could move to a more practical house. She won't do these things now because of the extra expense. She thinks it is a crime she has to make constant calculations. She bears a grudge because of the small amount with which she has to finance the care. She is of the opinion that this is not the way the older generation, who also lived through a war, should be treated.

Her evaluation of the housing situation is not a prominent one in the consideration of environmental factors. She says that the staircase and not having a toilet upstairs are not practical, but that on the other hand, the house has a beautiful garden and her husband still knows his way around it.

The behaviour of her son and her daughter-in-law are no longer a problem to her. She can find understanding for them because of their age and the phase of life they are in:

> My son is busy with his career and let him enjoy his wife and baby. They don't reflect on things, they are swallowed up by other matters. The new man goes his own way. In the old days maybe I was like that. There are times when I think about my own mother and wonder if I should not have done this or that.

In the early stages of her husband's disease she had hopes of being able to count on their understanding and support, but by and by she has had to let go of that expectation. The situation being what it is does not make her bear a grudge.

> I had hoped for something else, but I have come this far and I don't need their support anymore. Not that I am mad, mind you, but I don't want it

any more for it is better if I don't have it, I know I don't have it. Then I can't miss it either. With me, I think it has already died a little. I sometimes think: luckily I'm partly dead already where that is concerned. If they kick me in the head it may hurt, but I won't die of it anymore. Because I've already gone through that. Of course I used to worry about it in the past. I'd lie if I said I never did. I have also been very sad about it at times, so much so that I cried to myself. Until I thought everything over and said to myself, listen, if it is not there, it is not there, but I no longer bear a grudge, and furthermore I know, and that is also from experience, that for children it is very difficult to carry the load of the care for the parents. That restricts your life somewhat.

Not speaking with her sisters about her husband's situation is not seen as a problem by her. People who don't understand are better off without knowledge of the situation she says. With her sisters she does not discuss her husband's situation because they do not believe her, and because they do not react to her story. In some ways she can understand her sisters' reaction, she says, because when one of her sisters began having trouble with her brother-in-law she herself sometimes thought that her sister was making up the stories. Furthermore, she does not see the point in talking about him to them, because it does not change the situation anyway. Another reason for not discussing it with her sister is that she supposes that her sisters think that she is only nagging because she herself still looks so good. Furthermore, she thinks that her sisters (two have cancer and one is paralysed) have enough problems of their own.

Not having anyone within her social network to discuss the situation with, somehow makes it easier for her, she says:

If you tell others about the situation, you very easily become a pitiful figure, and the underdog is never a celebrated person. Besides, the situation changes so much each day, that it is impossible for anyone to imagine themselves in the other person's situation.

The reduced number of social visits do not bother Mrs W because visits cause their own problems. She would have to divide her attention among too many people. For, she does not want to show her husband to anyone like this, she would have to constantly interrupt a conversation when he did not understand something.

The way in which the contacts with the GP take place is not notably problematic she says. Mrs W does not want more contact than she has at present; she prefers not to discuss the situation with the GP for he might think she is no longer able to handle the situation. She assumes that this may lead to a hospitalization of her husband, which she does not want. Then she says about the GP that it would have been better if he would have told her more about the disease and its symptoms, which was a problem for her in the beginning. Now she has had to learn by bitter experience. She is glad of the GP's assurance that her husband will be hospitalized if she can no longer look after him. This gives her the feeling that she has not been 'sentenced to life'. On those days she thinks how can I keep going with this, it gives her strength to know that there is a solution if things would really become impossible at home. Mrs W remarks that the GP and the specialist do not really understand the situation. Her husband acts as if everything is normal in a conversation with them, and they buy that. Also they pretend her husband is normal and they cut her off if she wants to take over from her husband in order to place her experiences against his social facade. She has the impression that her problems and her credibility are thus diminished. The change in specialists in the hospital is a nuisance because she has to tell her story over and over again.

Having to do the caring all by herself and not receiving any help from the district nurse or a home helper is no problem for her. District nursing and home help have been offered to her but she does not want this. She forsees problems with these services. Mrs W thinks that she herself does not have a suitable character for district nursing or home help. She assumes these professional care-givers expect a helpless attitude from her. They would mother her and take over from her. She hates feeling dependent on others. Also, she thinks these care-givers are too young to understand what she has been through. Moreover, she does not have a high opinion of the care rendered by the home helper's association. She heard what they do from other people in her neighbourhood and she does not think that amounts to much; she can make coffee and tea by herself.

She would have liked to have private help, which she 'buys' because then she can keep her distance and give orders. She indicates that this would help her, but that unfortunately her finances are not sufficient.

Mrs W indicates that, if nothing changes, she could continue caring for her husband for a long time, which she wants to do. Extra financial resources would be experienced by her as a clear lightening of the burden, as the possibility to go on a supervised vacation with her husband would be.

Continuation of the intervening factors

In the previous pages a number of intervening factors were mentioned, which gave subjective significance to the separate variables and components of the objective burden. Thus, for instance, objectively speaking there is an increase in burden because there is no help from a district nurse or a home help, while on the other hand her husband needs continuous supervision and care. For this care-giver, however, it is no problem that there is no district nurse and home help, because she doesn't want them to help. She thinks she is better off without them because of her independent tendency and her (untested) expectations of this help. Other intervening factors also appear to play a part in the burden she experiences.

About her character, Mrs W says that she likes to take things in hand and not to despair. She always analyses where the problems lie and tries to find the solution. In this way with the help of her strongly developed coping mechanisms she battles the objective burden she is faced with.

Furthermore, she says that after she had totally drunk her 'cup of gall' she had come to accept the situation completely. She takes reality as a starting point and she faces the situation: 'That man happens to be like that, nothing can be done about it.' She says that in the beginning she was angry with others and that her disturbed expectations for the future were prominent.

Mrs W has been taking care of her husband for 7 years now. The duration has decreased her burden, she says, because through time she has learned to deal with the situation. She says that she has gone through it as a total process of trial and error. In the beginning she was mad at her husband because she was unfamiliar with the disease, and she felt insecure. She kept asking herself: 'Who is mad here?' She spared him in everything and started to mother him. Because she did not pay any attention to herself she began to feel whiny and overwrought. Because she did not understand the situation at the time, she did not develop effective coping mechanisms and, for instance, began to eat too much and to eat candy in order to have something pleasant in her life. Examples of effective coping mechanisms that she developed over time (see also p. 372) included: paying some attention to oneself, speaking to oneself and encouraging oneself (one self keeping the other self in balance), bringing back the situation to acceptable proportions by considering both the negative and the positive sides, and by emphasizing the positive side, placing the situation in another perpective. (If that man happened to be my child I would also want him to be taken good care of, it might have been worse when I was young, when I was unaware of the disease, etc.) Other coping mechanisms include: experimenting with pills and vitamins, establishing priorities and not bothering with things that are not really important, keeping oneself busy and no brooding or grieving, thinking away the situation as if it does not exist, living for each day (no memories, no expectations) and compensating (if you cannot go on vacation, read a book about the country). The ways and insights she has gained to deal with the situation and the satisfaction she experiences as a result of this, are a central theme in the interview. She worked hard to reach this equilibrium and is very content with the achieved result.

Being able to deal with the situation she finds herself in, is, according to her, also a result of her former relationship with her husband. Her husband was very busy and very dominant, so she has always had to compromise. Because her husband was also away at sea a lot, she always had to take care of herself. She says she never had much support from him. The problems she has had to overcome in the past made her strong enough for the present. About it she says: 'If things had always been easy, it would be more difficult now.' The fact that not only is she able to care for her husband, but is also strongly motivated to continue to do so relates also to some extent to what she has been through with her husband in the past. About it she says: 'I was not yet 18 when I met him, there was a war going on and in such a situation a different relationship develops. You never leave someone with whom you have been through terrible times. It gives you a feeling of solidarity you never get rid of.'

The wish to keep her husband at home is also related to the fact that, at the moment, she feels pity for him.

> When he sits on the couch with all those wrinkles and when he says 'Yes mommy' to me, I can no longer be mad at him. I just let him be for god's sake. I cannot possibly have him hospitalized. He is so skinny already, his teeth no longer fit well and he has trouble urinating. At least ten times a day, and another four times at night. It is absolutely impossible for me to let someone like that down. That is just a fact.

Mrs W also wants to take care of her husband as long as possible because she hates nursing homes. 'They smell of ammonia and you are confronted with other people's misery in them.' She also mentioned that her husband would get worse, if institutionalized. She would expect negative reactions from people for hospitalizing her husband. She would have to visit him continually and bring clothes, and it would be unpleasant for her son to have a father in a nursing home.

THE SIGNIFICANCE OF THE STUDY FOR PRACTICE

It is expected that with the help of the information gathered in this study the effectiveness of professional care rendered to primary care-givers of the demented patients can be increased. To achieve this, it is necessary that professional care-givers can make a correct estimate of the contents and the value of the subjective burden of the primary care-giver. The study provides techniques for this.

First of all, the study provides a survey of the different objective variables and components that play a possible part in the burdening of the primary care-giver. Insight into this series is a first requirement to make a realistic estimate of the burden.

The distinction this study makes between objective and subjective burden emphasizes that in order to estimate the burden of the primary care-giver, at least two persons are required, namely the primary care-giver and the professional care-giver. Hopefully professional care-givers will realize that the primary care-giver possesses valuable information which is not only supplementary to the information gathered by professionals, but necessary and indispensable. Only with such information can a true estimate of the burden of the primary care-giver be made. Specific answers as to the question of which type of professional care could reduce the burden of a given primary care-giver, or keep it at an acceptable level, must take into account objective and subjective burden.

Attention for, and insight, into intervening factors that, together with the objective burden, play a part in, and which therefore could explain subjective burden, also offer insight into the way which, and to what extent, it is possible to influence the burden of a primary care-giver.

ACKNOWLEDGEMENTS

The author gratefully thanks Prof J. Munnichs and Dr A. Smaling for their valuable suggestions, comments and advice throughout the research project.

REFERENCES

Bevers, A.M. (1982) *Oudere mensen en hun kinderen, een tweezijdig onderzoek naar de besefcontext van een verwantschapsrelatie*, Nijmegen: Sociologisch Instituut.

Brody, E.M. (1981) 'Women in the middle and family help to older people', *Gerontologist* 21: 471–9.

Cantor, M.H. (1983) 'Strain among caregivers: a study of experience in the United States', *Gerontologist* 23 (6): 597–604.

Duijnstee, M. (1985) *Ze lacht nog wel als ze me ziet; gesprekken met familieleden van dementerende ouderen*, Nijkerk: Intro. (1987)

—— (forthcoming) 'The difference between objective and subjective burden', doctorate research on the burden of care-givers of demented patients at home.

—— Erkens, C. and Sipsma, D.H. (1987) *Psychogeriatrie thuis; een handreiking voor wijkverpleging en gezinsverzorging*, Almere: Versluys.

George, L.K. and Gwyther, L.P. (1986) 'Caregiver well-being: a multidimensional examination of family caregivers of demented adults', *Gerontologist*, 23: 253–9.

Gilleard, C.J., Boyd, W.D. and Watt, G. (1982) 'Problems in caring for the elderly mentally infirm at home', *Archives of Gerontology and Geriatry* 1: 151–8.

Grad, J. and Sainsbury, P. (1983) 'Mental illness and the family', *Lancet* 3: 544–7.

Greene, J.G., Smith, R., Gardiner, M. and Timbury, G.C. (1982) 'Measuring behavioural disturbance of elderly demented patients in the community and its effect on relatives: a factor analytic study', *Age and Aging* 11: 121–6.

Herz, M.I., Endicott, J. and Spitzer, R.L. (1976) 'Brief versus standard hospitalization: the families', *American Journal of Psychiatry* 133: 795–801.

Hoenig, J. and Hamilton, M.W. (1966) 'Elderly psychiatric patients and the burden on the household', *Internationale Monatschrift für Psychiatrie und Neurologie*, 152: 281–93.

Horowitz, A. (1985) 'Family caregiving to the frail elderly', *Annual Review of Gerontology and Geriatrics* 5: 194–245.

Johnson, C.L. (1983) 'Dyadic family relations and social support', *Gerontologist* 23: 377–83.

Kvale, S. (1983) 'The qualitative interview : a phenomenological and a hermeneutical mode of understanding', *Journal of Phenomenological Psychology* 14: 171–96.

Morycz, R.K. (1985) 'Caregiving strain and the desire to institutionalize family members with Alzheimer's Disease', *Research on Aging* 7 (3): 329–61.

Niederehe, G. and Frugé, E. (1984) 'Dementia and family dynamics: clinical research issues', *Journal of Geriatric Psychiatry* 17: 21–56.

Pai, S. and Kapur, R.L. (1981) 'The burden on the family of a psychiatric patient: development of an interview schedule', *British Journal of Psychiatry* 138: 332–5.

Poulshock, S.W. and Deimling, G.T. (1984) 'Families caring for elders in residence: issues in the measurement of burden', *Journal of Gerontology* 39: 230–9.

Shanas, E. (1979) 'The family as a social support system in old age', *Gerontologist* 19: 169–73.

STG, scenario-rapport (1985) *Ouder worden in de toekomst, scenario's over gezondheid en vergrijzing 1984–2000*, Utrecht: Van Arkel.

Thompson, E.H. and Doll, W. (1982) 'The burden of families coping with the mentally ill: an invisible crisis', *Family Relations* 31: 379–88.

Chapter 21

Expressed emotion and coping techniques amongst carers of the dementing elderly

Janice Whittick

SUMMARY

This chapter discusses the concept of expressed emotion (EE) (Brown *et al.*, 1958) and its application to carers of the dementing elderly. The EE literature is reviewed in brief, and the use of the patient rejection scale (PRS) (Kreisman *et al.*, 1979) as a reliable measure of hostility and criticism is addressed. The coping literature is also briefly reviewed with particular reference to carers. Expressed emotion and coping techniques were investigated in a pilot study with carers of the dementing elderly and results are reported here. Clinical implications of this research are discussed.

INTRODUCTION

While schizophrenia had been the original and main focus of EE work, Koenisberg and Handley (1986) observed that 'there is nothing intrinsic to the EE concept that should limit it to schizophrenic patients'. In spite of this there have been relatively few attempts to take EE into other areas. Depressives (Vaughn and Leff, 1976a; Hooley *et al.*, 1986), diabetics (Minuchin *et al.*, 1975), obese women (Havstad, 1979) and disturbed adolescents (Valone *et al.*, 1983) are among the chronic conditions that have been studied.

Until recently senile dementia has not been explored in this way despite a wealth of information on the impact of the disease on the carer (Gilleard, 1984; Gilhooly, 1984; Whittick, 1988). It seems likely that carers of the dementing elderly are more likely than the general population and also other patient groups to suffer from elevated levels of emotional distress (Whittick, 1988). Also the nature of the disease is not always clearly understood and the carer may feel resentment towards the dependant because of this. In the author's experience this negative attitude is sometimes expressed in clear unambiguous terms during interview but what effect this in turn has on the dependant is as yet unknown. Clearly the

notion of relapse is not applicable in dementia but maybe institutionalization, crises, or the breakdown of care are related to EE.

THE CONCEPT OF EXPRESSED EMOTION AND EARLY STUDIES

The concept of EE originated from work by Brown *et al.* (1958) and
his study on a group of male schizophrenics discharged from hospital
back in to the community. The patients' prognosis appeared to be related,
to an extent, to the emotional atmosphere within the family to which they
returned. A family with a high level of EE would be overtly critical and
hostile about their dependant and hold a blaming attitude towards him or
her. A family with a low level of EE would not express this overt criticism
and hostility and would be much more accepting of their dependant's
condition. In addition, the amount of direct contact the dependant had with
his or her caring relative also seemed to be an important variable. In a
further prospective study, Brown *et al.* (1962) obtained similar findings and
an assessment procedure to measure the EE concept was devised, namely,
the Camberwell family interview (CFI).

The CFI was further refined by Vaughn and Leff (1976a) and their
shortened version is still the most widely used instrument for measuring EE
to date. An interview is recorded with the primary caring relative, in the
absence of his or her dependant. The interview covers the onset and
development of the illness, events and activities in the home and how they
are affected by the dependant's illness. The aim is to ascertain the type of
emotional atmosphere within the home over the past 3 months prior to the
dependant's admission to hospital. The shortened version takes up to 2
hours to complete and 125–75 hours of training is said to be required if
good reliability is to be obtained. Following the interview, ratings are made
along the following dimensions.

DIMENSIONS RATED IN THE CFI

1   Criticism – this dimension refers to the content of comments and/or tone
    of voice during interview. A statement is rated critical if there is an
    unambiguous remark of dislike, resentment or disapproval. If, however,
    the remark is then qualified by the carer either blaming him or herself,
    e.g., 'He can be so annoying but I really should be more patient', or
    showing an understanding of the illness, e.g., 'He can be lazy but he
    can't help it because it's part of his illness', then it can no longer be
    judged critical. This qualification does not apply if the rating of
    'criticism' is made according to voice tone only. The criticism rating is
    the total number of critical comments made and it is the most
    important dimension of EE.

2   Hostility – this dimension refers to a more general statement of rejection and is judged by the rater on a 3-point scale.
3   Emotional overinvolvement – this is rated on a 5- or 6-point scale and concerns exaggerated emotional response towards the illness or the dependant, e.g., 'I can't leave him, I stay with him 24 hours a day.'
4   Warmth – this is judged from voice tone alone and rated on a 5- or 6-point scale. It seems to be a relatively unimportant component of the EE concept.
5   Positive remarks – these are unambiguous statements of approval or praise and like critical comments, the total number emitted during interview are counted. However, as with warmth, this is thought to add little to the total concept.

FACTORS INFLUENCING THE PATIENT–FAMILY RELATIONSHIP

Several studies have demonstrated that EE is unaffected by the patients' clinical state or his or her level of behavioural disturbance (Vaughn and Leff, 1976b; Brown *et al.*, 1972). The effect of EE on relapse does however seem to be modified by compliance with medication (Brown *et al.*, 1972; Vaughn and Leff, 1976b). Regular medication seems to have a protective influence against a high EE family.

Vaughn and Leff (1976b) also discovered that the risk of relapse was greater if the patient spent over 35 hours per week face-to-face contact with their relative. Furthermore, an accumulation of independent life events for patients in low EE families has more recently been associated with relapse (Leff and Vaughn, 1980).

Many of the EE studies in the 1970s were concerned with the effect of EE on relapse. Brown *et al.* (1972) found an association between EE and relapse at a 9-month follow-up on a group of schizophrenics. Vaughn and Leff (1976a) obtained similar results on a group of schizo-phrenics and to a lesser extent with a group of depressives. For the schizophrenic group, carers were assigned to a high EE group on the basis of > 7 critical comments and/or marked emotional overinvolvement. At a 9-month follow-up 50 per cent of the high-EE group had relapsed, compared with only 12 per cent of the low-EE group. When a lower critical-comments threshold was used, similar results were obtained for the depressives. Hooley *et al.* (1986) replicated this finding on a group of depressed patients and suggested that the lower threshold for critical comments was perhaps due to the typical self-critical nature of depressives. This association between EE and relapse was held up in the face of extended follow-up intervals (Leff and Vaughn, 1981) and also in other countries (Vaughn *et al.*, 1984).

Several intervention studies have also reported encouraging results. Leff *et al.* (1982) randomly assigned high-EE relatives to either an experimental or a control group. The latter received standard outpatient care while the experimental group received a course of educational input, relatives' support groups and family therapy. This intervention package successfully reduced levels of EE amongst the experimental group and relapse at 9 months was 9 per cent compared with 50 per cent for the controls.

In a larger study, Hogarty *et al.* (1986) compared the effect of various inputs namely, family psychoeducation, social skills training, combined family therapy with social skills training, while supportive psychotherapy served as a control. The combination of family therapy with social skills training proved to be the most successful with no cases of relapse at 1 year. Relapse rates were at 19 per cent and 20 per cent for the family treatment and social skills training respectively. The control group had a 41 per cent relapse rate.

Orford *et al.* (1987) assessed EE in four groups of carers with one of the following dependants, either an adult psychiatric patient, an elderly person with a functional disorder, an elderly patient with a chronic physical disorder or an elderly patient with senile dementia. Contrary to previous findings high levels of EE were not found in any of the groups. When the threshold for critical comments was lowered to > 2 remarks, 52 per cent of carers with an adult patient, 42 per cent with elderly functional patients, 17 per cent with a physically disabled patient and 17 per cent with a dementing dependant were then rated as high EE. Although the carers found many of the behaviours and characteristics of dementia irritating and frustrating they were usually described or qualified in a way which expressed compassion or understanding. This is an interesting and pioneering project, however, the subsample of the carers with a dementing relative (n = 12) was small. It may be that a larger group would demonstrate the effect of EE. Furthermore, the CFI may not in fact be the most appropriate instrument for this group. Orford *et al.* comment that it does not appear to be a particularly sensitive measure for the given sample and in particular the emotional overinvolvement component was thought to be inappropriate because of the caring demands of dementia. Low-EE scores were obtained for all groups and it may have been that the criteria used were stricter than those employed by other researchers.

Bledin (1987) using the CFI assessed EE on twenty-five daughters caring for a parent with dementia. Fourteen of the sample were rated high EE and had > 4 critical comments. Like Orford, Bledin did not feel that emotional overinvolvement was a useful dimension as it was absent in all of the carers. He found that high-EE carers reported greater levels of emotional distress and strain than low-EE relatives and they were also found to be using more maladaptive coping strategies than low-EE relatives.

Gilhooly and Whittick (1989) rated EE by frequency of critical comments on a sample of forty-eight carers and found that the greater the number of critical comments, the lower the carer's morale and the poorer his or her mental health. Females were more critical than males and those carers who had enjoyed a good pre-morbid relationship with their dependant were less critical. Also, there was a significant association between the amount of contact the carer had with friends and the frequency of critical comments.

For a more detailed review of the EE literature, the reader is referred to Hooley (1986).

THE PATIENT REJECTION SCALE (PRS)

In response to the lengthy and complex training time associated with using the CFI, Kreisman et al. (1979) developed a patient rejection scale which comprised an 11-item questionnaire for completion by carers. This scale measured feelings of rejection towards the patient and had moderately high reliability and test–retest correlation. Using this scale, Kreisman et al. (1979) found that PRS scores were predictive of risk of rehospitalization. Freire et al. (1982) similarly found a correlation between PRS score and face-to-face contact between carer and dependant. Interestingly, they found no association between PRS and the degree of psychopathology as measured by the 'brief psychiatric rating scale'. In a cross-cultural study, Watzl et al. (1986) administered the PRS to a German sample and obtained similar results to those of the original New York City sample.

The original scale was extended to a 24-item scale in 1980, to contain positive as well as negative attitudes and feelings of the carer towards his or her dependant. As before, the carer responds to the items on a 7-point Likert scale; no particular training is required in order to administer it and it is straightforward and non-threatening for the carer to complete. McCreadie and Robinson (1988) used this version on a group of carers of schizophrenics and compared it with the CFI. They found that while the PRS could differentiate between groups of high- and low-EE relatives, owing to the wide range of scores within the high-EE category, a cut-off point for individuals could not be ascertained. In light of this they concluded that the PRS was a useful research tool but had limited use clinically.

Snyder et al. (1988) also with a group of schizophrenics found a strong correspondance between traditionally rated EE levels and PRS scores. They concluded that the degree of convergence between the two scales was sufficiently high for the two measures to be considered interchangeable. The PRS was identified as a useful screening tool worthy of further investigation.

LITERATURE REVIEW OF 'COPING'

Within the coping literature, different researchers and writers have defined and classified the concept of coping in many different ways. A brief review of some of the more applicable theories is given below. For additional information, the reader is referred to the reference list at the end of this chapter.

Pearlin and Schooler (1978) differentiated behavioural versus psychological coping. The former refers to actively finding out and seeking help, the latter attempts to change, modify or control the meaning of the stressful experience via a variety of techniques, e.g., making positive comparisons, reordering life priorities, etc. Furthermore, they identify three major types of coping responses:

1   Responses that change the situation out of which the stressful experience arises. This may seem a logical solution but it is not commonly applied as individuals often lack the skill to recognize the source of the difficulty or lack the ability to change a stressful situation.
2   Responses that control the meaning of the stressful experience after its occurrence but before the emergence of stress, e.g., selectively ignoring the negative aspects of the situation.
3   Responses that function more for the control of stress after it has emerge, e.g., interpreting an unavoidable stress as a moral virtue: 'Parents have a duty to look after their handicapped children.' Furthermore, they showed that the efficacy of a coping mechanism varied according to the particular role the individual was in.

The majority of models of stress and coping have focused on the general adaptation aspects and this has been criticized by Coyne *et al.* (1981) as being too inflexible and static. They proposed a model of coping which was transactional, emphasizing relationships between variables, process, fluctuation and change. With this model coping serves two main functions, namely, a problem-oriented alteration of the ongoing relationship between the person and his or her environment, and the control of stressful emotions.

In this model coping is not simply a response to environmental conditions but an activity which shapes the course of the ongoing person–environment relationship. Coping processes are also dependent on the cognitive process of appraisal.

On the basis of this theory, Folkman and Lazarus (1980) developed a 'Ways of coping checklist'. This 66-item questionnaire covers a vast range of coping techniques, both problem-focused and emotion-focused, to be marked by the subject in accordance with a specific named incident. Using this scale, Folkman and Lazarus found that in most instances both problem- and emotion-focused techniques were used. They also discovered that over time individuals were more variable than consistent in their coping patterns. In general, situations which are perceived as able to be changed are dealt with in a problem-oriented way, while situations that are appraised as having to be accepted call for emotion-focused techniques.

Carers coping with disabled non-dementing dependants

Much of the coping literature is concerned with how an individual copes with disability or ill health. More recently, researchers have turned their attention to the carers of the sick dependants and attempted to identify how they cope with their unanticipated and frequently stressful role.

Some of the earlier work on families coping with disability comes from the schizophrenic literature on expressed emotion. EE may well be the result of coping ability such that high-EE families, with little perceived control, perhaps use more coercive coping strategies. By contrast, low-EE carers with higher levels of perceived control, exhibit lower levels of stress and closer family links (Smith and Birchwood, 1987). They go on to identify three themes which are commonly found in families with a schizophrenic member and seem to be related to coping efficacy:

1   Availability of alternatives – those families that are flexible and can try out different solutions tend to show greater confidence and be more effective.
2   Consistency – those families who maintain consistency when trying new solutions fare better than those who are disorganized and try something only once.
3   Making allowances – those carers who understand their relative's illness and make allowances cope better than those who try to normalize the behaviour.

Locus of control (Rotter, 1966) has also been studied as a variable in the coping equation. Internal versus external locus of control refers to the extent to which an individual perceives the events that happen to him or her as dependent on his or her behaviour and actions as opposed to the result of chance or powers beyond his or her personal control or understanding. Schoeneman et al. (1983), in studying a group of wives coping with husbands' kidney failure and dialysis treatment, found that external locus of control was related to poorer adjustment to the situation.

Just as the patients' pre-morbid personality has been shown to be related to coping and adaptation following illness, so too has the pre-morbid carer–dependant relationship been shown to be significant in a group of depressed patients and their carers (Vaughn and Leff, 1976b). If the pre-morbid relationship was good, then the situation was more favourable than if the relationship had been poor, in which case the situation was exacerbated by the onset of the depression.

Fadden *et al.* (1987) looked at the coping responses of carers with depressed dependants and found in general that carers coped with a short-term view but had no clear idea of what they should be doing or how they might get help. It is perhaps worrying for health professionals to learn that the vast majority coped by 'wishing the situation would go away' or 'looking for the silver lining'. The carers were also self-punitive by criticizing themselves or through overindulgence of alcohol or tobacco. From what we have learned from other coping studies they would certainly appear to be the more maladaptive strategies.

Moffat (1987) studied coping in families with brain-damaged dependants and classified coping into:

- Practical and motivational problem solving, e.g., rising to the challenge; making a plan and following it.
- Diplomatic problem solving, e.g., being sensitive to the person's mood that day.
- Reappraisal, e.g., rethinking what is important in life.
- Collective coping, e.g., seeking social support.
- Loyalty, e.g., maintaining respect for the person.
- Catharsis, e.g., crying, losing one's temper.

Moffat also realized the importance of the relationship between the carer and the dependant. Where the relationship is emotionally close, it is often the case that the couple will withdraw from social and professional help and maintain a rigid routine. By contrast, families with a more distant relationship may also maintain a greater physical distance, shy away from responsibilities, and tend to look at short- as opposed to long-term solutions.

One major drawback of the coping literature is that terminology and classifications change from study to study making firm and general conclusions hard to come by. It may be the case that generalizations from one care group to another cannot be made and in order to develop counselling implications we must look at individual studies of particular illnesses and go on to build better models.

Coping with a relative with senile dementia

Coping techniques used by the carers of the dementing elderly is still a relatively new study area, hence there are only a few published studies.

Gilhooly (1987), adapting Pearlin and Schoolers' (1978) model, differentiated 'behavioural' versus 'psychological' coping. The former refers to attempts by the carer to seek out help and information and to organize help from the social network. The latter refers to the effort to change the meaning of the stressful experience, e.g., by making positive comparisons, selective ignoring, reordering of life priorities and converting hardship into a moral virtue. Gilhooly found that those carers who used behavioural techniques had higher morale. Also, those who made no attempt to 'cognitively neutralize' the situation coped poorly. Male carers were more likely than females to utilize behavioural coping strategies.

Zarit (1982) also found that males employed more effective coping strategies because it was easier for them to accept outside help to conduct household chores owing to traditional sex-role stereotypes.

Archbold (1981) in a sample of daughters caring for elderly, functionally impaired parents differentiated coping techniques of 'care managing' and 'care providing'. The former refers to the identification and management of service provision by others, while the latter refers to the identification and provision of services by the carer him- or herself. She found care managers were more likely to come from a higher social class and have a wide ranging professional network. They were also more likely to be in highly valued employment thus reducing the potential conflict between their employment and their caring obligations.

Johnson and Catelona (1982) from a study of carers of the infirm elderly distinguished 'distancing' from 'enmeshing' coping strategies. 'Distancing' involves physically being apart from the dependant either by not visiting, or by introducing help from other sources. It may also refer to psychological distancing where the carer ignores the emotional aspects of caring but continues to carry out the practical caring duties. By contrast, 'enmeshing' techniques result in the carer and her dependant drawing closer together, sometimes to the exclusion of other social relationships and outlets. Caring may become the carers' new and sole purpose in life and intervention from helping others may be rejected as infringing upon this role.

Some conclusions on coping

Orford (1987) attempted to summarize the many and sometimes diverse findings on coping with disabled relatives. He concluded that any techniques which allowed for a positive attitude to the caring situation was most effective, e.g. reordering of life priorities, information seeking and being clear and assertive about one's own needs. A limited element of denial seems to be appropriate in many cases and flexibility and consistency seem to be important factors. Coping techniques which seem to be unhelpful or indeed harmful are those which involve blame, the person rather than the illness, or blaming oneself. Any coping techniques which are 'coercive', 'avoiding', 'controlling' or 'colluding' are also thought to be unhelpful.

THE PRESENT STUDY

The study described here incorporates both concepts discussed in the chapter so far. It was an exploratory pilot study looking at EE and coping techniques among carers of the dementing elderly.

The sample

A sample of twenty carers with dementing relatives, both resident and non-resident, was drawn from the records of two day hospitals in Tayside and Lothian regions of Scotland. They were asked to participate in this study which involved intensive, semi-structured interviews in their own homes in the absence of their dependant. As with previous samples the majority of carers were female (n=13) with a mean age of 65 years. The majority were from the lower social classes and none were employed on a full-time basis. Their dependants were also predominantly female (n=13) with a mean age of 79 years. Most of the sample had a moderate to severe degree of dementia and were maximally dependent on their carers as determined by the Clifton assessment procedures for the elderly (Pattie and Gilleard, 1979).

Method

The semi-structured interviews lasted between 1.5 and 2 hours, covering many different aspects of the caring situation. Among the questionnaires completed during this interview were the following.

1   EE was measured using the 'patient rejection scale' which was adapted from the original scale devised by Kreisman et al. (1979). This self-report scale measures both hostility/criticism and warmth expressed by the carer about his or her dependant.
    The author also made subjective judgements of critical comments, hostility, warmth and emotional overinvolvement, which are the traditional components of EE.
2   The 66-item 'Ways of coping checklist' (Folkman and Lazarus, 1980) was used to measure the range and repertoire of coping techniques used by the carer in his or her care-giving role.
3   The Beck depression inventory (Beck and Beamesderfer, 1974) was used to assess symptoms of depression in the carer.
4   The dependants were assessed using the Clifton assessment procedures for the elderly (Pattie and Gilleard, 1979) and the 34-item 'problem checklist' (Gilleard, 1984) was also completed by the carer.

Results

Level of expressed emotion

The mean score on the patient rejection scale was 68 (range 47–99). In a sample of carers with schizophrenic dependants, McReadie and Robinson (1988) obtained a mean score of 68 in a group of high-EE relatives, as categorized by the Camberwell family interview. Thus the level of hostility and criticism would appear to be high for this group of carers.

Critical comments were made by at least twelve of the carers. One of the caring daughters described her mother in the following way:

R: She sits in that chair all day from morning to night and doesn't lift a finger to help. She sees me running about mad getting things done but she'll not even dry a dish.
Another wife described the annoying behaviour of her husband:
R: He's just finished a shave and I see his hand going up to his face again and I think, 'Oh no, here we go', and right enough, he's away back up the stairs shaving himself again. And it doesn't matter how often I say to him.
JW: How do you deal with that?
R: Well I get right mad with him, he's never done with shaving.

The author's judgement regarding the extent of the critical comments correlated well with the PRS score (Pearson's correlation coefficients).

EE and the quality of the carer–dependant relationship

It was not unexpected to find a significant and inverse relationship between the PRS score and the quality of the pre-morbid relationship such that the poorer the relationship had been, the greater the current level of hostility and criticism. This association did not, however, hold regarding the quality of the current relationship despite the fact that in all but one case the carer judged the relationship to have deteriorated. This possibly illustrated some understanding of the disease process on the carers' behalf. Indeed, compared with the author's experience in earlier studies, this sample in general had a good understanding of the dementing process, often from information gleaned through media coverage and relatives' support groups.

This finding was replicated in another study by Gilhooly and Whittick (1989).

EE and carers' psychological wellbeing

High levels of criticism were also expected to have an impact on the carers' psychological wellbeing and indeed the higher the PRS score the more likely the carer was to be depressed, as measured by the Beck depression inventory (Beck and Beamesderfer, 1974). Gilhooly and Whittick (1989) similarly found that the higher the carers' EE the lower was their morale and the poorer were their ratings of mental health. Bledin (1987) reported similar findings in his study.

EE and problem behaviours

As with studies of EE and schizophrenia, the level of hostility was not associated with the frequency or range of problem behaviours. In fact, the more demented the patient, the lower were the carers' levels of hostility and rejection. Perhaps then it is in the early stages when the carer is struggling to understand the dementing process that she is more inclined to be rejecting and hostile towards her dependant. One husband spoke of the early stages of his wife's dementing process:

R: In the early days I probably blamed my wife if things went, you know, not realizing that there was an illness. But I've come to realize over the last 2 years that it's outside of any control, and I've just got to accept that she's got this problem and it's not likely to improve.

Unlike the previous schizophrenic studies the hours of face-to-face contact were not associated with the PRS score. By the very nature of dementia the time spent together was high, on average, 52 hours per week.

Table 21.1 Categories of coping techniques used in response to specific stressful incidents

Coping technique	Example	Col. 1*	Col. 2†	Total no.
Direct action (verbal)	Correction of facts	14	6	20
Acceptance	Accept your lot and face up to your responsibility	5	15	20
Direct action (non-verbal)	Practical solution to the problem	9	10	19
Express feelings	Get angry at dependant	5	6	11
Inhibit feelings	Keep feelings to self	3	8	11
Physical distancing/ avoidance	Go out to garden and leave dependant	3	4	7
Use of tea/cigarettes		4	2	6
Psychological distancing	Change the subject	2	4	6
Maintain patient's independence	Leave him or her to dress him or herself	1	3	4
Hope/positive thinking	Realize the situation will be over one day	0	3	3
Create dependency	Shave dependant as it's quicker	0	3	3
Turn to other activities	Go out to the club	0	2	2
Other		0	3	3

Note: *Col. 1 represents those carers who mentioned technique in response to a specific stressful incident. †Col. 2 represents those carers who mentioned technique as a general way of coping.

COPING IN CARERS

The range of coping techniques

There was an association between the measure of rejection and the range of coping techniques the carer reported he or she used such that the wider the repertoire, the lower the hostility and criticism. This finding has clear implications for intervention. Although the direction of causality is not known, teaching adaptive coping techniques would possibly have the beneficial effect of lowering the level of hostility as has been found in the schizophrenic studies.

Verbal and non-verbal coping techniques

So, for better or worse, how were these carers coping? When asked how they dealt with either a specific stressful incident and more generally how they coped with dementia, a wide variety of responses were made. The categories of methods reported are shown in Table 21.1. All carers at some point took some form of direct verbal action, frequently to argue with their dependant or to correct confused thinking. An elderly caring wife described the following incident with her demented husband:

R: It's just the fact that, he wants to go out to Ann's, his daughter. He wants to go out at night, well he can't go out at night.
JW: Does this happen every night?
R: It happens most nights. He'll take off his slippers and he says to me 'Will you tie my laces?' Next thing, I say 'What are you wanting your shoes on for?' He says 'I'm going to see Ann.' He says 'Are you going?' I say 'I'm not going to see Ann at this time of night.' I say, 'How are you going to get up to the Grange Road from here?' 'Oh', he says, 'it's just round the corner.' So I say, 'Around a few corners?'

Taking direct non-verbal action and finding a practical solution were also usually stated with reference to a specific stressful incident. One daughter described how she had found a practical solution to her mother's wandering.

R: So my mother was wanting out to go home – she's always wanting home, she doesn't realize this is her home, and I have to lock the doors sometimes, both doors in case, because she has run out, so I wouldn't give her the keys.

Coping by acceptance

There was also a general feeling of coping by acceptance but more as a means of dealing with the whole situation as opposed to a specific stressful incident. A husband described his attitude to the caring situation:

R: I take a philosophical sort of view – these things happen and you can't really do much about them.

A wife summed up her general coping strategy as follows:

R: I just accept it because there's nothing one can do except struggle away, and I say, well, he's my responsibility now and you can't put it on other people's shoulders.

Expression and inhibition of the carers' emotions

Expressing feelings or holding back feelings were equally common and reported by about half the carers. Expression of feelings included getting angry and shouting at the dependant while inhibition of feelings included such things as keeping one's feelings to oneself.

The most common ways of coping

The most frequently endorsed items on the 'ways of coping checklist' are shown in Table 21.2. It is interesting that these commonly used techniques tend to be emotion-focused as opposed to practical or problem-focused. At this stage it is not known to what extent these cognitive strategies may be beneficial. They perhaps reflect a feeling of helplessness with regard to their situation and a feeling that in practical terms little can be done to resolve the situation. More practical techniques, e.g., 'I'm making a plan of action and following it' or 'I think about how a person I admire would handle this situation and use that as a model' could be used but are perhaps difficult to implement without some instruction. If this transpires to be so, then there would be a strong case for counselling and training in specific coping skills.

Coping and carers' psychological wellbeing

There was a relationship between the range of coping techniques the carer endorsed and depression such that the narrower the carer's repertoire the more likely he or she was to report symptoms of depression. This suggests that educational interventions may be beneficial in the treatment of the depressive symptoms, in the form of training carers in a variety of adaptive coping techniques.

Those carers whose dependants were the most severely demented seemed to use the widest range of coping techniques indicating that carers can adapt to the deteriorating condition of their relative. Experienced carers may also have a lot to offer novice carers beyond general support and understanding.

Table 21.2 The most frequently endorsed items (n > 15) on the 'ways of coping checklist'

Item	n
1. Maintain my pride and keep a stiff upper lip	20
2. I try to keep my feelings from interfering with other things too much	20
3. I try to see things from the other person's point of view	19
4. Look for the silver lining, so to speak; try to look on the bright side of things	19
5. I remind myself how much worse things could be	18
6. I wish that I could change what is happening or how I feel	18
7. I accept it, since nothing can be done	18
8. I'm getting professional help	18
9. I try to keep my feelings to myself	18
10. I just concentrate on what I have to do next – the next step	17
11. I try not to burn my bridges but leave things open somewhat	17
12. I accept the next best thing to what I want	17
13. I try not to act too hastily or follow my first hunch	17
14. I pray	16
15. I know what has to be done so I am doubling my efforts to make things work	16
16. I make light of the situation; refuse to get too serious about it	16
17. I go along with fate; sometimes I just have bad luck	16

CONCLUSIONS

Studies like this are now establishing that high EE does exist among carers of the dementing elderly. Where EE is high the carer's psychological wellbeing tends to be poor. Furthermore, in high-EE carers the range of coping techniques used seems to be limited and this also seems to be related to poorer mental health.

Although the direction of causality is not known, it seems likely that intervention by education and counselling could offer a great deal to reduce emotional distress in carers by teaching good coping techniques and reducing high EE. There is much to be gained from looking at the successful interventions with families with schizophrenic dependants.

As is the case with schizophrenia, high EE has little to do with the level of dependency or problems of the dementing person. EE may have more to do with an existing personality type and further exploration of the locus of control concept and EE may be helpful.

It now seems clear that the pre-morbid relationship is influential in determining the level of EE.

Finally, the exploration of coping techniques is new and further clarification of adaptive versus maladaptive strategies is needed. As the number of informal carers in the community is increasing answers to these questions are urgently needed.

ACKNOWLEDGEMENTS

The author would like to thank the Alzheimer's Disease Society for sponsoring the ongoing research and Dr Mary Gilhooly for her helpful supervision of the project. The author is also grateful to the carers who gave up their valuable time to participate in the project.

REFERENCES

Archbold, P.G. (1981) 'Impact of parent caring on women', paper presented at the Twelfth International Congress of Gerontology, Hamburg, West Germany.

Beck, A.T. and Beamesderfer, A. (1974) 'Assessment of depression: the depression inventory', *Psychological Measurements in Psychopharmacology. Modern Problems in Pharmacopsychiatry* 7: 151–69.

Bledin, K. (1987) 'Expressed emotion in daughters of people with dementia', paper presented at the British Psychological Society Conference, London.

Brown, G.W., Monck, E.M., Carstairs, G.M. and Wing, J.K. (1962) 'The influence of family life on the course of schizophrenic illness', *British Journal of Preventive and Social Medicine* 16: 55–68.

—— , Birley, J.L.T. and Wing, J.K. (1972) 'Influence of family life on the course of schizophrenic disorders: a replication', *British Journal of Psychiatry* 121: 241–58.

—— , Carstairs, G.M. and Topping, G.C. (1958) 'The post hospital adjustment of chronic mental patients', *Lancet* 2: 685–9.

Coyne, J.C., Aldwin, C. and Lazarus, R.S. (1981) 'Depression and coping in stressful episodes', *Journal of Abnormal Psychology* 90 (5): 439–47.

Fadden, G., Bebbington, P. and Kuipers, L. (1987) 'The burden of care: the impact of functional psychiatric illness on the patients' family', *British Journal of Psychiatry* 150: 285–92.

Folkman, S. and Lazarus, R.S. (1980) 'An analysis of coping in a middle-aged community sample', *Journal of Health and Social Behavior* 21: 219–39.

Freire, M., Roy, A., Blake, P. and Seeman, M.V. (1982) 'Rejection in parents of schizophrenic outpatients correlates with time spent together', *Comprehensive Psychiatry* 23: 190–3.

Gilhooly, M.L.M. (1984) 'The social dimensions of senile dementia', in I. Hanley and J. Hodge (eds) *Psychological Approaches to the Care of the Elderly*, London: Croom Helm.

—— (1987) 'Senile dementia and the family', in J. Orford (ed.) *Coping With Disorder in the Family*, London: Croom Helm.

—— and Whittick, J.E. (1989) 'Expressed emotion in caregivers of the dementing elderly', *British Journal of Medical Psychology* 62: 265–72.

Gilleard, C.J. (1984) *Living with Dementia: Community Care of the Elderly Mentally Infirm*, London: Croom Helm.

Havstad, L.F. (1979) 'Weight loss and weight loss maintenance as aspects of family emotional processes', unpublished doctoral thesis, University of Southern California.

Hogarty, G.E., Anderson, C.M., Reiss, D.J., Kornblith, S.J., Greenwald, D.P., Jauna, C.D. and Madonia, M.J. (1986) 'Family psychoeducation, social skills training, and maintenance chemotherapy in the aftercare treatment of schizophrenia', *Archives of General Psychiatry* 43: 633–42.

Hooley, J.M. (1986) 'Expressed emotion: a review of the critical literature', *Clinical Psychology Review* 5: 119–39.

Hooley, J.M., Orley, J. and Teasedale, J.D. (1986) 'Levels of expressed emotion and relapse in depressed patients', *British Journal of Psychiatry* 148: 642–7.

Johnson, C.L. and Catelona, D.J. (1982) 'A longitudinal study of family supports to impaired elderly', paper presented at the 35th Annual Scientific Meeting of the Gerontological Society of America, Boston, USA, November.

Koenisberg, H.W. and Handley, R. (1986) 'Expressed emotion: from predictive index to clinical construct', *American Journal of Psychiatry* 143: 1361–73.

Kreisman, D.E., Simmons, S.J. and Joy, V.D. (1979) 'Rejecting the patient: preliminary validation of a self-report scale', *Schizophrenia Bulletin* 5: 220–2.

Leff, J. and Vaughn, C. (1980) 'The interaction of life events and relatives' expressed emotion in schizophrenia and depressive neurosis', *British Journal of Psychiatry* 136: 146–53.

—— and Vaughn, C. (1981) 'The role of maintenance therapy and relatives' expressed emotion in relapse schizophrenia: a two year follow up', *British Journal of Psychiatry* 139: 102–4.

——, Kuipers, L., Berkowitz, R. Eberlein-Uries, R. and Sturgeon, D. (1982) 'A controlled trial of social intervention in the families of schizophrenic patients', *British Journal of Psychiatry* 141: 121–34.

McCreadie, R. and Robinson, A.O.T. (1988) 'The Nithsdale schizophrenia survey: VI. Relatives' expressed emotion: prevalence, patterns and clinical assessment', *British Journal of Psychiatry* 150: 640–4.

Minuchin, S., Baker, L., Rosman, B.L., Liebman, R., Milnan, L. and Todd, T. (1975) 'A conceptual model of psychosomatic illness in children: family organization and family therapy', *Archives of General Psychiatry* 32: 1031–8.

Moffat, N. (1987) 'Brain damage and the family', in J. Orford (ed.) *Coping with Disorder in the Family*, London: Croom Helm.

Orford, J. (1987) (ed.) *Coping with Disorder in the Family*, London: Croom Helm.

——, O'Reilly, P. and Goonatilleke, A. (1987) 'Expressed emotion and perceived family interaction in the key relatives of elderly patients with dementia', *Psychological Medicine* 17: 963–70.

Pattie, A.H. and Gilleard, C.J. (1979) *Manual for the Clifton Assessment Procedures for the Elderly*, Sevenoaks, Kent: Hodder & Stoughton Educational.

Pearlin, L.I. and Schooler, C. (1978) 'The structure of coping', *Journal of Health and Social Behaviour* 19: 2–21.

Rotter, J.B. (1966) 'Generalized expectancies for internal versus external control of reinforcement', *Psychological Monographs: General and Applied* 80: 1–28.

Schoeneman, S.Z., Reznikoft, M. and Bacon, S.J. (1983) 'Personality variables in coping with the stress of a spouse's chronic illness', *Journal of Clinical Psychology* 39: 430–6.

Smith, J.V.E. and Birchwood, M.J. (1987) 'Specific and non-specific effects of educational interventions with families of schizophrenic patients', *British Journal of Psychiatry* 150: 645–52.

Snyder, K.S., Jenkins, J.H., Nuechterlein, K.H. and Mintz, J. (1988) 'An expeditious technique for estimating the expressed emotion of relatives of recent onset schizophrenic patients', unpublished paper.

Valone, K., Norton, J.P., Goldstein, M.J. and Doane, J.A. (1983) 'Parental expressed emotion and affective style in an adolescent sample at risk for schizophrenia spectrum disorders', *Journal of Abnormal Psychology* 92: 399–407.

Vaughn, C.E. and Leff, J.P. (1976a) 'The measurement of expressed emotion in the families of psychiatric patients', *British Journal of Social and Clinical Psychology* 15: 157–65.

—— and Leff, J.P. (1976b) 'The influence of family and social factors on the course

of psychiatric illness', *British Journal of Psychiatry* 129: 125–37.
Vaughn, C.E., Snyder, K.S., Jones, S., Freeman, W. and Falloon, I. (1984) 'Family factors in schizophrenic relapse', *Archives of General Psychiatry* 41: 1169–77.
Watzl, H., Rist, F. and Cohen, R. (1986) 'The patient rejection scale: cross-cultural consistency', *Schizophrenia Bulletin* 12: 236–8.
Whittick, J.E. (1988) 'Dementia and mental handicap: emotional distress in carers', *British Journal of Clinical Psychology* 27: 167–72.
Zarit, J.M. (1982) 'Predictors of burden and distress for caregivers of senile dementia patients', unpublished doctoral dissertation, University of Southern California.

Chapter 22

Families and the institutionalized elderly

Carolyn Rosenthal and Pam Dawson

SUMMARY

This chapter focuses on the families of institutionalized elderly. Families are an important source of assistance to the community-dwelling elderly and continue to be important in the lives of institutionalized elderly. The chapter has two objectives: (1) to provide an overview of the importance of families to both community-dwelling and institutionalized elderly and (2) to examine the experiences of wives following the institutionalization of elderly husbands. In pursuing the second objective, while the empirical examination will be confined to wives, the findings apply to spouses of institutionalized elders, whether wives or husbands. A conceptual model, developed from a pilot study, will be presented. The model depicts four stages in the process experienced by wives. The major characteristics of each stage lead to calling stage I 'Ambivalence/uncertainty', stage II 'Assisting/action', stage III 'Relinquishing/augmenting' and stage IV 'Adaptation/resolution'. The distinctive characteristics of each stage imply that different types of interventions are appropriate at different stages.

INTRODUCTION

The chapter begins with a literature review of the families of older people in three distinct contexts: (1) when older family members are relatively healthy; (2) when the health of older family members deteriorates but the elder remains in the community and (3) when the elder is in a long-term care facility, that is a type of continuing-care facility in which the majority of clients are expected to remain as residents for the duration of their lives. In such settings, paid health workers, rather than family members, are the 'official' care-givers. The chapter then turns to its second focus: the experiences of wives of institutionalized elderly men. The discussion, however, applies in most instances to spouses of institutionalized elders, whether wives or husbands. The focus of interest is the process of adaptation experienced by spouses following the institutionalization of their mate. We call this process 'quasi-widowhood' to indicate the paradoxical situation of being without a spouse, in many respects, although one's spouse still lives. This process is viewed in terms of a conceptual model consisting of four stages. The study from which the model was derived is described with respect to setting, methodology and results. Then, the conceptual model derived from the study is presented, with each of the four stages described in detail. Finally, interventions appropriate to each stage are suggested.

It is the argument of the chapter that, when a spouse is institutionalized, the experiences of family members follow an overall predictable pattern, and it is on this broad pattern that we focus. We recognize that there will be variations based on the care-giving situation prior to entering the institution. For example, a wife who has provided a high level of care to a severely impaired elder for a long period of time will probably be more physically and emotionally exhausted but in less of a state of shock than a wife whose husband suffered a sudden, severe stroke and entered the long-term care facility following a period of time in an acute-care hospital. We also expect that variations in the process will be related to different health conditions of the institutionalized elder. For example, a wife whose husband has severe physical impairment will still be able to communicate and talk things over with him. Her sense of loss of a person she once knew will likely be less than in the case of a wife whose husband has severe cognitive impairment. There are undoubtedly numerous ways in which the process will differ among individuals, but we argue that the broad outlines of the process, such as we describe in our model, should be very similar. For this reason, in keeping with the general focus of this volume, we suggest that the model is applicable to, but not limited to, the spouses of persons with Alzheimer's disease. Further, while the discussion in the chapter focuses on wives, or, somewhat more generally, on spouses, it provides a basis for considering the process experienced by other types of relatives, particularly adult children of institutionalized elderly.

THE IMPORTANCE OF THE FAMILY IN THE LIVES OF THE ELDERLY

The great majority of older people are embedded in families. For most older people, their spouse and their grown children are the most important family members in their lives. Grandchildren are important, too, as are siblings, but the key relatives in terms of various kinds of social meaning and social support remain spouses and children.

Families are important to people for a variety of reasons and in a variety of ways. Families are important symbolically in that it is through one's family that one maintains ties to the past and the future. Families provide a sense of personal meaning in life. At a very practical level, family members help one another in innumerable small and not-so-small ways.

A large body of research has documented the importance of the family in the lives of both the healthy and impaired community-dwelling elderly (e.g. Brody, 1985; Horowitz, 1985; Rosenthal, 1987; Shanas with Heinemann, 1982). In contrast, very little research has focused on the families of institutionalized elderly (for exceptions see: Bowers, 1988; Montgomery, 1982; Rubin and Shuttlesworth, 1983; Smith and Bengtson, 1979). Perhaps this neglect reflects an implicit assumption that, following institutionalization, families cease to be important because paid health workers take on the care-giving role. An additional assumption may be that people in institutions have families who do not care about them, or, indeed, who have abandoned them. Ironically, both assumptions are profoundly misguided.

While it is true that families are one of the key mechanisms in preventing or postponing institutionalization of elderly persons, it is also the case that most institutionalized elders have relatives, and for this reason knowing more about the family relationships of institutionalized elders is important. The small body of research that has focused on families of institutionalized elderly has recognized the continuing importance of family members in the lives of these older persons, and, moreover, has recognized the importance of family members as providers of patient care as well as potential recipients of care. Research has also recognized that the family can be perceived as a 'problem' by the institution's staff.

We turn now to a brief review of literature concerning the families of older people, first in the context of the relatively healthy or 'well elderly', then in the context of impaired elderly in the community, and finally in the context of institutionalization.

Families and the relatively healthy elderly

While much recent research has focused on the highly impaired elderly, it should be remembered that most older people are quite healthy. Even at advanced ages, only a minority are in poor health (Chappell et al., 1986: 33–52). Most older people, then, can be viewed as relatively healthy, although there is a considerable range of health status and accompanying health needs. We feel it is important to distinguish between this group and elderly who have experienced serious health losses and require high levels of care.

Much recent research has examined the role of adult children in providing assistance to elderly parents. Norms of filial obligation specifying the obligations of children to help their parents are widely held by family members of older and younger generations alike (Brody et al., 1984). The actual role of norms in children's helping behaviour, however, is complex. Cicirelli (1983), drawing on attachment theory (Bowlby, 1979; 1980), found that the adult child's attachment behaviours to the elderly parent were a function of feelings of attachment, the needs of the parent, and norms of filial obligation. Helping behaviour was a function of attachment behaviours and the dependency needs of the parent. Both feelings of attachment and norms of filial obligation had only an indirect effect, through their effect on attachment behaviours.

In focusing on the help adult children provide to older parents, we should not lose sight of the fact that adult children and their parents are involved in mutual exchanges of assistance throughout the adult life course (for reviews, see Lee, 1980; Rosenthal, 1987). This assistance may take the form of financial aid, gifts, services such as baby sitting, help with transportation or errands, doing home repairs or yard work, providing advice, personal care, care in illness such as providing home nursing care during convalescence from an operation, helping out in a crisis, helping out during a move to a new home and so on. Another type of help – emotional or 'moral' support – is less tangible but very important and very common.

One important type of help provided in families is health care assistance. A number of studies have shown that most routine health care assistance to the elderly is provided by families (Brody, 1978; Comptroller General of the United States, 1977; Rakowski and Hickey, 1980; Shanas and Maddox, 1976; Tobin and Kulys, 1980). This may involve providing direct service or obtaining needed services by acting as a 'linkage' between the older person and the health care system (Sussman, 1977).

The overall pattern for help between parents and children is one of reciprocity, although with advancing age there is a decrease in the proportion of older people who help children and an increase in the proportion who receive help. It is important to note, however, that even among people aged 75 and over, a majority still report helping children, according to a national survey in the United States (Shanas with Heinemann, 1982). Similarly, a Canadian study of people aged 70 and older found that 84 per cent of older men and 71 per cent of older women who had children had given help to their children during the year preceding the interview and 80 per cent of the men and 84 per cent of the women had received help (Rosenthal, 1987). Each generation helps the other, although the specific type of help varies between the generations. In the Canadian study referred to above, older people gave more child care, financial assistance and advice than they received. Children provided more practical assistance, such as help with personal services, household chores, home repairs and personal care.

In western industrialized societies, the exchange of help among adult family members is ubiquitous. When people need help, they typically turn to family members. In the US and in Canada, the relative to whom one turns for help follows a principle of substitution (Cumming and Schneider, 1961; Shanas, 1979a). People tend to turn first to a spouse. Lacking a spouse, they turn to an adult child. Lacking kin in either of these categories, they will turn to a sibling, followed by other relatives, friends and neigh-bours. It seems likely that a similar pattern of help-seeking would be found in Britain. In Canada, Britain and the US, family care is typically provided by women – wives, daughters, daughters-in-law and sisters (Walker, 1983).

Over the life course, then, families provide help to their members, including older members. The amounts may be small or large, depending on the needs and resources of the particular family. Social-class differences are relevant, as are differences among ethnic groups. The overall picture, however, is one of lifelong patterns of mutual assistance and of support. In the normal course of aging, people tend to require increased assistance because of health losses and changes such as widowhood, among others. We view this kind of help as being part of normal family life. Adult children may today anticipate that they will at some point have a widowed mother who will need increased emotional support and perhaps tangible services such as help with yard work and home maintenance. With longer life, couples may typically anticipate a period of time when they provide small but vital kinds of help to one another that are required because of declining health.

However, there is another stage beyond what we have been considering. This occurs when an elderly person suffers serious health losses and comes to require a high level of care. Here we are no longer talking about helping out with household chores but rather about round-the-clock nursing care, tending to an elder who cannot leave the house or who is bedridden, who perhaps cannot look after his or her own toilet and so on. This brings us to a consideration of families and care-giving to impaired elders.

Families as care-givers to the community-dwelling impaired elderly

Health losses that are consequential in terms of daily functioning and the need for assistance tend not to occur until fairly advanced ages – in the late seventies for men and the mid-eighties for women (Marshall et al., 1983). When serious decrements in health occur, family care-giving emerges as a pivotal concern. Research suggests that in the UK for every institution-alized elder there are two equally disabled people living in the community (Shanas, 1979b). In Britain, the ratio is even higher, with three disabled elders in the community for every one person in an institution (Townsend, 1981:96). While the figures in other countries may be higher or lower, the underlying point is that it is the presence of a family member (or members) able to provide a high level of care that enables such older persons to remain in the community.

The care-givers to the impaired elderly are primarily women – wives, daughters and daughter-in-law. The burdens of care-giving are extensive. In a national survey in the US, Stone et al. (1987) found that, on average, care-givers spent 4 extra hours per day on care-giving tasks. Most care-givers had been providing assistance for 1 to 4 years, but one-fifth had been caring for the disabled person for 5 years or more. Spousal care-givers were the most likely to provide assistance every day.

The burden on adult daughters who become care-givers to impaired elderly parents has been well documented (Brody, 1985; Horowitz, 1985; Walker, 1983). Daughters in this situation are often referred to as 'women in the middle', the 'caught generation' or the 'sandwich generation' to denote the competing obligations to family members in different generations experienced by middle-aged women, many of whom are also in the paid labour force.

Concerns about 'women in the middle' should not deflect attention from the fact that many care-givers to the elderly are, in fact, spouses (Stone *et al.*, 1987). While care-giving spouses may experience fewer competing commitments than adult children do, they are more vulnerable because they are in their later years, and are more likely to themselves be in poor health or vulnerable to health loss. Indeed, as Fengler and Goodrich (1979) pointed out, they are often the 'hidden patients'. Some studies of care-giver burden have found that burden is greater for spouses than children (Cantor, 1983; George and Gwyther, 1986), although other studies have found no differences in burden between spouses and children (Robinson, 1983; Zarit *et al.*, 1980).

While the burdens of providing care to a severely impaired elder are great, families none the less strive for as long as possible to avoid placing the relative in an institution. In some families, though, a point is reached where institutionalization can no longer be avoided. What is it that tips the balance, that leads to a breakdown in the care-giving situation and the institutionalization of a loved one? The answer appears to be more strongly related to characteristics of the care-giver, including deteriorating health and perceived burden, than to the objective condition of the care-receiver (Chenoweth and Spencer, 1986; George and Gwyther, 1986; Zarit *et al.*, 1986).

The families of the institutionalized elderly

While most studies of care-giving have focused on care-givers to community-dwelling elderly (for exceptions, see George and Gwyther, 1986; Chenoweth and Spencer, 1986), there is no reason to assume that family care-giving ceases once an elder is institutionalized. Thinking beyond the confines of care-giving as a concept, we should assume that family relationships continue beyond institutionalization. While relationships may change due to changing circumstances, and while care-giving, too, may be altered, overall we may think of institutionalization as a point on a continuum of family caring.

One of the first studies to consider family relationships following institutionalization was conducted by Smith and Bengtson (1979). They found that in the great majority of cases the relationship between adult children and their institutionalized parents was viewed either as having improved, in terms of emotional closeness, or having remained the same. Improvement generally was related to relief from the former strain resulting from the parent's problems.

Glaser and Strauss (1965), studying families of dying patients in acute-care hospitals, were among the first social scientists to document the work that family members contribute to the care of hospitalized patients. In another study in the acute-care setting, Rosenthal *et al.* (1980) found that these contributions by families could be problematic in that they sometimes led to conflict with staff. Shuttlesworth *et al.* (1982) (see also Rubin and Shuttlesworth, 1983) showing that some of this conflict stems from ambiguity concerning whether the family or the health professional should be responsible for various tasks.

Studies have also recognized that family members of institutionalized persons have needs of their own to which health workers should attend. Support groups for family members are premised on recognition of these needs. When health workers in an institution focus on the needs of the family member of a patient, they are viewing the family member as a patient or client.

Thus, some research has concentrated on the family as worker or resource, while other research has concentrated on the family as client. That is, while most research implies that the role includes both dimensions, studies have tended to emphasize either one or the other, and to develop recommendations based on the emphasized theme.

Several studies emphasize the family as client and suggest a variety of approaches to meet family members' needs. Montgomery (1982) explicitly states that family members must be actively served as clients in order to achieve positive family relations. Additional recommendations include involving families in care-planning, providing specific activities and meetings for family members, ensuring availability of social work and administrative personnel during peak visiting hours, and creating rules, regulations and practices that provide a message of welcome to families. Strow and MacKreth (1977) feel that approaching the family as a client would have positive effects on the patient. They argue that effective family support will assist patients in the transition to institutionalization. They also recommend that families be more actively involved in a true partnership through which they can explore and verbalize their feelings. Greene (1982) feels that families can be assisted by examining the process leading to institutionalization through ongoing case work and group discussion, and by assisting staff in making the environment conducive to family interaction.

Other studies emphasize the role of family as resource and make recommendations accordingly. Shuttlesworth *et al.* (1982) suggest that a close partnership between families and institutions may depend on the degree of clarity regarding subdivision of their tasks and the degree to which institutions encourage and support family involvement in appropriate aspects of care (see also the idea of a family contract, Chapter 7, this volume). Rubin and Shuttlesworth (1983) recommend orientation sessions to clarify the subdivision of task between staff and families in five categories: personalizing care, monitoring and ensuring provision of care, clothing needs, grooming and providing reading material. They also recommend that periodic conferences take place between staff and family. Smith and Bengtson (1979) feel that the role of the family as resource would be enhanced by the incorporation of children and grandchildren into programmes within an institution. They suggest that this could be accomplished through the inclusion of families in activities, instruction in ways that they could give care, and the provision of orientation sessions and education programmes.

From the family-as-client perspective, a variety of planned approaches are regarded as necessary to enable professionals to help family members. From the family as resource perspective, it is viewed as necessary to develop the role of the family through purposeful collaboration and enlightened involvement. Most studies imply that families may be viewed from the perspective of both client and resource, but they do not specify which family role should be emphasized at any point in time and how this might be assessed. In order to make such assessments and decisions, Clark and Rakowski (1981) call for exploration of the psychological and interpersonal stages of care-giving. On this basis, a 'fit' between programmes and participants needs to be established. With such needs in mind, we undertook the study and developed the model described in the following sections.

THE PROCESS OF THE FAMILY MEMBER'S ADAPTATION TO THE INSTITUTIONALIZATION OF A RELATIVE

The pilot study

Background

As indicated in the previous section, a number of scholars have urged that greater attention be given to the needs of family members of institutionalized elderly, and have emphasized the role of the family as resource or client or both. Missing from these works, however, was a sense of process and timing.

Based on our analysis of existing literature as well as on the clinical experience of one of the authors, we felt that the adaptation of family members to the institutionalization of a relative and the family member's assumption of an altered care-giving role should be viewed as a process. Further, in the course of this process, we hypothesized that there might well be periods when the client role should take precedence over the resource role, while at other periods the resource role might take precedence. We feel that identifying the patterns in this process would enable practitioners to design and administer interventions at appropriate times, enhancing both the wellbeing of family members and the wellbeing of patients to whom these family members continue to provide care. With such goals in mind, we decided to conduct a pilot study of family members' experiences following the institutionalization of a relative.

Questions

Specifically, our questions were: (1) Is there an identifiable process experienced over time by a family member of an institutionalized elderly relative following the relative's admission? (2) What are the components of this process?

Methods

The study was conducted in the Extended Care Department of Sunnybrook Medical Centre, University of Toronto, Canada. Most patients in the hospital's 400-bed, chronic care unit are elderly; 90 per cent are male veterans, 49 per cent of whom have wives. About 70 per cent of the patients have cognitive impairment. Patient-related costs are covered by a combination of provincial health insurance and benefits from the Department of Veterans' Affairs. As a result of these arrangements, there are no direct charges to patients and families.

In-depth interviews, lasting on average 1 hour and 30 minutes, were conducted with fourteen wives of patients. The participants had been identified by the head nurses as appearing to have successfully adapted to the situation of institutionalization. The interviews were retrospective and focused on respondents' feelings, actions and perceptions at given periods of time. Questions were open-ended and probed specified areas for elaboration if necessary. Specifically, the interview content enquired about the feelings of the wives at the time of admission (e.g. guilt, depression, exhaustion, grief, uncertainty, denial), the factors which contributed to or hindered a resolution of earlier perceived problems, and when and how these problems were resolved.

Results and discussion

Wives were asked about their feelings at the time of admission. As Table 21.1 shows, almost all respondents reported at least one negative feeling at the time of their husband's admission, and indeed half reported two or more such feelings. Guilt and sadness were most frequently reported, followed by loneliness, a sense of shock or devastation, depression, anxiety, anger and resentment. In addition to the prevalence of negative feelings, a majority of wives said they had been in poor health at the time of the husband's admission. Although far more negative than positive feelings were reported, wives did recall some positive feelings. Primarily, almost all said they had experienced feelings of gratitude that their husband had been placed in this particular institution and was receiving good care. While these comments implied feelings of relief, some wives specifically said they felt relief at the time of admission.

One theme to emerge from the analysis of wives' feelings at the time of admission was ambivalence. That is, wives were both relieved and saddened at the same time. They were relieved or pleased that the husband was in a good institution and was receiving quality care. They recognized that they were no longer able to provide the kind of care their husband required. At the same time, they still wished they could keep their husband at home and felt a variety of negative emotions surrounding the institutionalization. A second theme that seemed to characterize the period around admission was uncertainty. Some wives explicitly said that they had been worried about how they would manage alone. Another type of uncertainty concerned whether the husband might indeed improve enough to return to living at home; that is, some wives at admission retained hope that the institutionalization would be temporary rather than permanent.

In the hospital setting, all wives provided instrumental support to the husband, and most also provided socioemotional support. Some wives specifically described a process suggesting that, once the initial period of exhaustion was over, they had tried to resume the care-giver role at a level that was unrealistic. Over time, however, they lowered the levels of support in order to achieve an appropriate balance between their own needs or abilities and the needs of the husband.

Similarly, visiting frequency was high but had decreased over time, in many cases. Initially, wives tended to visit very frequently, often as much as every day. Many soon found they simply could not manage to maintain that frequency because of health, distance and cost factors. Ultimately, the modal pattern was to limit visits to three or four per week.

Despite the intense emotions and life changes at the time of admission, the wives in the sample had made their adjustments to their altered lives. Most specifically described how they had eventually come to accept their situation. Almost all had come to feel comfortable in the hospital, and most knew some wives of other patients with whom they could share their experiences. Some wives had adapted by building new lives for themselves quite separate from the husband and the hospital, while slightly more reorganized their lives to centre around the husband and the hospital.

These data were highly qualitative in that the interviews were guided by very general questions. The fact that a respondent did not mention feeling

Table 22.1 Wives' reports of feelings, health, activities and adaptation to husbands' institutionalization (n = 14)

	Number and percentage of wives reporting each feeling, etc.	
	n	*(%)*
Negative feelings:		
Guilt	8	(57)
Loneliness	5	(36)
Anxiety	4	(29)
Depression	4	(29)
Anger, resentment	2	(14)
Devastation, 'in shock'	4	(29)
Sadness, wish husband could be at home	9	(64)
Number of negative feelings expressed: 0	1	(7)
1	6	(43)
2	4	(29)
3	0	(0)
4	3	(21)
Expressed one or more negative feelings	13	(93)
Health:		
Own health poor, especially at time of husband's admission	10	(71)
Positive feelings:		
Relief	4	(29)
Grateful for placement/grateful for good care	13	(93)
Ambivalence:		
Wife expressed both relief/gratitude for placement and wish that husband could remain at home	8	(57)
Uncertainty:		
Uncertain about patient's prognosis	2	(14)
Uncertain about ability to manage on own, live alone	3	(21)
Visiting patterns:		
Visits every day	3	(21)
Visits 3–4 times a week	5	(36)
Visits 1–2 times a week	6	(43)
Visiting declined somewhat over time, to a more manageable level	7	(50)
Helping patterns:		
Gives husband instrumental support	14	(100)
Gives husband socioemotional support	11	(79)
Amount of assistance/support declined somewhat over time to more realistic level	4	(29)

Comfort and integration in hospital:		
Feels comfortable in hospital	13	(93)
Knows wives of other patients	11	(79)
Acceptance:		
Expressed eventual acceptance of situation	9	(64)
Adaptation:		
Built new life centring around hospital	8	(57)
Built new life separate from hospital	6	(43)

lonely, for example, did not mean that she did not experience that feeling but only that she did not think to mention it. Thus, the summary of findings in Table 22.1 should be interpreted as showing the minimum rather than actual number of respondents experiencing the various feelings or other indicators.

Wives were also asked to describe how their feelings and situations changed over time. From the analysis summarized in Table 22.1, and from wives' descriptions of changes over time, we constructed a tentative model of the process of response and adaptation to the institutionalization of an elderly spouse (see Figure 22.1). The process appeared to fall into four stages. We turn now to a description and discussion of the model.

The model

The four stages of the model reflect a particular emphasis or adaptive task of the wife. Stage I is one of ambivalence and uncertainty in which attention is focused on one's own feelings. The predominant feeling is that of being 'at the end of one's rope'. In stage II, feelings shift to an interpersonal focus, directed toward the institutionalized spouse. Attempts to perpetuate past patterns in the spouse–patient dyad result in a pattern of assistance. In stage III, relinquishing and augmenting thoughts and behaviours occur. The interpersonal focus is broadened or augmented to incorporate staff as well as other patients and their families. There is an acceptance of altered family norms and relations in which some tasks or responsibilities are relinquished. Stage IV is characterized by resolution or adaptation and the interpersonal focus begins to extend beyond the long-term care setting. New norms continue to be established, both in relations with the patient and hospital and with respect to the wife's own needs and life beyond the institutional setting. These four stages reflect predominant themes which emerged from the interviews. However, within each stage numerous concerns and feelings were identified; we now describe these stages in more detail, using verbatim quotations from the respondents as illustrations. In developing the model, we also drew upon existing literature, as the reader will note.

Figure 22.1 Tentative model

PROCESS EXPERIENCED BY FAMILY MEMBERS AFTER ADMISSION OF A RELATIVE

STAGE I	STAGE II
END OF ROPE: *LEADS TO* POSITIVE AND NEGATIVE RESPONSES	PERPETUATION OF FAMILY NORM/RELATIONS: *LEADS TO* ASSISTING PATIENT WHERE POSSIBLE AND WITHOUT GUIDANCE
AMBIVALENCE/UNCERTAINTY	ASSISTING/ACTION
INTRAPERSONAL FOCUS	SHIFT TO INTERPERSONAL FOCUS (PATIENT CENTRED)

STAGE III	STAGE IV
ACCEPTED ALTERED FAMILY NORMS/RELATIONS AND ROLE OF HOSPITAL: *LEADS TO* DIFFERENTIATING AREAS OF PATIENT ASSISTANCE WHERE FAMILY MOST APPROPRIATE	ESTABLISH NEW NORMS/ RELATIONS WITH PATIENT AND HOSPITAL: *LEADS TO* BALANCING OWN NEEDS WITH PATIENT'S NEEDS
RELINQUISHING/AUGMENTING	RESOLUTION/ADAPTATION
BROADENING OF INTERPERSONAL FOCUS (STAFF, OTHER PATIENTS)	INTERPERSONAL FOCUS EXTENDS BEYOND SETTING

Stage I: ambivalence/uncertainty

At admission, intrapersonal concerns predominate: depression, low morale, isolation, loneliness, precarious health, guilt, resentment, anger and sorrow (Crossman *et al.*, 1981; Fengler and Goodrich, 1979). One wife described her condition this way: 'I felt devastated. I just didn't know what to do. I felt terribly depressed ... withdrawn.' The wife is uncertain both about her own future and the patient's prognosis. Ambivalence arises from feeling relief and gratitude that the patient is receiving a level of care the wife could not provide, yet sorrow over the loss of love and companionship and over the need for institutionalization. All these feelings are mixed with guilt, as respondents' comment show.

> I felt terrible. I was thinking I shouldn't have to do this. The day I brought him in, I felt like bundling him up and taking him home. Then, I realized that I was doing the best thing I could for him.
> I'm happy he's here. I don't feel he could get better care. But why did this have to happen to us?

Ambivalence also arises from simultaneously feeling optimistic yet apprehensive about the future. The major task is working through emotional states and beginning to seek resolutions of ambivalent feelings.

Stage II: assisting/action

With improved physical and mental health (Godkin *et al.*, 1983), wives begin to focus on interpersonal concerns. The wife–patient relationship, while not previously dormant, increases in salience. Depending on the patient's cognitive status, positive affect in the relationship is likely (Montgomery, 1982; Smith and Bengtson, 1979). Mutuality in the relationship influences wives' morale (Hirschfeld, 1983). Visiting is frequent but not enjoyable (York and Calsyn, 1977). Our data suggest that in stage II wives visit more often than they can comfortably manage. For example, one wife said: 'When he first came, I visited every day, but I had to cut it down. Now I come four times a week.'

This same excess often characterizes tasks performed for the patient, as the wife seeks to perpetuate the relationship and role expectations that existed prior to admission. Emerging from the emotional and physical debilitation of stage I, the wife may overzealously devote herself to the patient, perhaps to cope with the guilt or the uncertainty which persists through this stage. Differing norms regarding role tasks may be held by wives and staff, leading to conflict as wives seek to re-establish control over their situation (Shuttlesworth *et al.*, 1982).

Stage III: relinquishing/augmenting

In this stage, wives negotiate with themselves and staff towards altered definitions of responsibility, appropriate behaviour and task performance. Feasible patterns of visiting and assistance become established. Although affect between wife and patient remains positive, the wife's interpersonal focus broadens as she expands socially within the institution. A growing acceptance of an altered spousal relationship and of the staff's role enables the wife to relinquish some tasks. For example, one 90-year-old wife in the study said: 'I used to take his clothes home to be washed – then the nurse told me it wasn't necessary, that I shouldn't trouble myself.' An altered role definition enables the wife to set more reasonable visiting patterns. With staff, role clarity increases as, optimally, do confidence and trust.

Stage IV: resolution/adaptation

In this stage, the wife achieves a balance of her own needs with the patient's needs, feels comfortable in the institution, accepts the changed wife–patient relationship and the likelihood of decline in the patient's condition. She has accepted the loss of the person who was her full-time spouse, and learned to live with the situation of 'quasi-widow', a woman alone whose husband still lives. Emotional vulnerability has been overcome and guilt, while never eliminated, is understood and manageable. As one woman whose husband had been in the institution for several years put it:

> There's always guilt. Even to this day I can't help wishing I could do more. There comes a time though when you have to accept the fact that this is how it is ... nothing else can be done ... then the guilt starts fading and you worry less.

The wife's social life is being restructured. For some, this involves a new life outside the hospital, which includes an extension of social supports and involvement, with compartmentalization of the portion of life that still involves the spouse. One woman said: 'He's in one world and I'm in another.' Another woman described her feelings this way: 'This is his home and I have my home. I have to live my own life, separate from his. It's the only way.'

For other women, life is reorganized to centre around the hospital. Regardless of which form of resolution the wife chooses, in this stage uncertainty has given way to relative certainty, predictability and greater feelings of control.

Having described the four stages, we wish to emphasize that our use of the term 'stage' is not meant to imply that each stage is fully separate and distinct from the others. It is quite possible that some characteristics of stage I and stage II may be present simultaneously. As well, a crisis or change in the patient's condition may initiate movement back to earlier stages. While we do not argue that the four stages are inevitably experienced by everyone, nor that they are irreversible or qualitatively distinct from one another, we do feel they capture the predominant feelings and characteristics at periods during the process of adaptation to the spouse's institutionalization.

Figure 22.2 Client versus resource focus for interventions with families following admission of a relative

STAGE I	STAGE II	STAGE III	STAGE IV
AMBIVALENCE/ UNCERTAINTY	ASSISTING/ ACTION	RELINQUISHING/ AUGMENTING	RESOLUTION/ ADAPTATION
FOCUS:	FOCUS:	FOCUS:	FOCUS:
FAMILY AS CLIENT	FAMILY AS CLIENT	FAMILY AS CLIENT/ POTENTIAL RESOURCE	FAMILY AS RESOURCE/ CLIENT AS INDICATED

Interventions for family as 'client' and 'resource'

The stages or phases described in the model can assist nurses and other health professionals in evaluating the relevance of recommended approaches and interventions presented in previous studies for individual family members (see Figure 22.2). For example, a teaching programme during stage I, when an intrapersonal or self-focus predominates, would not be as effective as it might during stage II when the interpersonal focus is broadening. Thus, the model incorporates the need for ongoing assessment over time as well as a rationale for choosing specific interventions. Because the model is based on retrospective recall with a limited sample, it is only tentative and the 'fit' of the programme and participants at this point is primarily speculative. The usefulness of the model can only be determined through its actual application to practice. Keeping in mind the tentative nature of the model, however, we now offer some suggestions regarding interventions that might be appropriate to the various stages. Over and above specific interventions, we also argue that at some stages the wife should be viewed as a client, while at other stages she should be viewed as a resource.

During stage I when ambivalence, uncertainty and an intrapersonal focus predominate, the focus of intervention is primarily on the wife as a client. Encouraging the expression of ambivalent feelings may help the wife work through the conflict she is experiencing. Reminiscence may be of value at this stage. Staff demonstrations of interest in the patient are valued by wives and help to allay guilt. Ongoing meetings with family members permit validation of feelings and provide a basis for open communication. During this period information provided by the wife is kept confidential, rather than shared with the health care team, to facilitate the development of a therapeutic relationship. Although the resource role is not emphasized in this stage, the wife can contribute by providing personal belongings (for example, clothing, family pictures, radio) to the patient. The goal of care during this time is to decrease the ambivalence and conflict felt by the wife and to increase her trust in the new environment.

During stage II, the focus is still on the wife as client. However, since the interpersonal focus has expanded to incorporate the patient, and the wife is involved in assisting and acting on behalf of the patient, interventions can be focused differently. Wives can probably benefit from information related to the hospital such as where they can have privacy with their husband, when and how to arrange outings or passes, and planning and participating in activities. The wife's potential as a resource can be utilized, and her own needs to help the patient met, by her inclusion in care planning and conferences. This is enhanced by enabling the wife to understand the patient's therapeutic programme. When preoccupation with tasks is high, staff–wife division of responsibilities might be clarified. However, if relinquishing at this point is resisted, such clarification should wait until stage III. Meetings between the wife, patient and staff can be of assistance to all and allow the wife to contribute to the welfare of her husband. Because of a broadening interpersonal focus, a wife may now be comfortable expressing feelings and concerns within a wives' support group. The goal during stage II is to legitimize the participation of the wife, with the focus centering primarily on the patient–wife dyad.

During stage III, the focus is on the wife as client and potential resource. As wives begin to relinquish some roles and activities, and to augment or expand their interactions within the institution, they may continue to benefit from ongoing support groups. However, at this point, the role of staff may be that of facilitating a self-help group rather than providing a professionally led support group. Education programmes may be useful to families and may cover diseases of aging, the aging process and developments in gerontology. Further clarification and subdivision of tasks would be appropriate and staff, patient and family group meetings prepare the family to negotiate on an ongoing basis. This predictability for continued interaction through group meetings can free wives to acknowledge and meet their own needs in relation to the needs of others. The goals of stage III are to increase the insight and knowledge of families in regard to a broader context of aging, illness and the institution, and to increase their ability to conduct negotiations with each other, patients and staff.

During stage IV, the focus shifts to the wife as resource, while continuing to respond to the wife as client when necessary. In this stage the interpersonal focus may extent beyond the hospital setting and wives may be able to function more as a resource. Their needs as clients may be more transitory and secondary at this point. Teaching can be offered to enable wives to participate in productive visits. For example, teaching wives skills such as ambulation or reminiscence methods may enable them to make specific therapeutic contributions to the patient's care as well as fulfilling their own needs to offer something definitive to the patient. Regular group meetings will be helpful to sustain the wife's opportunities for negotiation and information sharing. This can create comfort in the relationship between the wife and the institution. Wives can be involved in and contribute to unit or ward activities such as parties or outings if such participation does not conflict with outside interests. When a wife develops outside interests, it is important that she perceive support since she has only learned to accept the guilt she feels, not overcome it. The goal at this stage is for the wife to contribute to the plan of therapy, and to continue to identify and negotiate for the meeting of her own and the patient's needs.

CONCLUSION

In this chapter, we first presented a literature review showing that families are highly involved in the lives of older members. Adult generations in families provide mutual assistance and support throughout adult life. As older members experience age-related health declines, families provide the majority of help enabling impaired elderly to remain living in the community. Families do not 'dump' their older members in institutions. However, should institutionalization become necessary and appropriate, families continue to be actively involved in the lives of institutionalized relatives.

To explore the experiences of families when a member enters a long-term care institution, we undertook a pilot study of wives of institutionalized elderly men. The chapter described this study which consisted of qualitative interviews with fourteen women. From the analysis of the study, we constructed a four-stage model depicting the process of adaptation to a spouse's institutionalization.

The model we presented focused specifically on wives of institutionalized elderly men. In most respects, it could be as suitably applied to men whose wives are institutionalized. Moreover, with modifications, it could be applied to the process experienced by adult children following the institutionalization of a parent. All these situations require research to investigate the validity of the tentative model. The authors are currently engaged in a longitudinal study of wives; the applicability of the model is being tested through data gathered over the 18-month period following the husband's institutionalization. We are encouraged by results from a small study (Hansen, 1988) that explicitly tested and found strong support for the first stage of our model and for the types of interventions we have suggested would be appropriate in that stage.

In suggesting interventions that would be stage-appropriate, we noted that individual therapy seemed appropriate in stage I, professionally led group therapy in stage II, and self-help groups in stages III and IV. This means that professionals need to assess which stage a wife is in prior to beginning therapy. Moreover, the implication is that, ideally, people in stage

II should not be in the same support group as people in stages III and IV.

The suggestions made in this chapter for supporting both the 'client' and 'resource' roles are by no means exhaustive. Rather, they indicate tremendous scope and direction for the professionals who provide health care to the elderly. Many family care-givers, such as those in our study, are themselves aging and require gerontological expertise. The incorporation of families in the planning and implementing of care, in both community and institutional settings, reflects a true gerontological perspective, and can only benefit both patients and their families. We hope that the model presented in this chapter will prove helpful in assisting health professionals to understand and respond to the situations and needs of family members of institutionalized elders.

ACKNOWLEDGEMENTS

The authors gratefully acknowledge the helpful comments of Donna C. Wiancko and Donna Wells. Preparation of this chapter was assisted by the Social Sciences and Humanities Research Council of Canada through a research grant to the authors, and by the Ontario Ministry of Health through a Career Scientist Award to Rosenthal.

REFERENCES

Bowers, B. (1988) 'Family perceptions of care in a nursing home', *Gerontologist* 28: 361–8.
Bowlby, J. (1979) *The Making and Breaking of Affectional Bonds*, London: Tavistock Publications.
—— (1980) *Attachment and Loss (vol.3): Loss, Stress and Depression*, New York: Basic Books.
Brody, E. (1978) 'The aging of the family', *Annals, American Association of Political and Social Science* 438: 13–27.
—— (1985) 'Parent care as a normative family stress', *Gerontologist* 25: 19–29.
——, Johnsen, P. and Fulcomer, M. (1984) 'What should adult children do for elderly parents? Opinions and preferences of three generations of women', *Journal of Gerontology* 39(6): 736–46.
Cantor, M. (1983) 'Strain among caregivers: a study of experience in the United States', *Gerontologist* 23: 597–604.
Chappell, N., Strain, L. and Blandford, A. (1986) *Aging and Health Care: A Social Perspective*, Canada: Holt, Rinehart & Winston.
Chenoweth, B. and Spencer, B. (1986) 'Dementia: the experience of family caregivers', *Gerontologist* 26: 267–72.
Cicirelli, V. (1983) 'Adult children's attachment and helping behavior to elderly parents: a path model', *Journal of Marriage and the Family* 45: 815–25.
Clark, N. and Rakowski, W. (1981) 'Family caregivers of older adults: improving helping skills', *Gerontologist* 19: 438–77.
Comptroller General of the United States (1977) *Report to the Congress: The Well-being of Older People in Cleveland, Ohio*, Washington, D.C.: General Accounting Office.

Crossman, L., London, C. and Barry, C. (1981) 'Older women caring for disabled spouses: a model for supportive services', *Gerontologist* 21: 464–70.

Cumming, E. and Schneider, D. (1961) 'Sibling solidarity: a property of American kinship', *American Anthropologist* 63: 498–507.

Fengler, A. and Goodrich, N. (1979) 'Wives of elderly disabled men: the hidden patients', *Gerontologist* 19: 175–84.

George, L. and Gwyther, L. (1986) 'Caregiver well-being: a multidimensional examination of family caregivers of demented adults', *Gerontologist* 26: 253–9.

Glaser, B. and Strauss, A. (1965) *Awareness of Dying*, Chicago: Aldine.

Godkin, M., Krant, M. and Doster, N. (1983) 'The impact of hospice care on families', *International Journal of Psychiatry in Medicine* 13: 153–65.

Greene, R. (1982) 'Families and the nursing home social worker', *Social Work in Health Care* 7: 57–67.

Hansen, L. (1988) 'Until death do us part: understanding the institutionalization process as it is experienced by the wives of institutionalized elderly men', paper given at the Gerontological Nurses' Association Conference, Kingston, Ontario, April.

Hirschfeld, M. (1983) 'Homecare versus institutionalization: family caregiving and senile brain disease', *International Journal of Nursing Studies* 20: 23–32.

Horowitz, A. (1985) 'Family caregiving to the frail elderly', in C. Eisdorfer (ed.) *Annual Review of Gerontology and Geriatrics*, vol. 5, New York: Springer.

Lee, G. (1980) 'Kinship in the seventies: a decade review of research and theory', *Journal of Marriage and the Family* 44: 217–24.

Marshall, V., Rosenthal, C. and Synge, J. (1983) 'Concerns about parental health', in E. Markson (ed.) *Older Women*, Lexington and Toronto: D.C. Heath.

Montgomery, R. (1982) 'Impact of institutional care policies on family integration', *Gerontologist* 22: 54–8.

Rakowski, W. and Hickey, T. (1980) 'Late life health behaviour: integrating health beliefs and temporal perspectives', *Research on Aging* 2: 283–308.

Robinson, B. (1983) 'Validation of a caregiver strain index', *Journal of Gerontology* 38: 344–8.

Rosenthal, C. (1987) 'Aging and intergenerational relations in Canada', in V. Marshall (ed.) *Aging in Canada: Social Perspectives*, 2nd edn, Markham, Ontario: Fitzhenry & Whiteside.

——, Marshall, V., Macpherson, A. and French, S. (1980) *Nurses, Patients and Families*, London: Croom Helm.

Rubin, A. and Shuttlesworth, G. (1983) 'Engaging families as support resources in nursing home care: ambiguity in the subdivision of tasks', *Gerontologist* 23: 632–6.

Shanas, E. (1979a) 'The family as a social support system in old age', *Gerontologist* 19: 169–74.

—— (1979b) 'Social myth as hypothesis: the case of the family relations of old people', *Gerontologist* 19: 3–9.

—— with Heinemann, G. (1982) *National Survey of the Aged*, Washington, D.C.: Administration on Aging, US Department of Health and Human Services, DHHS Publication No. (OHDS) 83-20425.

—— and Maddox, G. (1976) 'Aging, health and the organization of health resources', in R. Binstock and E. Shanas (eds) *Handbook of Aging and the Social Sciences*, New York: Van Nostrand Reinhold.

Shuttlesworth, G., Rubin, A. and Duffy, M. (1982) 'Families versus institutions: incongruent role expectations in the nursing home', *Gerontologist* 22: 200–8.

Smith, K. and Bengtson, V. (1979) 'Positive consequences of institutionalization:

solidarity between elderly parents and their middle-aged children', *Gerontologist* 19: 438–47.

Stone, R., Cafferta, G. and Sangl, J. (1987) 'Caregivers of the frail elderly: a national profile', *Gerontologist* 27: 616–26.

Strow, C. and Mackreth, R. (1977) 'Family group meetings – strengthening a partnership', *Journal of Gerontological Nursing* 3: 35.

Sussman, M. (1977) 'Family, bureaucracy, and the elderly individual: an organizational/linkage perspective', in E. Shaunas and M. Sussman (eds) *Family, Bureaucracy and the Elderly*, Durham, North Carolina: Duke University Press.

Tobin, S. and Kulys, R. (1980) 'The family and services', in C. Eisdorfer (ed.) *Annual Review of Gerontology and Geriatrics*, New York: Springer.

Townsend, P. (1981) 'Elderly people with disabilities', in A. Walker and P. Townsend (eds) *Disability in Britain*, Oxford: Martin Robertson.

Walker, A. (1983) 'Care for elderly people: a conflict between women and the state', in J. Finch and D. Groves (eds) *A Labour of Love: Women, Work and Caring*, London/Boston/Melbourne/Henley: Routledge & Kegan Paul.

York, J. and Calsyn, R. (1977) 'Family involvement in nursing homes', *Gerontologist* 17: 500–5.

Zarit, S., Reever, K. and Bach-Peterson, J. (1980) 'Relatives of the impaired elderly: correlates of feelings of burden', *Gerontologist* 20: 649–55.

——, Todd, P. and Zarit, J. (1986) 'Subjective burden of husbands and wives as caregivers: a longitudinal study', *Gerontologist* 26: 260–6.

Chapter 23

A carer's group for families of patients with dementia

Pearl Hettiaratchy and Jill Manthorpe

INTRODUCTION

This chapter describes an initiative in work with the informal carers of elderly mentally ill people; group work with carers. These carers, most of whom were related to the mentally frail people, looked after their relatives on a regular day-to-day basis except when the relatives were attending a day hospital. Most of these relatives or patients, as it would seem easier to call them, were dementia sufferers. The groups were a form of planned intervention by the NHS hospital and had specific objectives. They were held weekly at the day hospital for set lengths of time.

We divide the chapter into four sections, initially examining who carers are and their special needs. Second, we describe some of the particular 'mechanics' of the groups for carers, including comments on the organization needed within an agency in order to promote such initiatives. The specific role of the group facilitator and other associated staff are outlined, as well as how groups may be evaluated. The advantages and drawbacks of running a group are discussed. In the third section we describe one case history to illustrate how groupwork can positively affect an individual family, and in the final section we consider the implications of such groupwork for the carers, the patients and other support services. The potential of this approach in other settings, how best to communicate our results, and how to learn from others across the artificial divides of health and other welfare services, are explored.

SECTION ONE

The starting point for describing a new initiative in service delivery is to explore its aim. This is particularly important when describing work with relatives or carers[1] because the focus of attention within health services is traditionally the individual patient not the carer. Doctors and nurses rarely examine their relationships with carers. In some instances, carers may be seen as partners; sharing care, continuing treatment or as some form of unskilled 'minders' who have the potential to support or undo the work of professionals. But in many cases, carers are ignored or taken for granted.

The different views of hospital staff and carers are a possible source of tension. It is realistic to recognize this rather than to assume everyone has common aims. In supporting carers, for instance, it is important not to assume that what is good for the patient is good for the carer, or vice versa. This means that any agency or service considering establishing a group to support carers should clarify its aims, distinguish its targets and clearly specify the purpose of the proposed support group.

A dominant purpose must be to serve the needs of the carers: 'By definition, the basic and overall purpose of whoever conducts a helping group is to benefit its members' (Whitaker, 1985).

As these are needs as identified by hospital staff, not simply voiced by the carers, it may be useful to identify the sort of people who are likely to be carers and the types of need they will have. There is little doubt that the numbers of carers who look after elderly mentally ill relatives will increase. As numbers of very old people grow so do the numbers of very old people with illnesses such as dementia. The incidence of organic brain disease has been estimated at 6 per cent in the over-65 age group but among the very old, the over-80s, it is estimated at over 20 per cent (BMA's Board of Science and Education, 1986).

This affects carers in a number of ways. It means there will be more carers and that they are likely to be either elderly themselves, especially if the spouse or sibling are approaching retirement age. In her survey of carers who provided day-to-day practical assistance to dementing elderly relatives, Levin (1985) found that the average age of carers was 61 years. Almost half of these carers reported disabilities which limited their own activities and a quarter acknowledged that their health had not been good in the previous years. None the less, as many as 40 per cent of them had to cope with their relatives' heavy incontinence.

Most carers, like most elderly people, are women (Finch, 1989). Parker (1985) has said that: 'to talk about "care by the community" or even "family" care is to disguise the reality ... care by family members almost always means care by female members'.

Recent UK evidence has reminded us that a number of men do take on the caring role for their disabled wives (Arber and Gilbert (1989) estimated one-third of co-resident carers are male). For both genders it would appear that the role of primary carers is stressful. Their tasks are largely unshared; not only do they receive little help from services which tend to go to those living alone, but they also receive little help from other sources such as neighbours, friends or relatives. Gilhooly (1982), in her study of carers of relatives suffering from dementia, found that other relatives reduced their help once someone had assumed the caring role, while Nissel and Bonnerjea (1982) found 'near universal' factors of isolation, frustration and resignation among their sample of carers who received little help from any other family members.

The physical demands of caring are often exacerbated by difficulties in coping with unusual or unpredictable behaviour and changed interpersonal relations. These produce stress among the carers. Levin (1985) identified a number of factors which appear to correlate with strain, such as

- number of major problems
- number of trying behaviours
- severity of incontinence
- absence of normal conversation
- disturbance of carer during the night
- presence of dangerous behaviour

She found that a large number of carers showed signs of stress. Many (66 per cent) had lost their tempers with their relatives, 28 per cent thought there was tension in the household and 19 per cent admitted they had hit or shaken their relatives.

Such studies indicate the complicated relationship between carer and dementing relative. Gilhooly (1985) also examined a sample of elderly dementing patients most of whom attended a day hospital and tentatively suggested that: 'Willingness to continue giving care to a dementing relative is probably determined by factors beyond the control of service providers – things like the quality and nature of the relationship between the dementing person and the caregiver.'

Other researchers point out that the caring relationship also affects carers' other social and family bonds. Lewis and Meredith (1988) identified some of the effects on the carers' marital relationships, their relationships with their children and on the nuclear family as a whole. Frequently additional stress was caused when these relationships suffered from conflicting demands and the family's lack of privacy and peace. The 'non-co-operation' of an older person suffering from mental illness, such as dementia, was a particular concern.

Despite such difficulties in caring for an elderly mentally ill relative, this form of care is likely to continue and even grow. It is the preferred option of the Government (DHSS, 1978; 1981), of older people (see Salvage, 1986) and also of families and individuals who take on the caring role (Qureshi and Walker, 1989). Although the Equal Opportunities Commission (1982) points out the financial, social and emotional costs of caring for dependent relatives, and women's lack of any real choice of alternative acceptable care for their relatives; care for the overwhelming majority of elderly mentally ill people is likely to continue to be at home for the foreseeable future.

Summary of section one

Many people who care for their elderly mentally ill relatives suffer from physical and emotional strains. They are often aging themselves, in poor health and cope alone or with limited support. They may have problems in their relationships with their mentally ill relative and difficulties in reconciling their caring role with other roles.

A major objective of most support groups is to reduce strain and stress among carers by giving them an opportunity to share their experiences and talk about their feelings.

SECTION TWO

Setting up a carers' group

Contrary to widespread belief, group psychotherapy is not limited to the young. Although Freud argued that old people, those over 50, were not receptive to psychotherapy (see Hildebrand, 1982), in recent years many American psychogeriatricians have used psychotherapy on both an individual and group basis with older people (Goldfarb, 1956; Pfeiffer, 1971; Brody *et al.*, 1973). Their work has influenced UK developments both in work with people suffering from mental illness in old age (see Kapur, 1987; Kalus, 1987) and those older people who are under the stress of caring for them.

Hildebrand (1982) cites recent evidence which suggests that older people have learned considerable flexibility and have greater ego strengths than the young: 'They have been hardened and tempered by life and where their defences have not cracked they seem to have a good deal of capacity to delay gratification, allow problems to resolve and to take the long view.' Work with older carers can bring out these positive characteristics so that personal stress is reduced and feelings of guilt or aggression are expressed therapeutically.

The carers' support group to be described was set up in St James' Hospital, Portsmouth, and was a development from psychotherapy with hospitalized patients. Day patients' and inpatients' relatives were often being seen on a one-to-one basis, for periods of 15–20 minutes, usually weekly, so in order to use time more economically and efficiently, the carers were encouraged to meet together to draw strength from each other by sharing their problems and feelings within a group.

The group was built up slowly and a variety of health care staff at the day hospital were involved. Group membership was open to current and past carers. This meant that carers could attend irrespective of whether their elderly mentally ill relative was a current day-hospital attender, an inpatient on the assessment ward, or had moved to the continuing care ward or had recently died.

Within the organization of the day hospital, the psychiatrist had to resolve certain issues before the group could start. It was important to assure management that there would be no revenue consequences from the formation of the group, either in terms of extra staff time or by extra provision of care for the patients while their carers attended the group.

There are parallels in Smith and Cantley's (1985) study of a day hospital for elderly people with mental disorder. They found that hospital administrative staff were cautious about innovations such as relatives' support groups because 'This type of involvement with relatives entailed, for them, a departure from the customary model of hospital services in which relatives play no significant part and boundaries between the institution and the home are clearly defined and maintained.' At St James' Hospital, management and ancillary staff needed to be convinced of the potential benefits of the carers' groups to compensate for any administrative disruption.

The structure of the group

Participants in the carer's group met regularly at St James' for an hour once a week. The group's membership changed over time as patients' conditions deteriorated and as the carers' own feelings and needs altered. The size of the group fluctuated from eight to fifteen members. At any one time, some members had relatives who had been recently diagnosed as having organic brain disease, others were at the stage of giving up day-to-day care for their relatives, and a small number were recently bereaved. The members of the group were husbands, wives or children of the elderly patients. Individuals were referred to the group by any of a variety of professionals working within the local health service.

The role of the group facilitator or organizer included taking responsibility for organizing the group, finding a location, informing staff, contacting the carers, choosing the day and time, making refreshments available, clearing up and finding transport for carers who had no car. Transport could not be supplied through the hospital, nor was there any 'sitting' service that could be offered to carers who had other dependants or had the patient at home on the day of the support group meeting. MacCarthy et al. (1989) confirm the vital role of preparation before counselling in group settings.

Within the group, the facilitator had to decide how to direct the group, if at all. The psychiatrist and clinical assistant chose to take 'enabling' roles which meant they could steer discussion, indicate points of value that emerged, and sum up each meeting with a reference to significant remarks or issues that had been touched upon or explored. They did not set any agenda or direct discussion, and did not invite outside 'experts' to talk to the group. Their control was intentionally low-key and flexible. It varied according to the dynamics of each group session.

Two controls, relating to the introduction of new members were introduced because the group was always open to newcomers. First, the relatives' GP was notified and asked for permission for their attendance. This was a safeguard because the groups often entailed very emotional discussions. Second, to avoid newcomers feeling alarmed and anxious about what would be expected of them in a group, group members introduced themselves to the newcomers in turn and described the situation of the patients they cared for. They also described the various types of care received by the patients so that the newcomer could see the range of experience within the group. This sharing of experience often had an immediate effect. There would usually be a quick recognition by the newcomers that their apparently unique problems were common. In this way the tension of being a new member of the group was usually quickly eased.

Both the psychiatrist and the clinical assistant found it important to be up to date with the treatment and care of the elderly patients. This enabled them to explain any apparently puzzling changes in hospital routine to the relatives and alerted staff to any new difficulties that patients or carers might be encountering at home. For example, a carer might notice increasing incontinence and use the support group to explore whether this was being treated at the hospital and how other carers coped.

Keeping up with the minutiae of arrangements for a group was a time-consuming task but it was vital to its smooth running. It also had a symbolic effect. Participation in a group that was well managed, with adequate resources, was seen as a valued activity and was accepted more readily as part of the overall activities of the day hospital. Within 5 years a second group formed.

The benefits of the group

The benefits that participants gain from a group should be the major reason for the group's operation and the resources that are devoted to it. There are several possible ways to assess such benefits. Burnside (1986) lists possible benefits or help-giving activities from groupwork: empathy, mutual affirmation, explanation, morale-building, positive reinforcement and self-disclosure. We shall consider the costs and benefits together, based on the St James' group's findings.

The group existed to provide carers with the opportunity to share their feelings in a caring, uncritical and understanding environment. The aim of the group was to provide better psychological support for its members than could be provided simply by an *ad hoc* system of individual consultation.

It can be difficult to assess whether or not a group or individuals are deriving any benefits. It would be simplistic to say that if carers attended then they must have been deriving some benefit from the group. It might have been, for instance, that they saw the group as a way of influencing resources, such as the availability of a full-time bed or more time at the day hospital. It might have been that they found the group reinforced their feelings of depression or guilt.

The psychiatrist's definition of success for the group rested on a number of factors. One of these was individual members' reports of improvement. These reports were often couched in terms of feeling under less stress, feeling less guilty, feeling less isolated, such as, 'By hearing other people's problems I realized I was not the only one.' It was important to allow individuals time and opportunity to make such comments if they wished, either in the group or by talking to the psychiatrist or whoever was acting as the group facilitator afterwards. It was hoped that a number of relatives had been prevented from developing symptoms of stress-related mental illness by attending.

The existence of the group might have had a detrimental effect by depriving carers of the opportunity for private talk with members of the hospital staff. Carers might feel that other channels of communication were closed to them or that all dealings with carers would take place in the group. To preclude this possibility it was emphasized that the group was an additional resource, not an alternative. Another concern was that relatives who did not want, or were unable, to attend the carers' group might feel that they were being ignored or losing out on information. Although the carers' group was well attended, over 80 per cent of carers did not accept the initial invitation. Sometimes this was for practical reasons such as lack of transport, or the carers' own disabilities, such as hearing loss, and/or physical frailty.

Apparent benefits from the group were also assessed by monitoring individual behaviour in the group over a period of time. Some people attended several meetings but said little; they only slowly developed the confidence to talk about themselves, their situations as carers and their relationships with their relatives. This was particularly the case if they were deeply troubled by their relatives' excessive or inappropriate sexual behaviour, for example, or incontinence. Many carers' behaviour in the group changed gradually and it was important to listen to what was said, and also to watch out for shared laughter or shared tears and to realize their significance.

Pfeiffer (1971) stressed the importance of empathic understanding of older patients, and this was also relevant to the carers' group. He defined empathy as 'the process by which people understand one another's thoughts, feelings and actions. It is a complex psychologic process that makes use of multiple channels of verbal and non-verbal communication'. Group members collectively helped to empathize by sharing their common experiences and feelings, while the psychiatrist or group facilitator built upon this understanding to work towards individual and group goals. Pfeiffer, in his suggestions of limited goals, includes 'symptom relief' and 'adaptations to a changed life situation such as widowhood'. We would include reducing a carer's stress and adaptation to the situation of a carer as instances of the explicit goals of the group.

Eventually, group members began to express new insights into their caring relationship, or, about their feelings and concerns generally. People were often able to recall their feelings and put them into context. 'I realized I was very depressed then.' Gilleard and Watt (1983) give an example of the type of insight necessary in their discussion of the way a daughter might start to realize she had been patronizing her elderly relative by giving 'an exaggerated style of caring'. Sheldon (1982) gives an example of how such insight may need to refer back to events long past in people's relationships. She explains how guilt over past marital infidelity affected a husband's ability to share his care for his dependent wife with any professionals.

On a very practical level, carers became more familiar with the routine and practice of the hospital when they had spent some time there. Some began to take lunch there, for example. The general lack of involvement of many carers with the day hospitals attended by their relatives was remarked upon by Brocklehurst and Tucker (1980). They found little communication between the carers and staff. In some hospitals details about the chief carer were 'neither known nor recorded', while, on the other hand, few relatives interviewed had ever visited the day hospitals.

The group members benefitted from increased contact with the day hospital and the hospital as a whole, and several carers reported that they felt they had more trust in the staff. 'I feel I can ring them up at any time', and 'I feel I have someone to talk to'. The carers also reported that they felt happier about the type of care the patients were receiving because they knew what was going on at the hospital: 'It's a rather strange divided life we lead. One part at home trying to be normal, the other part wondering what's going on here.'

Conclusion

One of the problems in assessing new service developments is that the benefits are usually more acclaimed than the disadvantages. Little is written about why some carers' groups fail to attract members or why some cannot keep going. Most reports (e.g. Benson, 1987; Fuller et al., 1979) are still at the descriptive stage.

One exception to this is Smith and Cantley's (1985) study of a psycho-geriatric day hospital where they examined in detail the functions of the relatives' groups. They found that these could be broken down into an information role and an emotional role. Within the group relatives exchanged practical information about patients' treatment and future care with the hospital staff. They could discuss individual problems. The staff could explain treatment or how they allocated resources in return.

The emotional or therapeutic function of the group allowed relatives to express their feelings:

This kind of emotional release is not encouraged at other times or in other areas of hospital life where coping with distressed or irate relatives is viewed by staff as encroaching on their time and disrupting the smooth running of the hospital.

Smith and Cantley (1985) explain that this function of the group was the means by which the hospital staff could control the timing and setting of relatives' distress. In this way the group again had advantages for staff as well as benefits for the relatives, though these were not identical gains.

Such issues should be considered in the planning of a carers' group and regularly reviewed by the staff. It is important to acknowledge that groups have different benefits and disadvantages for carers and staff and that this should be recognized by professionals.

SECTION THREE

In this section we look in detail at the case of Mrs Joan Smith (all names have been changed). We will give brief details of her background and personal history, her mental state and diagnosis, and the involvement of her daughter with the relatives' support group at the day hospital.

Background history

Mrs Smith, then aged 75, was first seen by the psychiatrist when living in the house of her daughter and son-in-law. She had moved in with them as she was unable to cope any longer on her own, according to the daughter. The family had asked for a psychiatric assessment as they found Mrs Smith's behaviour increasingly difficult to manage.

In this initial interview the daughter described particular difficulties. Primarily, she was concerned about the effect of her mother on the young children in the household: 'Mother keeps shouting at the grandchildren for making any noise.' She also found her mother's muddled and confused state irritating. Her husband found Mrs Smith's conviction, that she owned the house, particularly aggravating.

Mrs Smith had lived abroad all her life; she was one of eight children who had scattered throughout various parts of the world. She had married at 18, and only returned to the UK in the 1960s. Her husband died soon after their return. Mrs Smith often spoke of her dead husband and according to her daughter had had an extremely close relationship with him.

The daughter said that her mother often reverted back to her life abroad, with her first husband: 'She often looks for her servants, the horses and the stables.' This 'living in the past' made the daughter very anxious that her mother was losing all touch with reality.

Mental state and diagnosis

When Mrs Smith was seen at home by the psychiatrist she appeared 'pleasant, communicative and co-operative' (case notes). She gave a good account of herself and looked younger than her 75 years. She was agile and looked well. After some discussion it became evident that her recent memory was very poor and her remote memory was patchy. Mrs Smith was assessed in more detail at a local day hospital, diagnosed as having pathological memory loss, and prescribed small doses of a transquillizer.

The daughter and her husband were also seen at the day hospital, to discuss short-term and long-term care plans for the care of Mrs Smith.

Five months later, it turned out that Mrs Smith was hallucinating and deluding, and that her memory had further deteriorated. On several occasions in the next 2 months, Mrs Smith had been found wandering in the local neighbourhood, inappropriately dressed and disorientated. Problems with the behaviour of Mrs Smith continued to accelerate, and a year after her initial referral she suffered a minor stroke and was admitted to hospital. Following her discharge, a period of relief care was arranged between the hospital and family, however, Mrs Smith's mental condition continued to deteriorate rapidly and she became hostile and aggressive.

Frequently, when writing about elderly people, the case study approach ends with the death of the subject. However, in this instance, 8 years after her referral Mrs Smith was still alive, living at home with her daughter and receiving regular hospital admission. Her physical agility greatly declined but she was still mobile, continent and able to do various self-care tasks despite her severe mental frailty.

The relatives' support group

Even though Mrs Smith's daughter, Sara, initially complained of her mother's behaviour as 'stubborn, belligerent and aggressive', Sara was not trying to shrink from providing care for her mother. In the initial interview it was recorded that the family was, 'at this stage unhappy to accept care'. Further discussion with Sara by the hospital registrar revealed that her 'Mother has always been dominant and autocratic. She is very bitter and resents her inability to cope. Guilty.'

It was concluded that these mixed feelings led Sara to being very critical of the care being given to her mother in the day hospital. Hospital staff found that she was making comments about the food, the attention, the cleanliness of the ward, which were not justified. Sara was unable to accept that anyone else could look after her mother.

During this time, several staff members spent time speaking with Sara on an individual basis. They tried to help her with her feelings of being a failure, and her guilt at letting other people care for Mrs Smith. Sara was particularly distressed at the incidents of wandering as she felt they reflected on her standards of care and supervision.

Initially, Sara refused all offers of help with her mother. The registrar commented in the case notes that Sara had not 'come to terms with her mother's progressive dementia'. However, following her mother's necessary admission to hospital after the stroke, Sara saw that shared care might be some solution to the stress of caring. She was helped again in this period by lengthy talks with hospital staff.

After this it was suggested to Sara by the registrar that she might like to attend the relatives' support group. There were practical difficulties to overcome as Mrs Smith and the young children had to be looked after. Arrangements were made to utilize other family members, neighbours and friends, so that Sara could attend the group regularly.

In the group, Sara was initially very cautious. She did not like to admit her difficulties as she felt it was a betrayal of her mother. She was also unable to verbalize that in spite of her loyalty and love for her mother, there were times when her mother was intolerably aggressive and cruel.

Two particular themes can be identified from Sara's comments and behaviour in the group. At first she was angry with the medical profession: 'What about brain transplants?' 'Why is cardiac surgery more attractive?' She questioned the standard of care within the hospital and the competence of individual staff. The other relatives in the group were able to gradually reduce this anger by detailing their own experiences or simply letting Sara make so many accusations that someone dissolved into laughter.

Associated with this anger was Sara's difficulty in allowing anyone else to care for her mother. In a letter to the hospital she stated: 'I thought about various offers, I am not ready to admit mother for any length of time'. She was anxious that she would be a failure, that other people would see her as an uncaring daughter, and that her mother would feel rejected. Sara's many anxieties about institutional life were alleviated when she visited the hospital regularly and talked to relatives who also had family members living in hospital.

The shared care-giving between family and hospital staff, was therefore only established once Sara had agreed to 'let go' partially. Once it began, she felt much more able to cope and her caring was a positive choice. The group had been of value to Sara and her family because it had enabled her to continue to care for her mother whilst working through some of her anger, guilt and bitterness.

SECTION FOUR

In this concluding section we examine the implications of carers' support groups for the people affected by them, and suggest that there are three possible models for carers' groups. The carers' group affected the relationships of carers with the staff at the hospital and hence carers' perception of the service. One consequence of the carers' group was that group members said they felt more recognized. Their roles as carers were acknowledged and their status enhanced. As they were increasingly 'recognized', staff began to know them individually. They were greeted by names instead of vaguely recognized as 'relatives'. Many group members commented that it was a change to be treated as individuals, and said that the attention they received in the group was an implicit acknowledgement of their work and its difficulties.

However, carers' groups are not the only way of reducing carers' stress nor the only method through which they can release their possible anger or resentment. For some carers, at some period, the groups may perform these functions, but the establishment of carers' support groups is not the only relevant service for carers (see MacCarthy *et al.*, 1989). Many need practical help with aids for disabled people or home adaptations; many need respite care or a reliable sitting-in service. Some carers have their own support systems worked out with friends and/or relatives and therefore have no wish to use hospital-based systems. Others have developed supportive relationships with professionals such as a nurse or a minister of religion. It is important to recognize that some carers do not wish to attend groups, and respect their reasons. None the less, work with the carers' group described confirmed our belief that such groups were beneficial to many carers. Even those who did not attend, saw the groups as a service they could use at a future date.

There are currently three main models that are used by professionals and carers themselves for carers' groups. The first is an educational model, such as briefly described by Trepka and Whittick. They established a 6 week programme for groups:

> designed to provide factual information about dementia, local resources and services available and practical advice about caring at home. While educational components are emphasized, the main function of the group is to reduce stress among carers by providing supportive contact.
>
> (Trepka and Whittick, 1987)

An alternative model is the 'peer support group' where groups operate without professional guidance. 'Such groups should have goals of mutual encouragement and not be used as therapy groups ... it is a group for mutual exchange and support.' (Mace and Rabins, 1985). These are based on a philosophy that carers benefit from sharing their experiences with other people, and the best people to understand are other carers (see Health Education Council, 1986). Some develop into groups which try to influence the provision of resources and the status of carers; getting involved in local service planning.

The third model can be described as a therapy group model, but it also contains elements of the other models. At times in the St James' group, many relatives wanted specific information about services and medical matters. They wanted 'education' about the nature of dementia, its causes and outcomes. Sometimes these questions could be answered factually by the co-therapists. This was obviously much appreciated as many carers said they did not feel they could trouble their GP with simple requests for information. However, there were many occasions where the educational elements of questions developed into discussion of deeper problems. Lazarus *et al.* (1981) studied the meetings of a group of relatives who were caring for Alzheimer patients. They found that the group members concentrated at first on hopes for a cure from experimental drugs. However, 'as group cohesion and trust developed, the focus shifted to more personal concerns ...'. The therapy group makes it possible to deal with feelings, such as anger and resentment, more elaborately than merely the ventilation of emotions.

Forster (1986), gives useful guidance about practical considerations such as publicity and recruitment for self-help groups. She also points out the need for group leaders to share their experiences in a network, pointing out that 'Providing a support system for people looking after a dementia sufferer is emotionally and psychologically exhausting and you will do it much better if you have a support system for yourself.'

It is clear that carers' groups raise many issues for professionals. They are not simply a service to relatives; the groups may often act as a valuable resource for professionals themselves.

Marshall (1984) points out that care for dementia sufferers is a rapidly changing and developing area, and that 'relatives are learning new skills of management as fast as any professional setting and these need to be collated and shared more widely'. Carers' groups also provide a valuable opportunity to put multidisciplinary beliefs into practice. This may be within one agency, such as a hospital, but may also be within a community setting under the auspices of a voluntary group or local care providers.

Last, we shall consider the implications of carers' groups upon the patients themselves. We discovered, from reports by carers themselves, that the quality of care they were providing had improved in two ways. Carers said they had learned numerous practical skills from each other, both in managing their relatives' behaviour and dealing with physical illnesses and disabilities. Such skills may be discovered and learned through publications (e.g. Health Education Council, 1986; Mace and Rabins, 1985) but it appeared that relatives appreciated being given specific personal advice by fellow carers.

They also felt less stressed and more tolerant. This resulted in more patience and less frustration by incessant, repetitive behaviour or questioning. They managed to see such problems as a symptom of the illness and not a personal attack.

Jacques (1984) has identified three possible groups of carers of ambulant, dementing older people:

- Those who like their relative, are willing to care and need support and encouragement.
- Those who care against their will.
- 'A groups of martyrs, often daughters, whose mothers have made them promise never to put them into a home. They feel such an obligation that they go on trying to cope far beyond the reasonable.'

He suggests that professionals should consider breaking through the 'barrier of martyrdom' characteristics of this third group and encourage them to accept help. This is a strategy which gives priority or equal consideration to the carer and demands deliberate intervention from the professional. It also has resource implications. Professionals may be accused of creating demand for services that cannot be provided or encouraging unrealistic expectations of help. They may be accused of putting the needs or demands of the carer above those of the patient. In the St James' group, sharing care was encouraged, as in the example of Sara, by allocating a day-centre place, or a relief bed in hospital.

There is no simple order of priority for tackling carers' problems in relative support groups. The challenge to professionals is to work together to identify and provide the most appropriate sources of help for carers. This will mean crossing traditional service and institutional boundaries, it will mean involving and listening to staff dealing with all levels of patient care, including the voluntary and commercial sectors. Above all, we will have to be guided by carers themselves about the type of support they need and want.

ACKNOWLEDGEMENT

We would like to thank Dr Andy Alaszewski, University of Hull, for his helpful comments on drafts of this chapter.

NOTE

1   We shall refer to those people who undertake the practical day-to-day support of elderly mentally ill people in their own home as *carers*, rather than family members or relatives. However, as the Equal Opportunities Commission (1982) points out, no satisfactory term exists for these individuals who care for dependents on an unpaid basis (p. viii).

REFERENCES

Arber, S. and Gilbert, N. (1989) 'Men: the forgotten carers', *Sociology* 23 (1): 111–18, February.

Benson, S. (1987) 'Caring for the Carers', *Community Care* pp. 25–7, 11 June.

British Medical Association's Board of Science and Education (1986) *All Our Tomorrows: Growing Old in Britain*, London: British Medical Association.

Brocklehurst, J.C. and Tucker, J.S. (1980) *Progress in Geriatric Day Care*, London: King Edward's Hospital Fund for London.

Brody, E.M., Cole, C. and Moss, M. (1973) 'Individualizing therapy for the mentally impaired aged', *Social Casework* pp. 453–61, October.

Burnside, I.M. (1986) *Working with the Elderly: Group Process and Techniques*, Monterey: Jones & Bartlett, p. 241.

Department of Health and Social Security (1978) *A Happier Old Age*, London: DHSS.

—— (1981) *Growing Older*, London: DHSS Cmnd. 8173, p. 6.

Equal Opportunities Commission (1982) *Caring for the Elderly and Handicapped: Community Care Policies and Women's Lives*, Foreword, p. iii.

Finch, J. (1989) *Family Obligations and Social Change*, Cambridge: Polity Press.

Forster, A. (1986) 'How to start a support group for relatives looking after a dementia sufferer', in A. Osborn (ed.) *Reaching Out to Dementia Sufferers and their Carers*, Edinburgh: Age Concern Scotland, p. 21.

Fuller, J., Ward, E., Evans, A., Massam, K. and Gardner, A. (1979) 'Dementia: supportive groups for relatives', *British Medical Journal* (1): 1684–5.

Gilhooly, M. (1982) 'Social aspects of senile dementia' in R. Taylor and A. Gilmore (eds) *Current Trends in Gerontology*, Aldershot: Gower.

—— (1985) 'A study of caring for the dementing elderly in Aberdeen' in *Dementia – Research Innovation and Management*, Edinburgh: Age Concern Scotland, p. 19.

Gilleard, C. and Watt, G. (1983) *Coping with Ageing Parents*, Edinburgh: Macdonald, p. 106.

Goldfarb, A.I. (1956) 'The rationale for psychotherapy with older persons', *American Journal of Medical Sciences*, pp. 181–5, August.

Health Education Council (1986) *Who Cares? Information and Support for the Carers of Confused People*, London: Health Education Council.

Hildebrand, H.P. (1982) 'Psychotherapy with older patients', *British Journal of Medical Psychology* 55: 19–28.

Jacques, A. (1984) 'Coping with the care of ambulant dementing older people: key issues for carers', in '... *the slow death of the intellect*', Edinburgh: Age Concern Scotland, p. 7.

Kapur, R. (1987) 'An application for group psychotherapy with older adults', *PSIGE Newsletter*, no. 22, pp. 7–10, March.

Kalus, C. (1987) 'Psychotherapy and the elderly – a case study', *PSIGE Newsletter*, no. 22, pp. 11–13, March.

Lazarus, L.W., Stafford, B., Cooper, K., Cohler, B. and Dysken, M. (1981) 'A pilot study of an Alzheimer patients' relatives discussion group', *Gerontologist* 21 (4): 353–8.

Levin, E. (1985) 'Problems and outcomes for carers of confused people', in *Dementia – Research Innovation and Management*, Edinburgh: Age Concern Scotland.

Lewis, J. and Meredith, B. (1988) *Daughters Who Care*, London: Routledge.

MacCarthy, B., Kuipers, L., Hurry, J., Harper, R. and Le Sage, A. (1989) 'Counselling the relatives of the long-term adult mentally ill', *British Journal of Psychiatry* 154: 768–75.

Mace, N.L. and Rabins, P.V. with Castleton, B.A., Cloke, C. and McEwen, E. (1985) *The 36-Hour Day*, London: Hodder & Stoughton.

Marshall, M. (1984) 'Strategies for planning a better future for carers' in '... *the slow death of the intellect*', Edinburgh: Age Concern Scotland, p. 37.

Nissel, M. and Bonnerjea, L. (1982) *Family Care of the Handicapped Elderly: Who Pays?* London: Policy Studies Institute, p. 43.

Parker, G. (1985) *With Due Care and Attention: A Review of Research on Informal Care*, London: Family Policy Studies Centre, p. 30.

Pfeiffer, E. (1971) 'Psychotherapy with elderly patients', *Postgraduate Medicine*, pp. 254–8, November.

Qureshi, H. and Walker, A. (1989) *The Caring Relationship – Elderly People and their Families*, London: Macmillan.

Salvage, A.V. (1986) *Attitudes of the Over-75s to Health and Social Services*, Final Report, Research Team for the Care of the Elderly, Swansea: University of Wales College of Medicine, p. 39.

Sheldon, F. (1982) 'Supporting the supporters: working with the relatives of patients with dementia', *Age and Ageing* 11: 114–88.

Smith, G. and Cantley, C. (1985) *Assessing Health Care: a Study in Organisational Evaluation*, Milton Keynes: Open University Press.

Trepka, C. and Whittick, J. (1987) 'A clinical psychology service for the elderly', *Health Bulletin* 45 (2): 84–7, March.

Whitaker, D.S. (1985) *Using Groups to Help People*, London: Routledge & Kegan Paul, Preface, p. x.

Part V

Summary

Chapter 24

The need for an interdisciplinary core curriculum for professionals working with dementia

Gemma Jones and Bère Miesen

SUMMARY

In this chapter, a plea is made for the establishment of a multidisciplinary 'core curriculum' for professionals working with persons with dementia. The need for such a programme arises not only out of the multiplicity of professionals coming into contact with persons with dementia and their families, but also from the often vague delineations between professional roles.

The lack of 'profession-specific' and 'shared' models and theories about dementia and care-giving impede progress in care-giving, and are a major focus of the core curriculum. Inadequacies in specific knowledge and surpervised practice relating to dementia within current nursing, social work and clinical psychology curricula are discussed within the context of five global problem areas: (1) limited educational resources, (2) specific problems within a profession, (3) interdisciplinary problems, (4) limited resources in practice and (5) difficulties in the dissemination of research.

The 'core curriculum' presented in this chapter comprises a sample curriculum based on a hierarchy of information, starting with normal aging processes and working through common physiological conditions treated in geriatric medicine, through to old-age psychiatry, and finally, specifically dementia. The curriculum also comprises a sample: interdisciplinary philosophy statement, specific interdisciplinary goals statement, a philosophy statement specific to a profession (the nursing example is used), nursing-care objectives derived from the nursing philosophy statement and, a nursing-management philosophy statement.

INTRODUCTION

Several of us, from very different backgrounds, have all found ourselves working with the mentally frail elderly. Between us we represent the professions of nursing, social work and psychology. None is the exclusive territory of any one of us. Because gerontology and geriatrics are newly developing disciplines, our routes into the fields of gerontology, geriatrics and old-age psychiatry have been anything but direct! This puts us in the position of wanting to talk about how we would like to have been prepared for the work we do, and how we would like to see educational programmes develop for our colleagues and students so that they will be more prepared for their work than we were. Presented here is an amalgam of our joint perceptions from clinical and educational settings. To introduce the subject, definitions of old-age psychiatry (otherwise known as psychogeriatrics), gerontology and geriatrics will be given.

Old-age psychiatry, geriatric psychiatry or psychogeriatrics is defined by Brice Pitt (1974) in two ways. Notice that the first definition is congruous with geriatric medicine and that the second one falls within the scope of psychiatry. (1) Psychogeriatrics 'is the assessment, treatment and management of elderly people suffering all kinds of mental disorder. These include depression, paranoid states and troublesome quirks loosely labelled personality disorders, as well as confusion.' (2) Psychogeriatrics is 'that branch of psychiatry which is concerned with the whole range of psychological disorder developing in the senium (i.e. after the age of 65)' (Pitt, 1974:1).

Gerontology in its broadest sense, is the study of the aging process in man. Havighurst (1974) started making the distinction between medical and social gerontology. Medical geronotology has three components: the treatment of the elderly patient, the prevention of disease and disability in the elderly and preservation of vigour in the elderly. Social gerontology considers the financial support of the elderly, their housing and living arrangements and ego support of the elderly.

Geriatrics is a term applied to the medical treatment of disease in the elderly. Geriatrics has been most simply defined as the positive approach to the preservation and restoration of human ability in old age.

From Figure 24.1 and the above definitions, it is already apparent that the definitions and terminology overlap and could be problematic for a discussion of questions such as: What is the 'overlap' and 'unique' territory of medical gerontology, geriatrics and psychogeriatrics?, and: Which health care professions are responsible for providing specific and joint services for the elderly? This issue of overlapping definitions arises again under the section about multiple disciplines converging upon a shared domain. It is the main reason for our emphasis on an 'interprofessional' approach to working with the mentally frail elderly, which ideally would be based on a common *Core Curriculum*.

The need for specialized training, is apparent from the following descriptive profile of the elderly by Pitt (1974). In Britain, there are more than 8 million persons over the age of 65, and 40 per cent of this population is estimated to suffer from some type of psychiatric disorder. In 1971 the elderly constituted only 12 per cent of the population, yet they formed 33 per cent of those who committed suicide.

Figure 24.1 The overlap between disciplines specializing in work with the elderly, which causes conceptual and practical difficulties in establishing old-age psychiatry as a speciality area in its own right

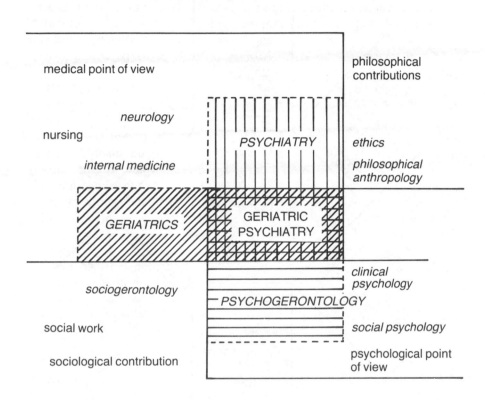

Source: adapted from Engelen, 1984:572.

WHO WORKS WITH THE MENTALLY FRAIL ELDERLY?

The elderly person/patient's 'care-giver network' is a very complicated organism, constantly growing and changing, and heavily dependent upon particular members. One study estimated that family, nurses and volunteers provide 90 per cent of all contact time with elderly persons and patients. Figure 24.2a and Figure 24.2b show the myriad of professions that comprise the 'care-giver network' and the 'organizational network' that a person with dementia and their family might have to deal with. This complexity necessitates careful organization, training, and some common

Figure 24.2(a) Care-giver network

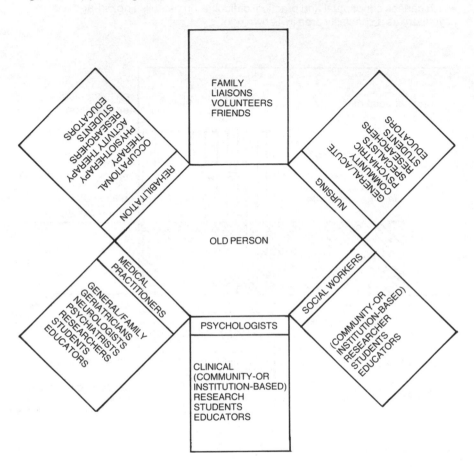

basis of professional knowledge. Note that even within a given profession there are many levels of expertise required, including educators, researchers and students. Additional specialization occurs when the distinction between work in the community or institutions is made. At present there is no common educational base for all of these different professions providing care, although their concerns and responsibilities often overlap.

How is this care-giver network organized? Does it work for the elderly person, their family, health care members and for the health care system at large? All indications are that care facilities are not keeping up with the rate of increase in the numbers of elderly persons and it is rare to find anyone; patient, resident or health care professional, who is totally satisfied with the care system.

Figure 24.2(b) Organizational network

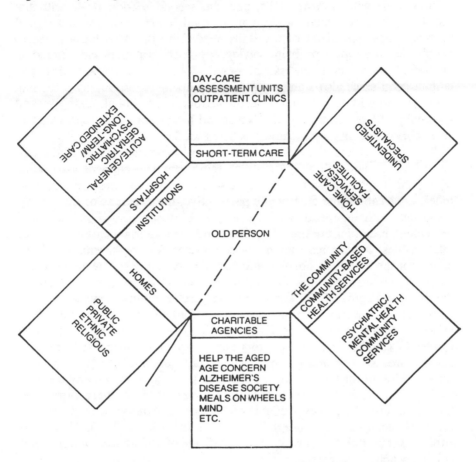

EXISTING CURRICULA FOR NURSING, SOCIAL WORK AND PSYCHOLOGY

Nursing

Within nursing, the general, mental health and postgraduate training will each be discussed briefly. In the general training programme, a short period in psychiatry and geriatrics is undertaken. However, the psychiatric module usually takes place in an acute environment rather than in a unit for the elderly mentally ill. The general nurse may complete her training without gaining any experience in the management of a difficult demented elderly person or an elderly dehydrated depressive person. In 1982, a new syllabus of nursing for registered mental health nurses came into being. The first section deals with nursing skills, and the second section deals with the knowledge base on which the skills are learned. The first section is designed to give a clear statement of the skills needed by the psychiatric nurse to enable her to adopt a problem-solving approach to patient care including intellectual, personal, interpersonal, practical and organizational skills. The emphasis on skills also stamps psychiatric nursing as essentially a 'human activity', responding particularly to behavioural, emotional, cognitive and spiritual problems. In theory, this is a sound base from which to develop an excellent curriculum, and headway is being made.

Within the studies of the care of the elderly, the learner studies the theories of aging, gerontology, patterns of aging, physical changes associated with normal aging, psychosocial aspects of old age, cultural aspects, attitudes, myths about the elderly, life perspective, the activities of the elderly associated with independence, housing, employment, nutrition, finance, retirement, use of leisure time, loneliness and the importance of meaningful relationships. Nurses also learn about services for the mentally infirm, caring for the elderly in hospital and community settings. The value of the elderly to younger persons and society in general is emphasized. Care of the dying and bereavement and counselling are also units of study.

Where are we now in practice? Nurses find themselves working in a variety of settings where the elderly are being cared for: in the community, residential (public- or private-sector) care, hospital geriatric wards, general acute wards or psychiatric units. They may continue to work in these settings without further specialist training in the care of the elderly mentally frail person. The available post-basic courses open to these nurses are limited in terms of places available and funds to sponsor them. Currently, the qualified nurse can undertake an English National Board Course for either 6 weeks' duration, leading to a certificate of attendance, or a 6-month course, which is recordable.

The aims of postgraduate courses are to enable the nurse to:

1   demonstrate an awareness of the need to promote positive health in elderly people,
2   function skilfully in the initial and ongoing assessment of the physical, psychological and social needs of the elderly in the community and hospital,
3   plan, execute and evaluate nursing care plans for elderly people in the community and hospital,
4   function effectively as a member of the multidisiplinary team providing care for the elderly.

The courses cover health education, demographic, sociological, psychological and cultural aspects of normal aging. Management of violent patients as well as their mental/psychological care. Students are taught to observe, interpret and assess the mental and emotional state of the elderly patient while providing the care needed by such persons. Support for the family members caring in the community is also dealt with. At the conclusion of the course, nurses are also expected to have acquired some basic teaching skills.

In summary, although the curricula for nursing since 1982 are adequate in theory, there are not enough courses or subsidy available to meet the need for post-basic training; neither for nurses wishing to specialize nor for staff in acute-care settings.

Social work

The role of the social worker with the frail elderly is extremely challenging because it often necessitates creative work with the family and community in situations for which there is no formula or experiential precedent. This profession is the key one in arranging the support and services for continued independent living for a fragile person without family. The picture in social work is similar to that of nursing; few programmes, much need, great demand and little funding. Two offical postgraduate training programmes for work with the elderly exist in Britain. One is newly established at Ulster University, and the other has been running at University of Southampton since 1977, filled to capacity. The second programme provides 60 days of theory and fieldwork for ten students. Contrary to projected expectations of the 1970s the number of social workers taking postgraduate training has decreased by 50 per cent, rather than increased. This will be discussed in more detail in the section on problems (pp. 444–6).

Psychology

The field of old-age psychiatry is in its infancy and no-one would deny that research of all types is critical for its progress. In particular the assessment and interventions for dementia and depression. Repeated measurements of mnemonic, attentional and cognitive ability should ideally be accompanied by detailed life histories in addition to traditional medical/social histories if good epidemiological and 'individual differences' research is to progress. Specialized training for both neuropsychological assessment and interpersonal therapeutic interventions is urgently required. Britton (1983) refers to the findings of a study of applicants for training in clinical psychology, such that work with the elderly did not seem at all appealing to them and was among the lowest rated of the areas for prospective training. Since then, special-interest groups for psychologists concerned with the care of the elderly have formed, and these persons will be instrumental in stimulating more permanent and stable forms of interest in psychology students.

At present several institutions offer MA programmes in clinical psychology with an optional rotation in a geriatric or psychogeriatric setting. The one at the London Institute of Psychiatry has sixteen positions filled each year. About half of these students choose a placement with the elderly.

The placement offers a variety of types of work. Some cognitive assessments are carried out. Treatment strategies and management planning is done in conjunction with other staff members. Many of the patients are depressed or anxious so that verbal behavioural psychotherapy is often appropriate, and adapted to meet the needs of the particular elderly person. With patients suffering from dementia, the focus is more on retraining and management of the problem behaviours in addition to counselling and support of the families and other carers involved through relative support groups, for example. Students often participate in reality orientation and reminiscence groups for the confused patients. Because the area is changing rapidly, project work, piloting and evaluating innovation are encouraged. Weekly seminars for psychologists and students are held, covering academic and applied aspects of assessment and care.

SYNOPSIS

In briefly reviewing graduate education programmes for nursing, social work and clinical psychology, the absence of a common pool of basic knowledge and principles of care for the mentally frail elderly is absent. Particularly missing are specific references to interpersonal care interventions. A core curriculum is recommended, not as a replacement for the specialized training required by each profession, but rather as an adjunct for each profession, to which can be added a specialized knowledge base specific to each profession. Problems within each profession will be considered next, and will make the necessity for a 'core curriculum' more obvious.

PROBLEMS IN PRACTICE

The problems of each of these health care professions can be subsumed under five broad categories. We will give some specific examples under each heading; they will not likely be new to you. The five problem categories identified are as follows:

1   limited educational resources
2   specific problems within a profession
3   interdisciplinary problems
4   limited resources in practice and
5   dissemination of research findings.

Limited educational resources

Under the first heading come difficulties such as decreased educational budgets, reduced subsidy for postgraduate training and the lack of formally trained educators. In a very real sense, everyone working in this area is a pioneer. The limited availability of programmes, the absence of interdisciplinary curricula, and the lack of specific training for research gerontology are additional problems.

Problems within a profession

Within any given profession are the problems associated with semi- or unskilled persons who are doing work that requires speciality training. The absence of guiding philosophies, theories and models about old age, and diseases causing mental decline have resulted in inappropriate use of the medical model. Within nursing specifically, there is still great debate concerning the status of geriatrics. Is it a speciality field or does it fall naturally under the care of the adult? The unspoken notion that 'work with the geriatric and psychogeriatric population lacks prestige and is a second-class career choice' haunts every profession. Lack of esteem felt by students is perhaps reflected by the limited numbers of young persons wanting to specialize in geriatrics and gerontology, and in the remuneration they receive. In the social work programme for example, Professor Coleman (see Acknowledgement) relates that the median age of students is 45 as opposed to 35 for all other post-basic programmes averaged together.

Interdisciplinary problems

Within interdisciplinary problems fall a whole range of misunderstandings arising from not sharing common metaphors, models, theories and vocabulary. It is increasingly obvious that each profession must have specialized models and theoretical approaches of its own, but that some global framework and philosophy should also guide the overall direction for care and research at the interdisciplinary level. If such a scheme were adopted, the boundaries of unique and shared roles and responsibilities of the professions could be collaboratively developed and respected. (In a recent survey of nursing homes, Jones (1991) found that less than 20 per cent of health care professionals had heard of more than three interpersonal interventions for dementia.)

Limited resources in practice

The increasing austerity in clinical and research resources is the most striking of the day-to-day problems for health care professionals. Government and health care planners are not responding quickly enough to the demographic projections, geriatrics gets the bulk of the budget cuts and the system aims to meet custodial needs rather than rehabilitative ones. The increasingly shorter stay in hospital for acute care episodes places increasing demands on the community health care services. The shortfall in the number of community-based staff also makes it very difficult for them to be released to attend post-basic training courses. How can highly trained and motivated persons be attracted, continually upgraded and kept? How can the atmosphere be created in which they feel challenged to utilize new methods to improve the 'system' and perhaps even undertake research themselves?

Dissemination of research

The dissemination of research and the development of new innovations is a slow process. Research in the area of care-giving is still seen as a luxury, ancillary to basic care. There is no vehicle for, or mechanism in place to screen the bulk of research that does exist, in the form of pilot projects. The entire responsibility falls onto exceptional, dedicated persons who try new techniques under their own initiative. Until health care professionals release their hold on using only existing methods of performing tasks and providing care, they will remain technicians, not responsible professionals involved in the process of evolution that allows for the advancement of care, and the development of a speciality of care-giving for dementia.

THE IDEAL CURRICULUM

We have provided the groundwork for you to appreciate our approach to presenting the ideal curricula. We would recommend that such a curricula be based upon these guiding principles.

1 The development of basic shared *core* education for all professions before they undertake further specialization within their profession.
2 The use of interdisciplinary (shared) and unique philosophies about health and illness throughout the aging process.
3 The development of *core* curriculum should be based on current knowledge about adult education techniques and curriculum development theory.
4 A *core* curriculum should address current and perceived future needs as determined by demography, existing health care services and, especially, by the experience of practising professionals and the elderly persons and families they care for.

The following sample curriculum is developed in a hierarchical fashion, that is from the general, to the specific. Normal aging topics precede illness and geriatric issues. Concepts about mental limitations and impairments are left to the end. In this way the idea of interactions between concepts and variables is enhanced. Note that loss theory, and theories of chronicity, and material on sensory deprivation are essential components of this core programme. A review of the known interpersonal therapies and approaches with both the elderly and their families and friends is essential.

Here is a sample programme. It incorporates some the suggestions of Gunter and Estes (1979) and Gray and Isaacs (1979).

Sample core curriculum

Perspectives on normal aging

    Demographics
    Common problems in normal aging:
        sensory/perceptual changes
        losses of independence, support systems, health
        adaptation to losses
        social adaptation to role changes
        loneliness/bereavement
        common mental health complaints
    Services available (government and voluntary)

Geriatric care

    History of geriatric care (nursing, medicine, psychology, social work)
    Common geriatric physiological problems:
        metabolic
        gastrointestinal/ nutritional
        urological
        cardio- and peripheral vascular
        bronchopulmonary
        musculoskeletal
        problems associated with medicating the elderly
        substance abuse/ alcohol misuse
        acute delirium
    Hospice care
    Adapted housing
    Relief/respite services available for chronic conditions
    Information needed for placement into institutions
    Services available
    Shared and unique professional responsibilities in providing care in the community, in acute settings, day care and long-term care settings.

Old age psychiatry

History of old age psychiatry
Incidence and description of specific psychiatric problems leading to institutional assessment and care:
depression
suicide
paraphrenia
mania
neurosis
personality and behaviour disorder
dementia
Pharmacological, psychosurgical, and interpersonal interventions
Effects of impoverished environments/ sensory deprivation

Dementia

Types of, incidence, assessment, diagnosis, progression of, theories of, individual differences in progression, language changes in
Dementia/depression complex and differential diagnosis
Drug treatment approaches to dementia
Interpersonal approaches to communication and interaction
Environmental considerations/ functional design and decoration to minimize confusion
Interaction with and support of family members
Services available for community care, in institutions
Legal considerations/ legal guardianship
Counselling and support services available to families

Biopsychosocial models and theories of aging, dementia and care-giving

Lifespan and development theories (Erikson, 1963; Peck, 1956)
Brain–behaviour correlations in dementia (Arendt and Jones, Chapter 2, this volume)
Loss theory (Crate, 1965)
Theory of chronic illness (Perdue, 1981)
Parent fixation/attachment theory (Miesen, Chapter 4, this volume)
Reminiscing disorientation theory (Jones and Burns, Chapter 5, this volume)
Model for communication (Jones, Chapter 6, this volume)
Nursing model for care of the elderly (Jones, Chapter 7, this volume)

Example of an interprofessional philosophy statement

1   We believe that persons receiving long-term care are members of the larger society and should be encouraged to retain active membership to the greatest extent possible. Individuals are members of families and as such should be encouraged to participate in family life and living as is feasible and desired by both the family and the older person.
2   We believe that all persons receiving care, and their families, have rights and privileges that must be respected, regardless of past or existing limitations. Value is placed on maintaining the ability to take an active role in decision making. Individuality, dignity, independence and a sense of self-worth are valued and supported.
3   We believe that persons involved/receiving care experience a variety of needs including physical and psychosocial. We want to provide assistance to meet those needs only if (or until) individuals are able to do so unassisted.
4   We believe that a team comprising of health professionals and a variety of support staff is the best method of delivering care. We value interprofessional collaboration as a means of ensuring effective management of care-giving within our present health care system resources.
5   We believe in the maintenance of an environment and climate that promotes learning, facilitates the teaching of individuals, students and families, and stimulates the ongoing education of all staff. We believe that as team members we have a responsibility to share both successes and failures with our colleagues and with other community-based agencies, and to provide a leadership and consultative role as required. We value the spirit of inquiry and support.
6   We see the need to initiate and conduct research appropriate for the advancement of care for the elderly, preventative and rehabilitative. We believe that planning and evaluation are essential for learning and growth and should be an integral part of the day-to-day activities of our work.

(Adapted from the philosophy statement of the University of British Columbia Extended Care Unit; developed by the department heads in 1977.)

Specific interdisciplinary goals arising from the interdisciplinary philosophy statement

The specific goals that are from this philosophy are:

1   To provide care designed to:
    (a) promote an optimal level of health and wellbeing for each individual

> (b) maintain abilities acquired by each individual for as long as possible, and
>
> (c) to prevent further disabilities and/or limitations.

2   to identify the changing needs of the long-term care-delivery system, to develop the best means of meeting those needs, and to provide assistance to the community.

3   to demonstrate interprofessionalism in the provision of care.

4   to ensure appropriate teaching–learning experiences for a variety of students.

5   to facilitate research directly and indirectly related to the care of the elderly.

6   to act as responsible, contributing members of the professional and academic community.

Nursing will be used to give an example of a philosophy statement specific to a given profession.

Sample philosophy statement specific to nursing

1   Nursing views each person as a member of society with rights, privileges and obligations. Some of these rights and privileges include the right to refuse treatment, to refuse service, to refuse to be cared for by students, to expect to be treated with dignity, to be treated as adults with decision-making ability and the right to expect quality nursing care at all times. People receiving long-term care have a right and an obligation to remain, to the extent possible, active members of society; nursing has the privilege of assisting them to meet this obligation.

2   Nursing views 'family' in its broadest context; i.e. any person or pet of significance is considered family and therefore becomes an integral part of the nursing care planned and provided to persons involved in the long-term care continuum.

3   Nursing views each persons receiving care as continually learning and developing and also constantly striving to meet basic needs. Nursing perceives the needs as follows: (specify the particular needs according to the nursing model used) (see Jones, Chapter 5, this volume for a specific nursing model).

4   Nursing determines nursing care requirements in relation to these (specified) needs and organizes the nursing care required to have these needs met. Nursing accepts the responsibility:

> (a) to determine with each person and their family the extent to which each of these needs are being met as well as the manner in which they are being met (assessment: upon admission, initial visit and ongoing);
>
> (b) to establish with each person, family and other professions thera-

peutic, realistic and measurable goals and treatment plan(s);
(c) to implement nursing action relative to established goals and plan(s);
(d) to consistently and continually evaluate progress with a view to making changes as required.

5   Nursing shares nursing care *requirements* (i.e. basic needs attainment as per model) with other professions and in turn receives information about care requirements from them ensuring an interprofessional approach to care.

6   Nursing assumes accountability for the provision of nursing care. Nursing is responsible for making sound clinical nursing judgements on behalf of persons receiving care, based on sound clinical judgement. Nursing is responsible in collaboration with medicine, for ensuring that people receive acute care services when required, and for determining when a person is 'dying' in order to ensure that the dying process is as comfortable as possible for the person, the family, other patients, and staff. Nursing views dying as part of living and believes that dying persons should be cared for in their own familiar surroundings to the extent possible.

Nursing care objectives derived from philosophy statement

1   To determine with persons receiving nursing care and their families, acceptable, safe and successful methods of meeting basic needs.
2   To individualize nursing care to the extent feasible and desirable.
3   To contribute to the maintenance of the therapeutic, normal and supportive milieu.
4   To facilitate people's active participation as members of their own living community, as members of families and society.
5   To promote adult behaviour in terms of decision making involvement in their own care and future, learning and in continual psychosocial growth and development.
6   To be participating members of an interprofessional team.

Nursing management philosophy statement

Nursing administration believes that quality nursing care to patients and families is our primary goal and that the most desirable and effective method of achieving this is by means of a decentralized management system. Such a system facilitates expression of three essential professional behaviours, i.e. accountability, commitment and interprofessionalism.

Nursing administration accepts a 24-hours per day, 7 days per week accountability. The director is accountable for all activities of the nursing department. A care manager is accountable for the provision of nursing care in one area which should not exceed (number of patients, depending on setting).

Nursing administration believes there are at least two components of management exercised by the director of nursing and the nursing care managers; an independent component and a collegial component. The independent component of management is realized in decision making regarding nursing-care delivery methods, appropriate numbers and assignments of staff, establishment of nursing care goals, etc. The collegial component of management is realized by effective collaboration with other departments in attaining mutually agreed upon goals for the delivery of quality care to the person.

Objectives

The nursing department commits itself to:

1   facilitating a decentralized management system,
2   fostering a milieu in which accountability and leadership is demonstrated and rewarded,
3   maintaining an interprofessional approach to management and patient care,
4   developing the knowledge and skills of all nursing staff to meet expectations regarding management.
5   utilizing nursing-care delivery methods which ensure the provision of quality nursing care.

CONCLUSIONS

The enormous need for specialized education has been demonstrated within several health care professions. General categories of problem areas were discussed. A common core curriculum, to be taken by all health care professionals, was recommended as a foundation for more specialized training in a particular discipline. A sample core curriculum was described including interdisciplinary and specialized philosophy statements. We believe that such a programme is essential for assuming the shared care, responsibility and objectives required by interdisciplinary work and collaborative research in care for persons with dementia.

ACKNOWLEDGEMENTS

Sue Ely, independent consultant and geriatric nurse specialist, is thanked for her contributions to this chapter.

We wish to thank Professor P. Coleman of the Social Work Department, University of Southampton, UK, and Mr. R. Woods of the Department of

Clinical Psychology, Institute of Psychiatry, London, UK, for the material and assistance they provided.

REFERENCES

Britton, P.G. (1983) 'Psychological services for the elderly', in A. Liddell (ed.) *The Practice of Clinical Psychology in Great Britain*, London: John Wiley & Sons Ltd.

Crate, M. (1965) 'Nursing Functions in adaptation to chronic illness', *American Journal of Nursing* 65(10): 72–6.

Engelen, G. (1984) 'Psychogeriatrie: diskussie blijft nodig', *Medisch Contact* 18: 571–2.

Erikson, E.H. (1963) *Childhood and Society*, 2nd edn, New York, W.W. Norton.

Gray, B. and Isaacs, B. (1979) *Care of the Elderly Mentally Infirm*, London: Tavistock.

Gunter, L. and Estes, C.A. (1979) *Education for Gerontic Nursing*, New York: Springer.

Havighurst, R.J. (1974) 'Successful aging', in R.J. Williams, C. Tibbitts and W. Donahue (eds) *Processes of Aging*, New York: Atherton Press, pp. 229–320.

Jones, G.M. (1991) 'Survey of interpersonal therapies used in 25 London area nursing homes', in preparation.

Peck, R.C. (1956) 'Psychological developments in the second half of life', in J.E. Anderson (ed.) *Psychological Aspects of Aging*, Washington, D.C.: American Psychological Association.

Perdue, B.J. (1981) 'Teaching chronicity: in search of a theoretical framework' in B.J. Perdue, N.E. Mahon, S.L. Hawes and S.M. Frik (eds) *Chronic Care Nursing*, New York: Springer.

Pitt, B. (1974) *Psychogeriatrics: An Introduction to the Psychiatry of Old Age*, London: Churchill Livingstone.

Chapter 25

Care-giving in dementia: review and perspectives

Bère Miesen

Care-giving in dementia carries with it a challenge for the future of all human beings. In spite of the enormous implications of care-giving, the approaches for interpersonal care are relatively new and bearing in mind the increased care requirements of elderly persons with dementia, our expectations for the future are thus laden with anxiety. The field of care-giving must be able to 'hold its own' beside the field of neurobiological research into dementia whilst it has barely begun to evolve; in fact most interpersonal approaches are just beginning to develop and be utilized. Along with the desire to search for useful methods and approaches comes uncertainty arising from the hope that this goal is achievable, but not being sure. Besides this anxiety is the reality that many different disciplines, which have all been moulded separately, must work together in this field without any common vocabularly, theories, models or training as yet. The multidisciplinary approaches that are discussed in this book attempt to show the reader how care-giving in dementia is evolving, and to encourage each discipline to fill in some of the gap between research and practice. The result is like finding the focal point of a painting where all the lines of perspective meet. A book which is intended to be practical, for practical people, must dare to evaluate whether its goals have been met. The following synopsis and evaluative comments on each of the chapters are intended to help the reader to do that.

PART I: MODELS AND THEORIES

Clinicopathologic correlations and the brain–behaviour relationship in Alzheimer's disease (Chapter 2)

This chapter is a simple synopsis of the neurobiology of dementia in conjunction with its known links to behaviour. As far as advances in the field of neurobiology are concerned, there have undoubtedly been 'lucky shots' and individual successes although the total knowledge about the pathology of dementia is far from complete. The synthesis between brain structure and the biochemical approach to the behaviour of dementing persons thus will not provide a cure in the very near future. Pharmacological manipulation aimed at cognitive improvement of, for example, the cholinergic system, has not been particularly successful. That is not surprising. The psychopathology of dementing persons is more varied than the neuropathology of dementia alone. Considering the unlikelihood of finding a cure in the short term, the differentiation of character traits of persons during a lifetime, and individual differences in functioning and behaviour that occur in dementia, it seems most logical to try to activate the 'spared' functions through environmental and interactive manipulation, i.e. to manipulate care-giving itself. Neurobiological research could be more useful if its vision were expanded to include the dissemination of research findings to professional care-givers in the clinical setting, in other words, if it made a direct contribution to care-giving. The manipulation of intensive care-giving as a suitable method for creating individualized enriched environments for the psychosocial wellbeing of the person with dementia is actually supported by research into some biochemical parameters. The underlying message is about the apposition and individualization of neurobiological knowledge.

Learning and memory in demented patients (Chapter 3)

Memory disorders comprise, so to speak, the heart of clinical psychopathology of dementia. A true assessment thereof is important, not only for research but also for care-giving. This assessment is more important than has been recognized in the past and encompasses the individual's activities of daily living. A multi-stage model of memory processing is required to meet these assessment goals. Complete assessment leads to a better understanding and to realistic expectation of behavioural change. Thorough assessment helps, for example, in making decisions about whether to use reality orientation or validation therapy, but it can also help to prevent tragic emotional complications due to unrealistic expectations on the part of the family and care-givers. Emotional complications have been thought to pertain more to families of the person with dementia than to the sufferer him- or herself. This is strange because 'suspicious and aggressive behaviour' arises out of an awareness of one's own memory and mental deficits. This awareness is commonly accepted; even the World Health Organization in defining dementia refers to the awareness of the demented persons about what is happening to him (absence of clouding of consciousness) as a key feature in diagnosing dementia. Individualized and process-oriented assessment of the memory deficits can help to facilitate care-giving of dementia along the continuum of care required: at home, in the community and in institutions.

Attachment theory and dementia (Chapter 4)

Research on parent-fixation and dementia is partly built upon a process-oriented model of memory in which retrieval cues play an important role. There are many perspectives on the theoretical and empirical foundation of the attachment theory, which asserts that all aspects of the behaviour of demented elderly persons can be seen as individual reactions to loss. The process of dementia can be usefully understood in terms of the person experiencing a continuous, increasingly strange situation which triggers feelings of fear and anxiety. Similarly, the aggressive and blaming/clinging behaviour of the demented person towards the care-giver can be seen as a general human response occuring in conditions of multiple loss. Although it has not yet been empirically demonstrated, it seems obvious that besides an individual's life history, the ways in which a person coped with losses pre-morbidly are also apparent in behaviour occuring in dementia. Psychopathology is varied precisely because of the heterogeneity of behaviours that occur in older persons. Attachment behaviour occurs when persons find themselves in situations which feel unsafe. The feelings which occur in these situations function as retrieval cues which make early emotions feel real again. As feelings of being unsafe increase in dementia, old and new attachment figures are increasingly less at their disposal to give them security. The social interations of demented older persons could be described as attachment behaviour, complementary to care-giving behaviour. It becomes apparent thus that the individual life histories and attachment behaviours of the carers themselves, be they family members or health care professionals, come into play, and that validation workers, for example, can represent attachment figures for persons with dementia.

Reminiscing disorientation theory (Chapter 5)

Reminiscing disorientation theory provides a theoretical framework within which many of the interpersonal interventions for disorientation described within this book can be understood; it also provides an understanding of the psychological meaning of dementia to the person experiencing it. All sorts of behaviours of demented elderly persons, seen through the eyes of both reminiscing disorientation theory and attachment theory, make it possible to understand behaviour occurring with disorientation in general human terms rather than from the perspective of a particular disorder. This means that behaviour, which until now was labelled as 'psychotic', including parent-fixation behaviours, can now be used as norms for later stages of dementia and accepted as part of the dementia pattern, rather than attributed to additional generalized psychotic behaviour. Changes in the information resources and information processing gradually alter the threshold between the person's inner and outer world. The individual tries to make sense of, or find meaning within circumstances of increasingly threatening cognitive and emotional chaos. The person is in a disoriented state in which eidetic imagery is activated, namely seeing and hearing with the mind's eye and ears. Reminiscing disorientation occurs when a person cannot find the way back to the state of reality. It is a problem of transit between these states. This also explains how lucid moments are possible. The essence of the validation approach can be seen from this description. Disorientation in dementia cannot be viewed as a static situation. The pathology pertains precisely to the inability to make the transition between the state of reality and the state of reminiscing, voluntarily or automatically. A variety of factors, of which dementia is only one, influence the ability to transit between states. Care-givers must try to influence these other factors in providing optimal care, thereby creating optimal control of the transit between the states and thus reducing the negative feelings of loneliness and fear.

A communication model for dementia (Chapter 6)

One aspect of providing care for a person with dementia is verbal communication by the family or health care professionals. Improvement in communication is thought to reduce negative feelings; particularly feeling unsafe. The material presented in this chapter provides a communication model for individual nursing care plans. This model is especially practical to help care-givers understand the limitations in communication occurring as dementia progresses. The model provides guidelines for care-givers which help to maximize the communication potential at any stage, whether it be through reality orientation, the validation approach, music or reminiscing. Persons in long-term care institutions are particularly dependant on interactions by care-givers, precisely because of their extremely limited activities of daily living functioning. For example, in the study described it was found that: there was little communication during morning and evening care; that most communication was made in the form of commands; and that very few introductions were made by staff to residents. Neither were there many clear explanations of what staff were going to be doing for, or with, the resident. Naturally this results in an escalation of the insecurity that disoriented persons already experience. These limited and low-quality interactions arise in part because of the limited use of life-history information made by professional care-givers and also because of a lack of information about the pathology and the meaning of experience of dementia to the resident themselves.

A nursing model for the care of the elderly (Chapter 7)

In the same way that attachment theory shows that the feelings that persons with dementia have can be understood in terms of normal human emotions, this model shows that their needs can be best understood in terms of a universal human-needs framework. This model, developed for use in long-term care settings, provides guidelines for useful interactions and also gives structure to recording of care provided by all care-givers. It requires only that health care workers remember Maslow's universal 'needs' hierarchy as opposed to the more complicated conventional 'subsystem' models used in acute-care nursing settings. This model also helps to focus family members and care staff on the dementing person's 'needs' rather than 'problems'. Because every person has individual needs in addition to universal needs, this model provides scope for a person's individual needs to be negotiated and partitioned between family, friends and care-giving staff by means of a life history, avocational interest inventory, personal possessions inventory and a family contract. Family are more in tune with information about a person's hobbies, routines and personal habits whereas staff are more familiar with general care needs; both types of information are pertinent to complete, optimal care.

PART II: INTERVENTIONS FOR PERSONS WITH DEMENTIA IN CARE FACILITIES

What can be learned from studies on reality orientation? (Chapter 8)

Reality orientation is the most widely researched of any of the approaches for dealing with dementia to date. Although the goal for RO is the improvement of cognitive functioning and orientation through repetition and relearning, the research is not very encouraging in terms of concrete effects or outcomes of this method. This is because too much emphasis has been placed on improvements in general cognitive behaviour. The opening premise of this chapter is that although the potential for behavioural change in dementia is limited by cognitive learning potential, it is sensitive to environmental factors which family or care-giving staff can provide or control. The predominant difficulty seems to be that advice about enriching the environment for maximal benefit is always confounded by the slow inevitable deterioration of information-processing abilities and other cognitive functions. On the basis of the latter point, one ought to speak of minimizing random, non-meaningful stimuli for the person with dementia, as well as increasing environmental stimuli. A separate problem concerning the practice of RO is the advice that one must never agree with what the person says if the facts are clearly wrong. This is in juxtaposition to more current thinking which asserts that 'reality' should not be forced on a person, and that instead the underlying feelings should be recognized, even if the content or facts are garbled. In any event, focusing on the individual has the advantage of giving a person much needed additional attention, and to individualizing their care plan.

Reminiscence and life review with persons with dementia: which way forward (Chapter 9)

Reminiscing and life review are increasingly popular approaches for working with dementia. They are pleasant to use but have not been subjected to much evaluative research. The evaluative problems are considered in this chapter. Life review is a structured form of reminiscing. Old myths were exploded by the writings of Butler, who identified life review as a universal inner experience for everyone, including the elderly. This process also includes the review of negative experiences leading to feelings of despair and sadness, perhaps out of the awareness of one's finitude. Feelings of safety are required if the negative feelings are to be set aside and replaced with inner peace. This necessitates the presence of attachment figures or substitutes for them.

This chapter emphasizes that in order to measure the effectiveness of these approaches, individual norms and baselines must be established before individual goals are set. Furthermore, individual differences must be considered within the context of the different stages of dementia. Some behavioural differences can be related to life history and others to cohort influence. In compiling a life history, family can be invaluable in providing and corroborating information and they should be encouraged to help in this process as part of optimizing care. Family involvement in compiling a life history can also improve the relationship between professional caregivers and family. The emphasis on individual differences and the importance of individual care deserves treatment as a special topic in a curriculum on care-giving in dementia.

Music therapy in the management of dementia (Chapter 10)

Music therapy, as opposed to activities in which music is used for pleasure, involves the planned, systematic use of music specific to a person's stage of dementia and their life history. Personal experiences of all sorts, particularly a person's musical preferences, are used in planning music therapy sessions. Does this process facilitate the development of trust and feelings of security? Music therapy supposedly replaces the emphasis on cognitive goals (cortical functioning) with affective ones (subcortical functioning) and thus utilizes the spared abilities and functions. Most notably, even persons who have lost the ability to speak can often still sing. Music therapy can be classified as a specialized form of life review or reminiscing in which music functions as the retrieval cue or trigger. Persons with dementia generally react well to music, certainly on an individual basis it has been observed that agitation and aggression often are reduced. The goal of the therapy is to help demented elderly function at their best instead of their worst; in no way is it expected that cognitive functioning should improve or that cellular brain damage is reversed.

Dynamic psychotherapy with elderly demented patients (Chapter 11)

Dementia is conceived of as a stressful time of life, not only for the sufferer but also for their family who find themselves in a set of changed affective conditions. Psychotherapy seeks to intervene in the affective realm which dementia complicates. Instead of emphasizing external stressors, internal factors which determine the ability of the person with dementia to cope are dealt with. Life history and reminiscing are an integral part of the process of psychotherapy, and the content involves identifying internalized ways of coping with change. Everything is dependent on the relationship which the therapist has with the demented person, and on the presence of security, empathy and acceptance. The most common type of transference on the part of persons with dementia is that of placing the therapist in a parental role (attachment figure). The content of this chapter is similar to that used in the validation approach, although psychotherapy has been more extensively described because it has a much longer history and development. It is possible that this transference also relates to the model of internalized attachment previously described. The author suggests that: if an old person experiences change in the form of loss, earlier unresolved conflicts surface which the ego resources/defences tap; it is precisely these defences which are less available to the person with dementia. New losses crystallize old painful losses and hence the person with dementia develops loss feelings such as depression and anger, etc. In other words, the dementing elderly are elders with limited cognitive abilities who, in addition to having old pain and unresolved feelings of loss, suffer additional affective complications with fewer means to resolve them. Persons with dementia do not, by definition, have unresolved conflicts, although it can be assumed that many older persons reach old age with at least some losses unresolved. Taken together, this means that the behaviour of the care-giver can be of paramount importance in helping a person because of the associations and identifications they naturally make. Loss of control, no effective means of mourning, increasing fixation on the past as short-term memory fails, and increasing isolation, ... form a vicious circle. How a demented person copes is dependent thus on the individual life history, and the history of their affective attachments in life.

Validation therapy with late-onset dementia populations (Chapter 12)

The validation approach to care-giving in dementia encompasses a totally empathetic stance and skills in interpersonal verbal and non-verbal communication, and it can be performed one-to-one or in group settings. Although many aspects are not new and find common ground with other interpersonal counselling methods, this stage-specific approach to dementia however is completely new. The validation approach maintains that all behaviour has meaning and that the care-giver must work with the emotional content of communication rather than the factual content. According to validation theory, physical and emotional losses and the process of reminiscing all serve as retrieval cues. Current losses in present time often evoke (memories of) losses in the past. In spite of their cortical brain damage, and the awareness that something strange is happening to them, elderly persons continue trying to communicate. Behaviour in dementia is not regulated solely by brain damage, but by the person's life history and coping routines, including physical and psychosocial losses.

Although there is not yet much research about the validation method, it is important to teach this method to families and carers because it is the first systematic, stage-specific approach to the communication methods which are most likely to succeed.

This method is gaining popularity rapidly and is continuing to develop and be refined accordingly. The theory base is being strengthened by research into such areas as attachment, parent-fixation and the various stages of dementia. More subtle distinctions such as the difference between 'restoring the past in order to feel safe' versus 'restoring the past to tie up loose ends' are increasingly being made.

An evaluation of an occupational therapy service for persons with dementia (Chapter 13)

Occupational therapists have tried to determine what their role is in working with persons with dementia, in relation to other health care professionals, and in relation to activities used routinely with elderly persons. Several modest studies reported in this chapter indicate that demented elderly persons do benefit from increased attention by staff. This is in keeping with the previous work supporting the development of enriched environments. Of particular importance is the distinction between long-term effects versus behavioural changes during a course of sessions or research measurements. This issue of long-term effects leads to changed priorities in care. The final study, still in progress, is in line with the work presented by Duijnstee in Chapter 20, this volume. Her work emphasizes the importance of taking account of the well-being of family carers and supporting the work they do, as well as working with the person with dementia. It is important to find activities that the family and the person with dementia can do together; this is seen by families as being more useful than merely providing training in activities of daily living. Individual differences amongst family carers must be acknowledged before practical help is given to them routinely.

PART III: INTERVENTIONS FOR PERSONS WITH DEMENTIA IN THE COMMUNITY

The anticipation of memory loss and dementia in old age (Chapter 14)

This chapter describes a 'sociology of memory' and a model of memory which makes a distinction between different phases of information processing: input (attention), storage (consolidation), and output (retrieval). Insight into this model could help to diminish the negative stereotype of memory loss in old age, and allay some of the anxieties which many normal healthy elderly persons have, by realizing that there are multiple factors which have negative influences on memory. Many elderly persons and relatives of persons with dementia have internalized a negative image of memory loss in old age whilst such a decline never occurs in the vast majority of the elderly. It is important to explain to elderly persons how memory works because it helps put their minds at ease. Myths must be replaced by accurate information about which factors influence memory, and how some of these can be manipulated, for example, by consolidation strategies. Memory functioning is a very variable entity: even under normal circumstances memory capacity can be affected by biological rhythms and emotions. The focus of this chapter relates to teaching elderly persons that memory loss is not usually due to irreversible biological damage, but more often to the personal expectations governed by a societal myth of memory loss in old age and self-fulfilling prophecy.

Memory training for older adults (Chapter 15)

This chapter presents a practical approach for a home self-help memory-training method. Persons can be taught to train their mnemonic abilities more efficiently in order to remain functioning, confidently, at their maximum potential for as long as possible. There appears to be a big discrepancy between memory complaints and actual decline in memory performance, i.e. the relationship between these variables is not linear. Benefits are seen immediately and not in the long term. Unfortunately, to date, no long-term effects have been shown with this method. However research in this area is relatively new and ultimately many methods, samples and periods of follow-up must be compared. Possibly repeat sessions should be scheduled at regular intervals.

The structured life-review process: a community approach to the aging client (Chapter 16)

Elderly persons tend to consider the past and review their lives most when prompted by a current crisis or problem. At that moment, a participant observer can be helpful in listening to and helping persons come to terms with their life. This is a challenging job for a therapist or care-giver, let alone for elderly persons with dementia to do themselves. Life review done in the community setting can be a therapeutic means of helping persons whilst performing other interventions simultaneously. Research to date about the value of reminiscence has been ambivalent. Although it appears that interventions are usually of too short a duration, it is generally a pleasant experience for elderly persons. Life review conducted with non-demented elderly persons in their home environment led to an improvement in life satisfaction. Such work needs to be extended with a sample of persons with dementia, but provides an encouraging model for community work with dementia in conjunction with the COPA model.

Community care services for the elderly mentally infirm (Chapter 17)

The Leicester model for home care of demented elderly persons is a combination of day care, carer support groups, sitting services and released admission facilities. The model attempts to reduce the emotional strain of care-givers at home. The starting premise of this chapter is based on the statistic that about 90 per cent of all demented elderly persons are cared for outside of institutions, and that care-giving in the home is very stressful for family carers. It is supposed that the more carers are supported, the longer admission to an institution can be staved off. This model is a step forward because it is concrete and practical. The prescribed model is actually an integrated network of interdisciplinary, preventative care based on a clear philosophy which focuses on non-institutional care (unlike the present situation in the Netherlands). Many of the points mentioned are important for providing care to those still at home, particularly the differences between families who do not seek help (the silent copers) and those overtly distressed families who seek help. Family care-givers automatically interpret the dementing person's behaviour within the context of their historically meaningful relationship with the person, which naturally accompanies a sense of trust and security. This can become an impediment if family members cannot accept the gradual loss of the person who was familiar to them, and do not begin the mourning process because it is too painful.

Mourning is important if family members are to successfully use validation or other techniques presented in this book, because all these interpersonal interventions require that the carers' own emotions be put aside so that full attention and energy can be used to empathize with the person with dementia.

Day care and dementia (Chapter 18)

This chapter is discussed within the history of day care in the Netherlands and fits in well with the philosophy of community care presented by Gilleard. Day care for persons with dementia has three goals: the improvement or stabilization of the spared functions; caring for the carers; and the delay of institutionalization. Many points common to other chapters can be found in this chapter. Most noticeable are the plea for individual care programmes developed on the basis of life-history information, and interdisciplinary assessment. Little official research has been done on the effectiveness of day care; descriptive studies, however, generally conclude that most elderly demented persons and their families perceive day care as offering positive benefits.

The COPA project as a model for the management of early dementia in the community (Chapter 19)

This chapter also has features in common with Chapter 17 (the chapter by Gilleard). COPA is an experimental multi-goal programme to help elderly persons with alcohol problems. Whereas traditional anti-alcohol programmes do not reach elderly persons and are very confrontative in their methods, this programme was designed specifically for the elderly and avoids confrontation. Alcoholism, like dementia is seen as a hidden problem which, in the beginning is denied. The project is an inspired example for providing community care for demented persons and their families because it allows ancillary psychosocial and health care needs to be met simultaneously. In the application of this model to dementia, it is important to determine the degree of involvement of both the person with dementia and their family in the loss process. The whole COPA project is based on the development of individual treatment plans. Another parallel of alcholism to dementia relates to the key goal of the COPA project, which is to reduce alcohol intake, not to demand total abstinence; the dementing process likewise cannot be removed but its effects must be minimized. The suggestion that the COPA model could be made applicable to any elderly persons experiencing multiple problems is certainly worth further research.

PART IV: INTERVENTIONS FOR FAMILY

Caring for a demented family member at home: objective observation and subjective evaluation of the burden (Chapter 20)

As already mentioned, over 90 per cent of persons with dementia are cared for outside of institutional settings. The informal network, i.e. the primary care-giver is usually the spouse or daughter, and remains the principal source of support. They have both a leading and a suffering role. The demented person requires continuous supervision and proximity to the carer. Such demands radically change the life of the care-giver. This qualitative research is based on interviews of primary care-givers, and it asks: What determines subjective burden? Which factors play a role in the difference between objective and subjective burden? Professional care for carers must take into account what their needs are within a framework of evaluating both objective and subjective burden. The study described in this chapter tries to answer how and why objective and subjective burden differ. Help must aim itself at the individual experience of burden, specifically at the subjective perception of that burden as the carer experiences it. There appear to be large individual differences in this perception. The key issue involves finding out what psychological meaning the whole care-giving situation has for the carer. In terms of putting the material in this chapter into practice, first-hand information from the care-giver is essential for the assessment of the type and degree of burden experienced by them. Information about the perceived burden by the family member should be seen as key information, not as supplementary to the evaluation of burden made by a professional.

Expressed emotion and coping techniques amongst carers of the dementing elderly (Chapter 21)

Most of the expressed emotion (EE) literature has been conducted within the chronic illness framework of schizophrenia. Not surprisingly, carers suffer from heightened levels of emotional distress. This possibly influences their ability to provide care. Often there is much resentment, criticism, animosity and aggression directed toward the patient. The more emotional distress present, the higher the levels of EE, and the more aggression and displeasure occur in interactions. Coping techniques which help in these situations can be directed at either the problem or emotion. There is little research about coping techniques for carers of demented persons. Blaming behaviour seems purposeless, but is certainly understandable in view of the losses and grieving that are being experienced. This pilot study shows that animosity in contact and care-giving is related to the pre-morbid relationship between the carer and the person with dementia as well as with the stage of dementia. This confirms the importance of helping care-givers to realize that they are undergoing a grieving process because of the continuous changes and losses in their relationship with the dementing person. Findings indicate that an equilibrium exists between the expression and inhibition of emotions. The care-giver is focused more on emotional issues than on developing coping techniques for specific problems. The conclusion is that as well as educational information, counselling also reduces expressed emotions and thus the distress felt by care-givers. High levels of

EE seem to have the highest correlation with the personality of the care-giver and the lifelong pre-morbid relationship. Again we note that the life-history information is vital for providing care not only for the person with dementia, but also for the carer.

Families and the institutionalized elderly (Chapter 22)

Care-giving by family members is dependent on the health of the care-giver and of the person with dementia, whether they are living at home or not. Care-giving by children is directly related to the attachment behaviour of the parent with dementia. A lifelong pattern of mutual assistance and/or support of parents to children is related to support given in old age. There is no perceived burden when the care-giver is healthy, but when he or she is not, parents are institutionalized earlier than the objective condition or the severity their situation would suggest.

After admission there are often staff-versus-family care-giver conflicts. Staff can see family members as either patients or co-workers. A model is presented which was developed from spouses' experiences after admission in a long-term care setting with a husband without dementia. It is not yet known if this model is valid for families of someone with dementia. It is concluded that the experiences of spouses can be understood in terms of a predictable process comprising of several phases for which different inter-ventions are appropriate by professional care-givers. Spouses of persons with dementia are in a sort of quasi-widowhood after their admission even though their relationship continues.

A carer's group for families of patients with dementia (Chapter 23)

In the past, health care professionals used to work with persons with dementia to the exclusion of their families. This is changing fortunately. It is universally recognized that their plight is very stressful, and given that the population of care-givers themselves is getting older, they have an increased risk of experiencing deterioration in their own well-being and social-support environment. The enormous complexity of the care-giving situation must be emphasized. As already mentioned, this is influenced by the nature of the early relationship and the personalities of the persons themselves. Attachment theory maintains that if care-givers have worked through losses successfully in the past, then they are in a better position to work through new losses, and vice versa.

The goal of the group is to share the experiences and feelings associated with 'letting go'. The therapist has an informative and emotionally support-ive role. The feeling of security within the group also has positive effects. Again we note the importance of an empathetic attitude. It is in keeping with the difficulties of families in coming to grips with the loss process (i.e.

in denying it because it is too painful) that 80 per cent of carers did not accept the initial invitation to join the group. Many interactional situations, and care-giving, can be improved once the grieving process is acknowledged. If 'mother' is living in the past, and fixating on her own parents, it can be a very frightening situation for the daughter who is looking after her because of the anticipated further decline. Somehow the daughter must develop insight into the need for her own grieving. The three models presented, represent three goals for a carers' group: the presentation of information, peer support and therapy. Professionals will have to be guided by carers themselves in the type of support that they need and want.

PART V: SUMMARY

The need for an interdisciplinary core curriculum for professionals working with dementia (Chapter 24)

It is clear that everything that has preceeded this chapter has consequences for the development of educational and training programmes for professionals, particularly for nursing, social work, psychology and medicine. In the broadest sense, this information could be made applicable to anyone dealing with older persons. Care-giving in dementia must be placed within the continuum of scientific facts and the practical knowledge of care-giving. Precisely because care-giving is an interdisciplinary activity, it is necessary to have a common pool of basic knowledge and principles with which to direct care which can be personalized as much as possible. A core curriculum is the obvious way to strengthen interdisciplinary interactions and to build bridges between not only the science or neurobiology of dementia, but also between research and practice. These bridges can only improve the methods available to achieve the goals which professional care-givers have, which are the wellbeing of the person with dementia and their family members.

PERSPECTIVES

Most elderly persons, fortunately are quite healthy and happy. Dementia affects only a small minority of persons. None the less, the problems it poses when it occurs are enormous, for the person with dementia, their families, professional care-givers, and the community.

The goals of all of the approaches mentioned in this book, like the lines of perspective in a painting, lie close together. The most notable one is the improvement of the contact between demented persons and their social environment by way of improving and increasing the number of meaningful interactions with them. This goal involves the improvement of the quality of their existence which they cannot achieve without the help of those providing care for them. The differences between the approaches are more related to questions pertaining to 'how' and 'under what conditions', than to content. There are apparently many roads to the same goals. It would seem most sensible for care-givers to learn as many of these methods as possible, rather than familiarizing themselves with any specific one since there is no magic formula to working with dementia. A variety of skills are needed to interact with persons in the different stages of dementia. The real clinical value of these approaches must be sought in the individualization of care plans rather than in value reports of generalized group effects. Inter-individual differences are usually so great that it is not possible to obtain well-matched control groups. Group data often do not mean much because of small sample sizes and hence may not show any changes or effects. The only norm in old age is heterogeneity of behaviour which crytallizes out of the diverse life histories. This is precisely why we can speak of the need for individual care planning and the unique meaning of behaviour.

Many methods and approaches that have been tried with dementia were not originally developed for this population, but rather were borrowed from other populations in a desperate attempt to find something to do with dementia patients in long-term care settings. Early on it was already recognized that affective interventions were necessary. For example, even Folsom (1968), credited with the formalization of reality orientation for use in dementia, said that 'the emotional needs of individual patients required concentrated attention'. More recently, methods have begun to develop in response to increasingly specific knowledge about deficits in SDAT. The contributions to this book have looked particularly at those methods which have developed in response to cognitive deficits within the context of persons experiencing multiple losses (physical, psychosocial and environmental) simultaneously.

Interventions do not fundamentally change the nature of the dementia, but under the right conditions the person is helped to function at the highest level possible, which might be higher than the one at which they are presently functioning. Thus, interpersonal interventions do not act as a therapy or treatment for the primary symptoms of dementia, but rather the secondary ones. Functions which are related to the phylogenetic and onto-genetic, deep-brain structure remain intact longest. This is reflected in the frequency of behaviours, memories and emotions from early life which are evidenced in dementia behaviour and utilized in reminiscing activities.

In future, research must pay more attention to reporting case histories as well as stating clearly the stage of dementia and the interventions used. This is beginning to happen for such interventions as the validation approach, and its credibility benefits thereby. A general research plan and framework would be helpful, in which the pros and cons of all relevant approaches and methods for dealing with dementia, for each stage, were given, allowing for a given person to act as their own control. Strict assessment in terms of the stage of dementia and the impediments to information processing is needed to determine the degree of limitation and hence the extent of the emotional consequences of the cognitive impediments and to other losses. Persons are aware, well into the later stages of dementia that something 'is not right' with their thinking. Interventions can then be chosen and tried systematically. Life-history information, including attachment history, coping strategies and the personality of both the person with dementia and the family carers, is essential since all of these variables contribute to the heterogeneity of the psychopathology in dementia, perhaps even more than the neuropathology.

Important research topics for the future arising from the various interpersonal approaches include: the dilemma of reducing non-meaningful overstimulation while increasing salient beneficial forms of stimulation; determining whether enriching the psychosocial environment in specific ways maximizes remaining information-processing resources; and how often and for how long various therapies must be conducted at each stage for optimal effects. Along more theoretical lines, communication models, Bowlby's theory about attachment behaviour and the complementary care-giving behaviour, the concept of attachment history, the nursing care model, and reminiscing disorientation theory, are ready to be evaluated and used conceptually in practice settings. With regard to new conceptualizations, the daily, concrete interactions occurring between a person with dementia and a care-giver can now be thought of as a substitute attachment and as a junction of two or more attachment histories.

In general, the picture for specialized education in health care for aging and more specifically for dementia, is a bleak one, with widespread complaints about lack of money and resources for programmes. There is a great need for specialized multidisciplinary education.

Almost all of the authors of this book exhibit a personal drive, beyond that required of their respective professions. It is hoped that this book will be used as a vehicle to communicate some of their ideas, that it will contribute to the acceleration of the dissemination of knowledge and research about care-giving in dementia. We hope it will encourage other persons to further develop their own ideas or those presented herein.

REFERENCE

Folsom, J.C. (1968) 'Reality orientation for the elderly mental patient', *Journal of Geriatric Psychiatry* 1 (2): 291–307.

Name index

Subject index